Tibia and Fibula

Other books in the Musculoskeletal Trauma Series:

Humerus
Edited by E. Flatow and C. Ulrich

Radius and Ulna
Edited by M. McQueen and J. Jupiter

Femur
Edited by C. Court-Brown and J. Chapman

Series Editors

C. Court-Brown MD, FRCSEd (Orth)
Consultant Orthopaedic Surgeon
The Royal Infirmary of Edinburgh
Edinburgh, UK

D. Pennig MD
Professor and Director
Department of Trauma, Hand and Reconstructive Surgery
St Vinzenz Hospital
Cologne, Germany

Musculoskeletal Trauma Series

Tibia and Fibula

Edited by

C. Court-Brown MD, FRCSEd (Orth)
Consultant Orthopaedic Surgeon
The Royal Infirmary of Edinburgh
Edinburgh, UK

D. Pennig MD
Professor and Director
Department of Trauma, Hand and Reconstructive Surgery
St Vinzenz Hospital
Cologne, Germany

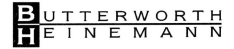

Butterworth-Heinemann
Linacre House, Jordan Hill, Oxford OX2 8DP
A division of Reed Educational and Professional Publishing Ltd

℞ A member of the Reed Elsevier plc group

OXFORD   BOSTON   JOHANNESBURG
MELBOURNE   NEW DELHI   SINGAPORE

First published 1997

British Library Cataloguing in Publication Data

Tibia and fibula. – (Musculoskeletal trauma series)
  1. Tibia – Fractures   2. Fibula – Fractures
  I. Court-Brown, Charles M.   II. Pennig, Dietmar
  617.1'5'8

ISBN 0 7506 0529 4

Library of Congress Cataloguing in Publication Data

Tibia and fibula / edited by C. Court-Brown, D. Pennig.
  p.   cm. – (Musculoskeletal trauma series)
  Includes bibliographical references and index.
  ISBN 0 07506 0529 4
  1. Tibia – Fractures.   2. Fibula – Fractures.   I. Court-Brown,
Charles M.   II. Pennig, Dietmar.   III. Series.
  [DNLM: 1. Tibial Fractures.   2. Fibula – injuries.   WE 870T552
  1997]
RD560. T52   1997   96–53900
617.1'58–dc21   CIP

Typeset by Wyvern 21 Ltd, Bristol
and printed and bound in Great Britain at The Bath Press plc, Avon

Contents

Contributors

S. Bonar
Department of Orthopaedics
University of Iowa Hospitals and Clinics
Iowa
USA

C. Court-Brown
Consultant Orthopaedic Surgeon
The Royal Infirmary of Edinburgh
Edinburgh
UK

J. Grünert
Professor and Head Department of Hand Surgery
and Plastic Surgery
Friedrich-Alexander University
Erlangen
Germany

J.L. Marsh
Associate Professor
Department of Orthopaedics
University of Iowa Hospitals and Clinics
Iowa
USA

M. McQueen
Consultant Orthopaedic Surgeon
Princess Margaret Rose Orthopaedic Hospital
Edinburgh
UK

D. Pennig
Professor and Director
Department of Trauma, Hand and Reconstructive
Surgery
St Vinzenz Hospital
Cologne
Germany

M. Saleh
Professor of Orthopaedics and Traumatic Surgery
The University of Sheffield
Clinical Sciences Centre
Northern General Hospital
Sheffield
UK

S. Sjolin
Consultant Orthopaedic Surgeon
West Suffolk Hospital NHS Trust
Suffolk
UK

J.P. Waddell
Division of Orthopaedics
St Michael's Orthopaedic Associates
Toronto
Canada

Series Foreword

Surgeons who deal with musculoskeletal injuries tend, on the whole, to use the methods of treatment practised at the units where they trained and served their apprenticeships. The more adventurous and intellectual of them also study other methods, but they are inevitably influenced by their earlier experiences. Those who trained where operative fixation was the norm are inclined to look down on those whose first choice of treatment is conservative; and the latter may in turn feel (if only unconsciously) that the 'always operate' merchants do so because 'fixation is fun'. Indeed, who can deny the joy of using skilled hands effectively.

What trauma surgeons need is a balanced view and here, in this series, we have precisely that. I was tempted to apply the initials NATO meaning, in the present context, the North Atlantic Trauma Organisation. Certainly the contents are a happy blend of North American and European views on fractures. Charles Court-Brown and Dietmar Pennig, the series editors, have earned great renown on both sides of the Atlantic for their work on the understanding and management of musculoskeletal trauma. They have collected a most distinguished set of authors and have been careful to ensure that the text does not read as if it was written by a committee; though it is clear that they have provided guidelines and minimized overlap,

they have wisely allowed each contributor to retain something of his national linguistic flavour.

The series consists of four volumes: Court-Brown and Pennig have themselves edited the volume on the tibia and fibula; the other three volumes are on the humerus (edited by E. Flatow and C. Ulrich), the radius and ulna (edited by M. McQueen and J. Jupiter), and the femur (edited by C. Court-Brown and J. Chapman). Each volume provides a comprehensive description of all the injuries discussed. Epidemiology, classification and fractures of the shafts as well as the upper and lower ends of each bone are described in detail; management includes authoritative accounts and clear illustrations of both operative and conservative treatment. Summaries of the literature are a notable feature of the text, and the lists of references will satisfy even the greediest reader.

This is the work which every trauma surgeon has been waiting for, using it to revise their knowledge of a particular field or to give practical guidance in approaching the individual patient. I wish it had been available when I was in active practice. I would have treated my patients better and slept more soundly at night.

The late Alan Apley

The death of Alan Apley after the publication of the first book in this series has deprived the orthopaedic community of one of its great teachers. He had a profound influence on all surgeons of our generation and all orthopaedic surgeons are in his

debt. Urbane, witty, charming and incisive he correctly questioned our more aggressive approach but always provided encouragement and support.

C. Court-Brown and D. Pennig

Series Preface

Our aims in editing a series of four books dealing with limb fractures were twofold. There has been an explosion of interest in the management of fractures in the last decade with the result that the large textbooks dealing with the management of fractures have tended to become reference books and we believe that there is a need for a series of short, concise texts describing the management of fractures in different bones. We have therefore been pleased to help with the production of four books detailing the epidemiology, classification, treatment and complications of fractures of the femur, tibia, humerus and forearm.

Our second goal was to try to combine the talents of North American and European editors and authors. Textbooks have tended to be based in one continent, often to their detriment. This collaboration has not always been easy or even possible but we are happy with the results of the enterprise and we are grateful to the volume editors and the individual authors for their contributions. We hope that the series will be of interest to all orthopaedic surgeons interested in trauma.

C. Court-Brown and D. Pennig

Preface

We have edited, and mostly written, this book as part of a series of books dealing with fractures of the long bones. Although all fractures are important we believe that the tibia has a special place in orthopaedic surgery. If one wants to court controversy or stir up an otherwise inactive meeting, merely discuss car parking or the management of tibial fractures. Most surgeons have problems with both and certainly have strongly held views on the subject of tibial fractures.

We have tried to present a complete overview of all of the fractures of the tibia and fibula. Little has been written in recent years about the epidemiology of these fractures and a section on this is included as well as chapters on the various treatment methods and complications. We are indebted to our guest authors for their valuable contributions which greatly enhance the book. Writing books is a time-consuming business and we are grateful to our families, colleagues and secretaries for their forbearance and help.

C. Court-Brown and D. Pennig

1

Classification of fractures of the tibia and fibula

C. Court-Brown

Introduction

Classification systems tend to be of two types: they are either morphological, describing the different patterns of fractures seen on X-ray, or they are aetiological and attempt to classify fracture patterns based on the direction and magnitude of the causative force. Most of the classification systems that have been devised for the different fractures of the tibia and fibula are morphological, having been devised following the analysis of a considerable number of X-rays.

The purpose of a classification system is superficially obvious but in practice difficult to define. It is usually stated that a classification is only useful if it defines the severity of a fracture with a view to determining the optimal treatment method and the eventual outcome. Obviously classification systems can never achieve this ideal as the treatment and outcome are as much determined by the age and general activity level of the patient, the degree of soft tissue damage associated with the fracture and the type and distribution of other injuries as they are by the individual characteristics of a particular fracture. Usually, therefore, too much is expected of classification systems. They do, however, have an important role in helping to increase surgical awareness of the importance of different fracture types and to highlight any particular characteristics of a fracture that will be important in its management. They should provide a broad correlation between increasing severity of fracture and worsening prognosis. Advocates of aetiological classification systems suggest that they are superior to morphological systems as they help to determine treatment, particularly if non-

operative treatment is being considered. However, as interest in operative fixation of fractures has increased, it has become clear that aetiological classifications are little better than morphological systems in determining either treatment methods or subsequent outcome.

The complexity of classification systems has increased with greater understanding of fracture epidemiology and pathophysiology. Early classification systems tended to be simple and easier to apply, although they conferred little benefit to the surgeon or the patient. The most comprehensive classification produced thus far is the AO classification of long-bone fractures produced in 1987 by Müller and his co-workers. This classification is based on more than 150 000 operatively treated fractures collected at the AO/ASIF documentation centre in Berne, Switzerland.

In the AO classification, each long-bone is specified by a number between 1 and 9. Each bone is subdivided into its component segments with the diaphysis being separated from the proximal and distal metaphyseal segments using the method of squares proposed by Heim (1987) (Müller *et al.*, 1990). Each fracture is then classified into types A, B or C. In the diaphyseal fractures type A represents simple fractures with two fragments and at least 90% cortical disruption, type B fractures have a wedge component and type C represents the more complex fractures.

In metaphyseal fractures the letters A, B and C are used differently. Type A metaphyseal fractures are extra-articular, type B are partial articular fractures, where the fracture involves part of the articular surface while the remainder of the joint is intact and connected to the metaphysis and diaphysis, and type C fractures contain complete articular fractures which are characterized by disruption of the articular surface and its separation from the diaphysis. All diaphyseal and metaphyseal fracture types are subdivided into three groups and each group is further divided into three subgroups. Many of the subgroups are divided into a number of specific fracture types so that every possible fracture the surgeon will encounter is specified. Each bone segment is therefore characterized by 27 different fractures, there being a total of 108 different fractures for the tibia and fibula, in addition to a considerable number of minor variants.

Superficially the AO classification is complex, but the underlying principles on which the system is based are straightforward and logical. When using the AO classification manual it is important to follow the text description of the fracture, rather than try to match the inevitably somewhat stylized pictorial representations with an X-ray of the fracture.

The most obvious criticism of the AO classification does not refer to its complexity, but rather to its forced compartmentalization of fractures into an alphanumeric system containing a previously determined number of groups. There is no doubt that some fractures fit the alphanumeric system better than others. The tibial diaphyseal segment (4.2) divides more comfortably into 27 types than does the distal metaphyseal segment (4.3). The system also does not take fracture displacement into account. This obviously has a bearing on both management and prognosis.

The AO group have also provided classification systems for skin damage, muscle/tendon injury and neurovascular injury. It is intended that all four AO classifications should be used together to provide an accurate classification for individual fractures.

Classification of tibial plateau fractures

Bradford *et al.* (1950) and Palmer (1951) formulated simple morphological classifications for tibial plateau fractures. Each had three types, these being unicondylar split and compression fractures and bicondylar fractures. Hohl (1967) extended the classification to six types, these being undisplaced unicondylar fractures associated with less than 3 mm depression, central depression unicondylar fractures, split depression unicondylar fractures, total unicondylar depression fractures, posterior unicondylar split fractures and bicondylar fractures.

Moore (1981) devised a classification of fracture-dislocations of the knee. This contained five types of fracture, these being split condylar fractures, total condylar fractures, rim avulsion condylar fractures, rim compression condylar fractures and bicondylar fractures. Subsequently Hohl and Moore (1983) combined their classifications to produce the revised Hohl classification system. This is shown in Figure 1.1. Hohl now classifies tibial plateau fractures into seven different types. His type 1 fracture contains all minimally displaced fractures, with minimal displacement being defined as less than 4 mm depression or displacement. The type 2 group contains all local or central condylar compression fractures and the type 3 group contains all split compression fractures. The total condylar depression fractures are type 4, and the type 5 group contains the split condylar fractures. Hohl recognizes that there are rim avulsion and compression fractures and includes both these categories in type 6. The last group of fractures, type 7, contains all the bicondylar fractures.

The Schatzker classification

Schatzker *et al.* (1979) were the first to introduce separate categories for medial condylar fractures and bicondylar fractures associated with significant metaphyseal comminution. Their six-category classification was based on both morphological and aetiological criteria and is shown in Figure 1.2.

Type I comprised the lateral condylar split fracture found mainly in young people with good quality cancellous bone and associated with bending and axial forces. The authors stated that the fracture could be associated with a peripheral meniscal tear or complete meniscal detachment with the meniscus being caught in the fracture.

Type II was a split depression fracture occurring in older people with mechanically inferior cancellous bone, while type III was a pure depression fracture of the lateral condyle, again occurring in older patients. The authors distinguished between peripheral and central depression fractures, but combined both in one group.

The type IV fractures involved the medial condyle. The authors separated type IV fractures into two subtypes, A and B: subtype A was a split fracture of the medial condyle such as occurs in young people as a result of severe trauma; subtype B was a depression fracture of the medial plateau, such as occurs in older patients, frequently as a

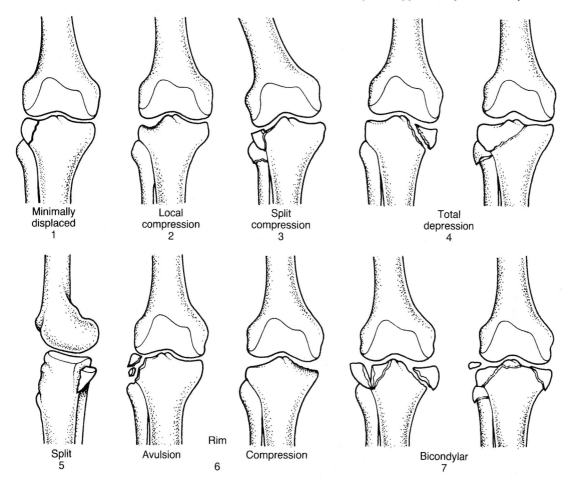

Figure 1.1   Revised Hohl classification of tibial plateau fractures

Type 1:   minimally displaced fractures. Less than 4 mm depression or displacement
Type 2:   displaced local compression fracture. Comminution of the tibial condyle with depression of the subchondral bone to a variable extent
Type 3:   displaced split – compression fracture
Type 4:   total depression of condyle without comminution of the articular surface
Type 5:   displaced condylar split fracture
Type 6:   rim fractures. These are either avulsion fractures where the fragments are raised, or compression fractures where the fragments are impacted downwards
Type 7:   bicondylar fractures

result of minor trauma. Schatzker and his colleagues also appreciated that it required greater force to cause medial condylar fractures than lateral condylar fractures and that the former were often associated with both intercondylar eminence damage and rupture of the lateral collateral ligamentous complex. The severity of the type IV injury is highlighted by the fact that they found many were associated with knee dislocations and therefore with both vascular and neurological damage.

The type V fracture was a bicondylar fracture without separation of the metaphysis from the diaphysis. Schatzker *et al.* described medial and lateral fracture lines running centrally from the joint surface to the medial and lateral metaphyses, with the gap between the proximal fracture lines being variable. Type VI fractures involved separation of the metaphysis from the diaphysis, with the lateral condyle usually more comminuted than the medial condyle.

The relationship between the Schatzker classification and the subsequent AO classification is

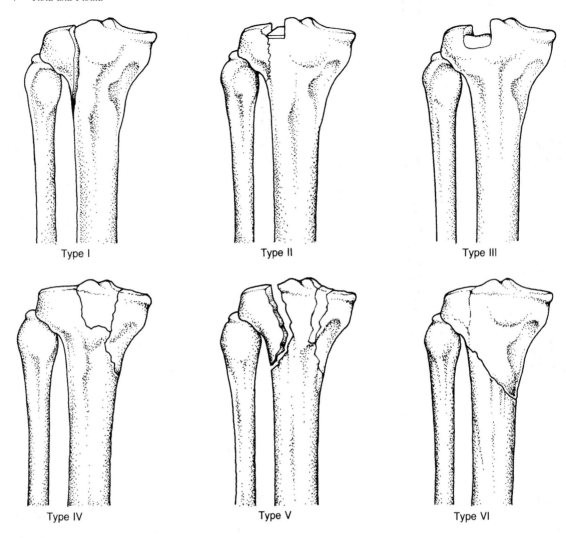

Figure 1.2   The Schatzker classification of tibial plateau fractures

Type I: a split fracture of the lateral plateau without associated joint depression. There may be a variable amount of displacement. More common in younger patients with better bone

Type II: a split depression fracture of the lateral condyle. This is usually associated with considerable articular and subchondral damage. More common in older patients with osteoporotic bone

Type III: a pure depression fracture of the lateral condyle. Depression may be central or peripheral and may be of variable extent. As with the type II fractures, they are more common in older patients

Type IV: a fracture of the medial plateau. This may be a split depression fracture. It usually occurs as a result of high energy injury

Type V: a bicondylar fracture. The intercondylar fracture lines may vary in location. There may also be a depression fracture of one of the condyles

Type VI: The essential feature of this fracture is the separation of the metaphysis and diaphysis. The intra-articular component may be a split or depression fracture. As with the type V fractures, the articular surface may be impacted into the subchondral bone for a considerable distance

obvious. Many of the subgroups mentioned by Schatzker are detailed in the AO classification. The major difference is that the AO classification includes extra-articular fractures and a much more detailed analysis of the bicondylar fractures, which increase from two types in the Schatzker classification to nine in the AO classification.

The AO classification

The AO classification details 27 fractures in their 4.1 bone segment group. It is shown in Figure 1.3. The inclusion of extra-articular fractures (type A) (Figure 1.3.1) is new and obviously open to debate. However, it seems reasonable to include the A1.2 and the more common A1.3 fracture as these are tibial plateau fractures. The A2 and A3 fractures must either be classified with the tibial plateau group or as a separate group of diaphyseal fractures. Ideally they probably should not be combined with diaphyseal fractures, as A2 and A3 fractures occur in cancellous rather than cortical bone and therefore have a different prognosis. Their inclusion in the same classification as intra-articular tibial plateau fractures is therefore not unreasonable.

The A1 subgroups are a mixture of fractures. They are all fractures which in other classifications tend to be grouped together with the appropriate ligamentous injury. Group A2 contains extra-articular simple metaphyseal fractures classified according to the direction of the fracture line. The A3 subgroups contain the multi-fragmentary metaphyseal fractures and are subdivided according to the number and extent of the intermediate fragments.

AO type B fractures (Figure 1.3.2) include the majority of fractures detailed in both Hohl's and Schatzker's classifications. They are the partial articular fractures and the separation into nine groups depends on their lateral or medial location, the presence of lateral or central depression and whether the fracture involves the intercondylar eminence.

Type C fractures (Figure 1.3.3) are all bicondylar, with the C1 lesions showing simple articular and metaphyseal fracture configurations. The C2 lesions have simple articular fractures, but multifragmentary metaphyseal fractures and the C3 fractures have complex articular and metaphyseal components.

Use of the AO proximal tibial classification is straightforward in clinical practice. Its use in the analysis of 225 proximal tibial fractures is detailed in Chapter 2. Two possible criticisms can be levelled at the classification. The revised Hohl classification (Hohl and Moore, 1983) includes a minimally displaced type. Displacement clearly affects subsequent prognosis and since many tibial plateau fractures do present with no or minimal displacement it is probably important that a complete classification system describes the amount of displacement of the fracture fragments. Secondly, it is well accepted that tibial plateau fractures are often associated with ligamentous or meniscal damage and obviously these soft tissue injuries will affect the prognosis of the tibial plateau fracture. Ideally, the extent of the soft tissue injury should also be detailed.

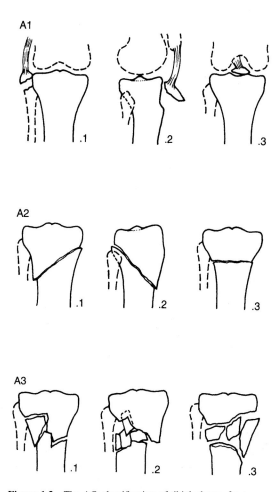

Figure 1.3 The AO classification of tibial plateau fractures

Figure 1.3.1 Type A fractures: extra-articular avulsion fractures and the metaphyseal fractures

Group A1	Extra-articular avulsion fractures
Subgroup A1.1	Avulsion fractures of the fibular head
A1.2	Avulsion fractures of the tibial tuberosity
A1.3	Avulsion fractures of the tibial eminence. Anterior or posterior cruciate insertions
Group A2	Simple metaphyseal fractures
Subgroup A2.1	Fracture line oblique in the frontal plane
A2.2	Fracture line oblique in the sagittal plane
A2.3	Transverse
Group A3	Fragmented metaphyseal fractures
Subgroup A3.1	Intact lateral or medial wedge
A3.2	Fragmented lateral or medial wedge
A3.3	Medial and lateral fragmentation

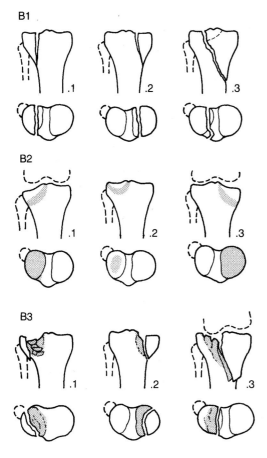

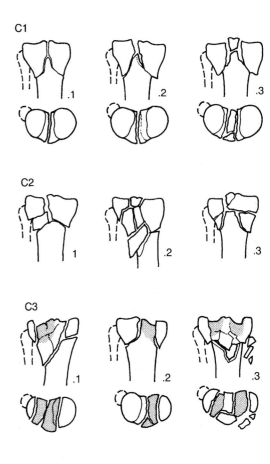

Figure 1.3.2   Type B fractures: fractures involving one condyle

Group B1		Split fractures
Subgroup	B1.1	Lateral condylar fractures
	B1.2	Medial condylar fractures
	B1.3	Fractures involving either condyle and the tibial spines
Group B2		Depressed fractures
Subgroup	B2.1	Total depression of lateral condyle
	B2.2	Limited depression of lateral condyle
	B2.3	Depression of medial condyle
Group B3		Split depression fractures
Subgroup	B3.1	Lateral condylar fractures
	B3.2	Medial condylar fractures
	B3.3	Fractures involving either condyle and tibial spines

Figure 1.3.3   Type C fractures: bicondylar fractures

Group C1		Simple intra-articular and metaphyseal fracture configurations
Subgroup	C1.1	Slight displacement
	C1.2	One condyle displaced
	C1.3	Both condyles displaced
Group C2		Simple intra-articular and comminuted metaphyseal fractures
Subgroup	C2.1	Intact medial or lateral wedge
	C2.2	Fragmented medial or lateral wedge
Group C3		Comminuted intra-articular and metaphyseal fractures
Subgroup	C3.1	Mainly involving lateral condyle
	C3.2	Mainly involving medial condyle
	C3.3	Both condyles

Classification of tibial diaphyseal fracture

A number of early workers realized that the severity of injury largely dictated the speed of healing of tibial diaphyseal fractures (Bohler, 1936; Carpenter *et al.*, 1952). However, the first major studies to distinguish between different types of

tibial diaphyseal fractures were documented by Ellis (1958) and Nicoll (1964).

Ellis analysed 535 fresh diaphyseal tibial fractures in terms of the degree of fracture displacement, the extent of the open wound and the severity of comminution. Based on these criteria, he was able to divide tibial diaphyseal fractures into three types or grades. These were:

1 Fractures of minor severity, these being fractures with undisplaced or angulated fragments, whether or not complicated by minor degrees of comminution or compound wounding.
2 Fractures of moderate severity with completely displaced fragments, whether or not complicated by minor degrees of comminution or compound wounding.
3 Fractures of major severity complicated by major comminution or a major compound wound.

It was found that in clinical practice all grade 3 fractures were completely displaced.

Nicoll (1964) analysed 705 adult tibial diaphyseal fractures and agreed with Ellis's findings. However, he went further and suggested that four factors, namely displacement, comminution, infection and associated soft tissue injury, all had an effect on the rate of union. He also stressed the importance of the degree of bone loss in subsequent prognosis.

Weissman *et al.* (1966) also used displacement to categorize tibial diaphyseal fractures. They suggested four types of diaphyseal fracture based on the degree of displacement and angulation. If there was less than one-eighth cortical diameter displacement and less than 10° of angulation, the fracture was defined as being minimally displaced. The second category included all fractures that showed displacement of between one-fifth and two-fifths of the cortical diameter and angulation of between 10° and 30°. The third category contained fractures where the displacement was more than half the cortical diameter, and the most severe, fourth, category contained all fractures that had no cortical contact at all.

In 1983 Johner and Wruhs produced a morphological classification of tibial diaphyseal fractures that was the forerunner of the present AO tibial diaphyseal classification. They used the alphanumeric system and divided tibial diaphyseal fractures into nine groups according to the degree of comminution and the mechanism of the injury. They also detailed the typical cause of each of the nine types. There are no important differences between the nine Johner and Wruhs fracture types and the nine basic AO diaphyseal groups, and the Johner and Wruhs classification will therefore not be reproduced here.

The AO diaphyseal classification (bone segment 4.2) is illustrated in Figure 1.4. The type A fractures (Figure 1.4.1) are simple fractures without any butterfly fragment or comminution. The A1

group comprise spiral fractures. The A2 group contains oblique fractures, the definition of obliquity being that the angle of the fracture line is

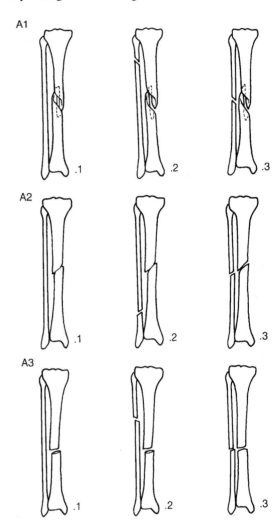

Figure 1.4 The AO classification of fractures of the tibial diaphysis

Figure 1.4.1 Type A fractures: simple fractures (one fracture line)

Group A1	Spiral fractures	
Subgroup A1.1	Intact fibula	
A1.2	Tibia and fibula fractures at different level	
A1.3	Tibia and fibula fractures at same level	
Group A2	Oblique fractures (fracture line >30°)	
Subgroup A2.1	Intact fibula	
A2.2	Tibia and fibula fractures at different level	
A2.3	Tibia and fibula fractures at same level	
Group A3	Transverse fractures (fracture line <30°)	
Subgroup A3.1	Intact fibula	
A3.2	Tibia and fibula fractures at different level	
A3.3	Tibia and fibula fractures at same level	

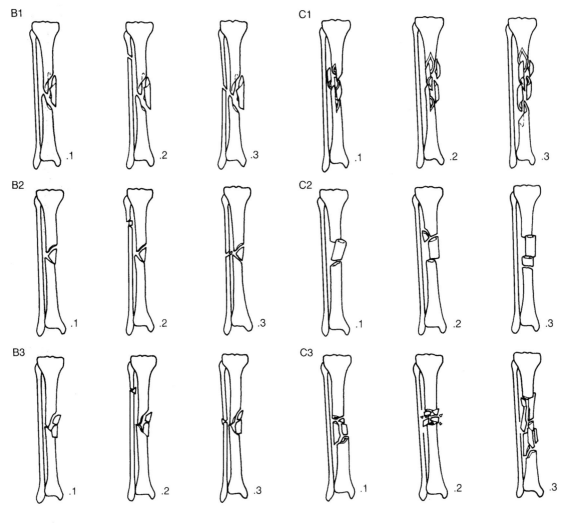

Figure 1.4.2

Type B fractures	Wedge fractures (intact or comminuted butterfly fragment)
Group B1	Intact spiral wedge fractures
Subgroup B1.1	Intact fibula
B1.2	Tibia and fibula fractures at different level
B1.3	Tibia and fibula fractures at same level
Group B2	Intact bending wedge fractures
Subgroup B2.1	Intact fibula
B2.2	Tibia and fibula fractures at different level
B2.3	Tibia and fibula fractures at same level
Group B3	Comminuted wedge fractures
Subgroup B3.1	Intact fibula
B3.2	Tibia and fibula fractures at different level
B3.3	Tibia and fibula fractures at same level

Figure 1.4.3

Type C fracture	Complex fractures (multi-fragmentary, segmental or comminuted fractures)
Group C1	Spiral fractures
Subgroup C1.1	Two intermediate fragments
C1.2	Three intermediate fragments
C1.3	More than three intermediate fragments
Group C2	Segmental fractures
Subgroup C2.1	One segmental fragment
C2.2	Segmental fragment and additional wedge fragment
C2.3	Two intermediate segmental fragments
Group C3	Irregular (comminuted) fractures
Subgroup C3.1	Two or three intermediate fragments
C3.2	Limited comminution (< 4 cm)
C3.3	Extensive comminution (> 4 cm)

greater than 30°. Where the angle of the fracture line is less than 30° these fractures are defined as transverse and are included in the A3 group. The type B fractures (Figure 1.4.2) are wedge frac-

tures that have an intact or fragmented butterfly segment. The subdivisions of both the type A and type B fractures are identical and depend on the presence of a fibular fracture and its location in relation to the tibial fracture. The type C fractures (Figure 1.4.3) are all complex comminuted fractures. The C1 group contains a number of variants of the spiral fracture with different numbers of intermediate fractures. The C2 group represents different types of segmental fracture and the C3 group shows different degrees of cortical fragmentation.

The AO diaphyseal classification is easy to use in clinical practice and its application to the 523 diaphyseal tibial fractures listed in Chapter 2 was straightforward. As with the AO classification of proximal tibial fracture, it does not consider the degree of displacement, this being one of the criteria that both Ellis and Nicoll found to be important in terms of prognosis. It does, however, deal with comminution and the use of the ancillary AO classification detailed later allows

assessment of co-existing soft tissue injuries to be made.

Classification of pilon fractures

Historically there is some overlap in the classification of tibial pilon or plafond fractures (see Chapter 13) and ankle fractures. Ashurst and Bromer (1922) described an aetiological classification of ankle fractures separating the causative forces into external rotation, abduction, adduction and compression (see Figure 1.7). In each group they defined first-, second- and third-degree injuries. All the third-degree injuries of the external rotation, abduction and adduction groups are extra-articular distal tibial fractures, which the current AO classification would include as type A

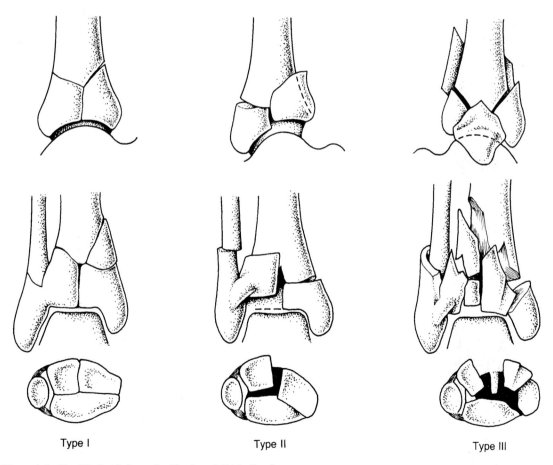

Type I   Type II   Type III

Figure 1.5 The Rüedi–Allgöwer classification of tibial pilon fractures

Type I: cleavage fracture of the distal tibia without major dislocation of the articular surface
Type II: significant fracture-dislocation of joint surface without comminution
Type III: impaction and comminution of distal tibia

pilon fractures. The Ashurst compression fractures are all variants of the pilon fracture. Lauge-Hansen (1948, 1950, 1952, 1953, 1954) also recognized the relationship between pilon and malleolar fractures, and his pronation dorsiflexion group includes different configurations of the pilon fracture (see Figure 1.8).

Rüedi and Allgöwer (1973) devised the first practical tibial pilon classification system. They recognized three types dependent on the degree of intra-articular comminution. Their type I group corresponds to the AO partial articular fractures without significant displacement of the articular fragments. The type II fractures involve greater damage to the articular surface and the type III fractures have considerable impaction and comminution (Figure 1.5).

Maale and Seligson (1980) pointed out that a benign variant of the tibial pilon fracture was the spiral fracture of the distal tibia in which a distal extension of the spiral fracture enters the ankle joint. Mast *et al.* (1986) drew together the relationship between ankle fractures and pilon fractures and incorporated both the Maale–Seligson fracture and Rüedi–Allgöwer classification in their pilon classification. They described three types of fracture: type 1 fractures of the pilon were malleolar fractures associated with a significant axial load at the time of injury and had large posterior plafond fragments; the type 2 fracture was the spiral extension fracture described by Maale and Seligson and the type 3 fracture included all of the fractures described by Rüedi. Mast and his co-workers suggested that the three types of fracture described by Rüedi and Allgöwer became subgroups A–C of the type 3 fractures in their classification.

The AO classification of the distal tibial fracture (bone segment 4.3) includes both extra-articular and intra-articular fractures in the same way as the proximal tibial fracture classification. It is shown in Figure 1.6. The type A fractures (Figure 1.6.1) are all extra-articular and are divided into subgroups 1–3 by the extent and location of the metaphyseal damage. The type B fractures (Figure 1.6.2) are all partial articular fractures with increased articular damage from B1 to B3. The type C fractures (Figure 1.6.3) show complete articular fractures with increased articular and metaphyseal damage from C1 to C3. Broadly, there is increasing morbidity from group A1 through to group C3, but it could be reasonably argued that B3 and even B2 fractures are more severe than the C1 fractures. In practice, the application of the AO

classification to the 66 pilon fractures detailed in Chapter 2 was not as easy as that of the tibial plateau, diaphyseal and malleolar fractures. Nevertheless, it encompassed all variants of the distal tibial fracture.

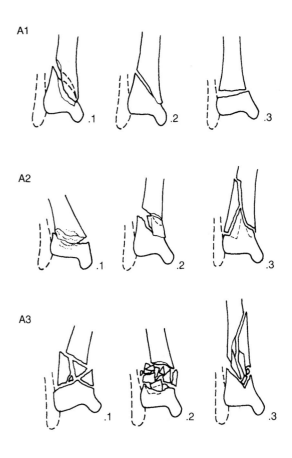

Figure 1.6   The AO classification of tibial pilon fractures

Figure 1.6.1   Type A fractures: extra-articular tibial fractures (regardless of fibular fracture type)

Group A1	Simple metaphyseal fracture configuration
Subgroup A1.1	Spiral fracture
A1.2	Oblique fracture
A1.3	Transverse fracture
Group A2	Wedge metaphyseal fracture
Subgroup A2.1	Posterolateral impaction
A2.2	Anteromedial wedge
A2.3	Wedge fracture extends into the diaphysis
Group A3	Complex metaphyseal fracture
Subgroup A3.1	Three intermediate fragments
A3.2	More than three intermediate fragments
A3.3	Comminution extends into the diaphysis

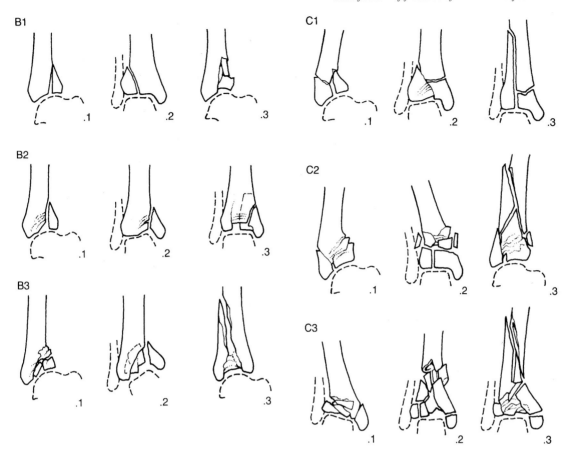

Figure 1.6.2 Type B fractures: partial articular fractures (regardless of fibular fracture type)

Group	B1	Pure split fracture
Subgroup	B1.1	Fracture in frontal plane
	B1.2	Fracture in sagittal plane
	B1.3	Associated metaphyseal comminution
Group	B2	Split depression fractures
Subgroup	B2.1	Fracture in frontal plane
	B2.2	Fracture in sagittal plane
	B2.3	Depression of central fragment
Group	B3	Multi-fragmentary depressed fractures
Subgroup	B3.1	Fracture in frontal plane
	B3.2	Fracture in sagittal plane
	B3.3	Severe metaphyseal comminution

Figure 1.6.3 Type C fractures: complete articular fractures (regardless of fibular fracture type)

Group	C1	Simple intra-articular and metaphyseal fractures
Subgroup	C1.1	Without impaction
	C1.2	With epiphyseal depression
	C1.3	Fracture extends into the diaphysis
Group	C2	Simple articular and complex metaphyseal fractures
	C2.2	Without asymmetric impaction
	C2.3	Fracture extends into the diaphysis
Group	C3	Complex intra-articular and metaphyseal fractures
Subgroup	C3.1	Epiphyseal fracture
	C3.2	Epiphyseal and metaphyseal fracture
	C3.3	Epiphyseal, metaphyseal and diaphyseal fracture

Classification of ankle fractures

Ankle fractures have been extensively studied and there are many eponymous terms associated with their description. These will not be used in this book as they are frequently confusing, but if more information on eponyms is required, the list-ing by Kelikian and Kelikian (1985) should be consulted.

The first major ankle classification was intro-duced by Ashurst and Bromer in 1922. This aetiological classification is shown in Figure 1.7. Ashurst's classification describes four deforming forces and three grades for injury for each force.

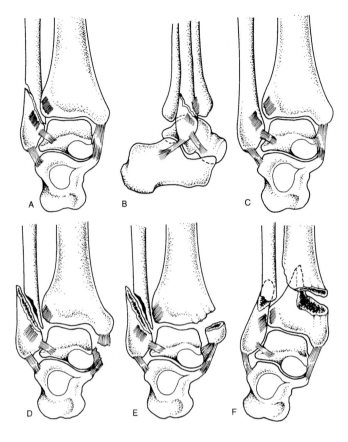

Figure 1.7 Ashurst classification of ankle fractures

Figure 1.7.1 External rotation injuries

A, B First degree external rotation injury with trans-syndesmotic oblique fracture of the distal fibula

C Alternative first degree injury with rupture of anterior tibiofibular ligament with or without a fracture of the proximal fibula

D Second-degree injury with rupture of the deltoid ligament

E Alternative second-degree injury with avulsion of the medial malleolus

F Third-degree injury. Metaphyseal pilon fracture with the distal fragment moving forward and rotating laterally

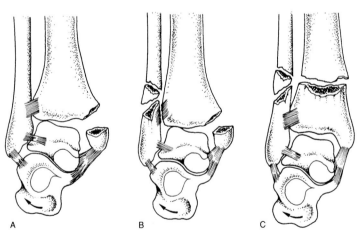

Figure 1.7.2 Abduction injuries

A First-degree injury. Transverse fracture of the medial malleolus

B Second-degree injury. Rupture of the deltoid ligament or avulsion of the medial malleolus followed by a fracture of the lateral malleolus

C Third-degree injury. Transverse metaphyseal pilon fracture with the distal fragment inclined laterally

The more popular aetiological classification is that of Lauge-Hansen (1948, 1950, 1952, 1953, 1954), shown in Figure 1.8. He divided the injuries of the ankle mortise into five main categories based on the position of the foot at the time of injury and the direction of the deforming force. Five injuries were described, these being supination-adduction,

supination-eversion, pronation-eversion, pronation-abduction and pronation-dorsiflexion. Lauge-Hansen used the term 'eversion' to mean external rotation.

Supination-adduction (SA) injuries (Figure 1.8.1) occur when the supinated foot is forced into adduction. This initially results in damage to the

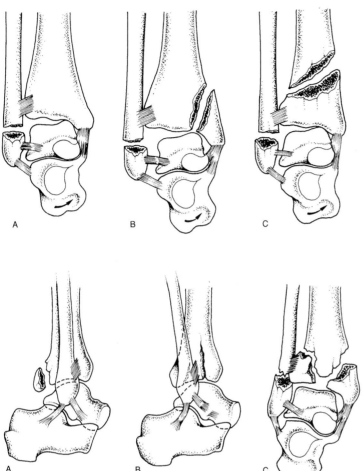

Figure 1.7.3 Adduction injuries

A   First-degree injury. Avulsion of the lateral malleolus or rupture of the lateral ligament

B   Second-degree injury. First-degree plus shear fracture of the tibial buttress

C   Third-degree injury. Oblique metaphyseal fracture of distal tibia and fibula

Figure 1.7.4 Axial compression injuries

A   First-degree injury. Isolated marginal fracture of the distal-bearing plate of the tibia

B   Second-degree injury. Comminution of the tibial plafond

C   T- or Y-fractures

lateral ligamentous complex or a transverse fracture of the lateral malleolus (SAI). Continuation of the deforming adduction force results in a vertical type of medial malleolar shear fracture (SAII).

Supination-eversion (SE) injuries (Figure 1.8.2) result from external rotation of the supinated foot. The initial damage is to the anterior talofibular ligament (SEI). Continuation of the deforming force produces the common spiral fracture of the lateral malleolus (SEII). Following this, there is division of the posterior tibiofibular ligament with or without detachment of adjacent bone (SEIII). Lastly, there is division of the deltoid ligament or a medial malleolar fracture (SEIV).

Pronation-eversion (PE) injuries (Figure 1.8.3) occur when an external rotation force is applied to the pronated foot. As the medial structures are under tension, the initial damage is either a deltoid ligament rupture or a medial malleolar fracture

(PEI). Subsequently, there is damage to the anterior talofibular ligament or an associated fracture of the anterior tibial tubercle (PEII). If the deforming force continues, there is a supra-syndesmotic fibular fracture followed by a rupture of the posterior tibiofibular ligament (PEIII) or a posterior malleolar avulsion fracture (PEIV).

Pronation-abduction (PA) injuries (Figure 1.8.4) result from an abduction force on the pronated foot. Initially there is rupture of the deltoid ligament or a medial malleolar fracture (PAI). Continuation of the deforming force causes rupture of the syndesmotic ligaments or fracture of the tibial tubercle to which the ligaments are attached (PAII). The interosseous membrane tears proximally and there is an oblique fracture of the fibula above the syndesmosis (PAIII). The pronation-dorsiflexion (PD) injury (Figure 1.8.5) results from forced dorsiflexion of the pronated foot. Lauge-Hansen detailed

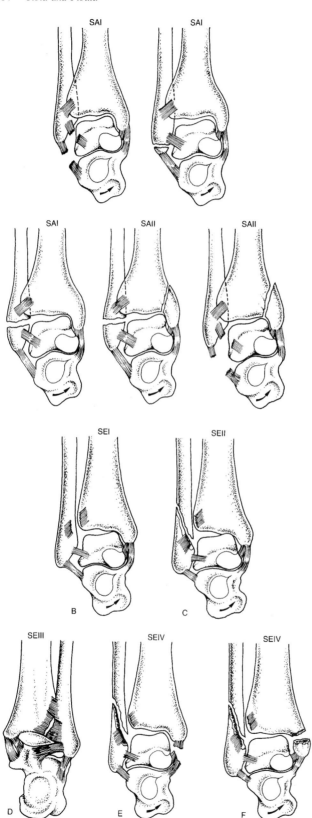

Figure 1.8   Lauge-Hansen classification of ankle fractures

Figure 1.8.1   Supination-adduction injuries

SAI   Rupture of the lateral ligament, avulsion fracture of tip of lateral malleolus or transverse avulsion fracture of the lateral malleolus

SAII   SAI plus compression fracture of medial malleolus

Figure 1.8.2   Supination-eversion injuries

SEI   Tear of the anterior tibiofibular ligament or avulsion fracture from one of its attachments

SEII   SEI plus trans-syndesmotic spiral fracture of the distal fibula

SEIII   SEII plus rupture of the posterior tibiofibular ligament with or without avulsion fracture from the corresponding tibial tubercule

SEIV   SEIII plus rupture of deltoid ligament or fracture of medial malleolus

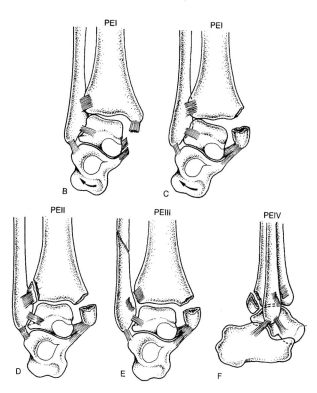

Figure 1.8.3 Pronation-eversion injuries

PEI   Disruption of the deltoid ligament or fracture of the medial malleolus

PEII   PEI plus tear of the anterior tibiofibular ligament or avulsion fracture of its attachment to tibia or fibula

PEIII   PEII plus supra-syndesmotic spiral fibular fracture

PEIV   PEIII plus rupture of posterior tibiofibular ligament or avulsion fracture from its tibial attachment

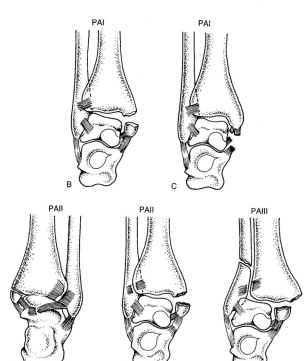

Figure 1.8.4 Pronation-abduction injuries

PAI   Avulsion of the medial malleolus or rupture of the deltoid ligament

PAII   PAI plus rupture of the anterior and posterior tibiofibular ligaments with or without avulsion fractures from their insertions

PAIII   PAII plus supra-syndesmotic fibular fracture

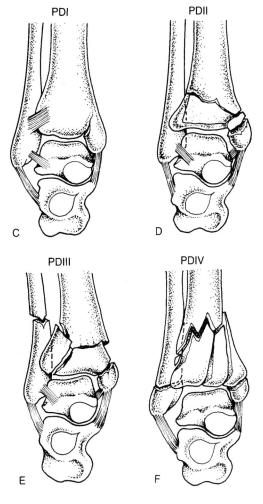

Figure 1.8.5   Pronation-dorsiflexion injuries
PDI   Fracture of the medial malleolus
PDII   Avulsion of anterior lip fragment of tibia
PDIII   Transverse fracture in fibula level with tibial fracture
PDIV   Comminuted intra-articular tibial fracture

In Group A1 the fractures are isolated infra-syndesmotic lateral fractures. The A2 fractures have an associated medial malleolar fracture and the A3 fractures have a postero-medial tibial fracture in association with an infra-syndesmotic

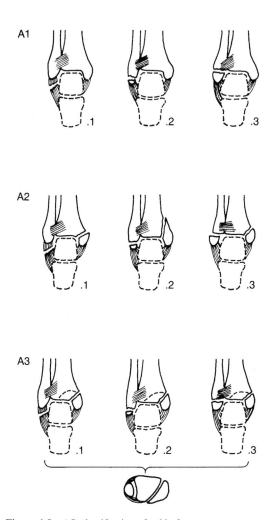

Figure 1.9   AO classification of ankle fractures

Figure 1.9.1   Type A fractures: infra-syndesmotic fractures

Group A1	Isolated lateral malleolar lesion
Subgroup A1.1	Lateral ligament rupture only
A1.2	Avulsion of tip of lateral malleolus
A1.3	Transverse fracture of lateral malleolus
Group A2	Lateral lesion with medial malleolar fracture
Subgroup A2.1	Lateral ligament rupture only
A2.2	Avulsion of tip of lateral malleolus
A2.3	Transverse fracture of lateral malleolus
Group A3	Lateral lesion with posteromedial fracture
Subgroup A3.1	Lateral ligament rupture only
A3.2	Avulsion of tip of lateral malleolus
A3.3	Transverse fracture of lateral malleolus

four stages, the first being a medial malleolar fracture (PDI). Following this, there is a fracture of the anterior lip of the distal tibia (PDII). This is followed by a supra-syndesmotic fibular fracture (PDIII). Lastly, there is comminution of the anterior surface of the distal tibial metaphysis (PDIV).

The AO classification of ankle fractures (bone segment 4.4) is shown in Figure 1.9. This is set out in the usual alphanumeric style with type A fractures being infra-syndesmotic (Figure 1.9.1), type B fractures trans-syndesmotic (Figure 1.9.2), occurring between the anterior and posterior syndesmotic ligaments, and type C fractures occurring above the syndesmosis (Figure 1.9.3).

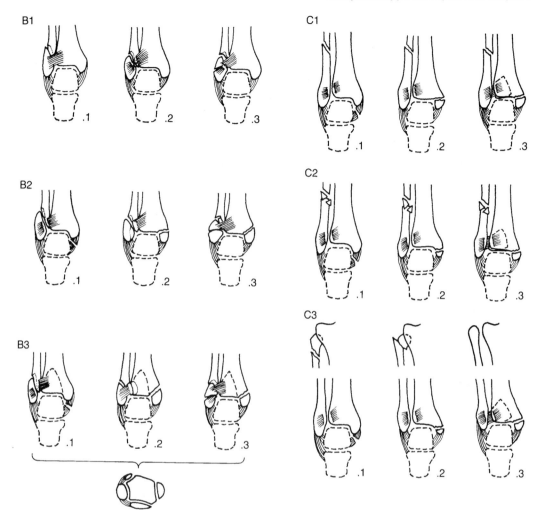

Figure 1.9.2   Type B fractures: trans-syndesmotic fractures

Group B1		Isolated fibular fractures
Subgroup	B1.1	Oblique fracture
	B1.2	With rupture of the anterior syndesmosis
	B1.3	Comminuted lateral malleolar fracture
Group B2		Fibular fracture with medial lesion
Subgroup	B2.1	Oblique fracture with deltoid ligament rupture and rupture of the anterior syndesmosis
	B2.2	Fracture of medial malleolus and rupture of the anterior syndesmosis
	B2.3	Comminuted lateral fracture and deltoid ligament rupture of fracture of the medial malleolus
Group B3		Medial lesion and Volkmann fracture (fracture of posterolateral rim)
Subgroup	B3.1	With rupture of deltoid ligament
	B3.2	With medial malleolar fracture
	B3.3	Comminuted lateral fracture with medial malleolar fracture

Figure 1.9.3   Type C fractures: supra-syndesmotic fractures

Group C1		Simple fibular diaphyseal fracture
Subgroup	C1.1	With rupture of deltoid ligament
	C1.2	With medial malleolar fracture
	C1.3	With medial malleolar and Volkmann's fractures (Dupuytren's fracture)
Group C2		Comminuted fibular fracture
Subgroup	C2.1	With rupture of deltoid ligament
	C2.2	With medial malleolar fracture
	C2.3	With medial malleolar and Volkmann's fractures (Dupuytren's fracture)
Group C3		Proximal fibular fracture including fractures through neck and head of fibula, proximal tibiofibular dislocation, rupture of the deltoid ligament, fracture of the medial malleolus or an articular fragment
Subgroup	C3.1	Without shortening or a Volkmann's fracture
	C3.2	With shortening but no Volkmann's fracture
	C3.3	Medial lesion and a Volkmann's fracture

lateral lesion. The B1 fractures show an isolated trans-syndesmotic lateral fracture. The B2 fractures have an associated medial ligamentous injury or fracture and the B3 fracture show an associated posterolateral malleolar fracture. The C1 fractures show a supra-syndesmotic fibular fracture associated with medial malleolar and posterior malleolar fractures. The C2 group have the same basic configuration as the C1 group, but are associated with fibular comminution. Different variants of the high fibular fracture are seen the C3 group.

This AO classification is logical and straightforward to use. It is easier to apply than the Lauge-Hansen classification and will probably become universally acceptable. The advantage of the aetiological Lauge-Hansen classification is mainly in understanding the causative force of the injury. This allows the surgeon to reverse the deforming force if it is wished to reduce the fracture and treat it conservatively. However, with modern fixation methods conservative management of all but the most minor ankle fractures is unusual, and therefore the ease of use of the more morphological AO classification will probably ensure its popularity.

Classification of fibular fractures

Isolated fractures of the fibula without ankle involvement are very unusual and no classification system has yet been devised.

Classification of epiphyseal injuries

The first classification of epiphyseal fractures was detailed by Poland (1898). He documented four epiphyseal injuries. First, he described a fracture through the physis without any involvement of the epiphysis or metaphysis. His second type involved a fracture through the physis with a metaphyseal extension. The third and fourth type were similar in that they involved both the physis and the epiphysis, with the third type leaving half of the physis intact. The fourth type showed a fracture of the physis in association with a complete epiphyseal fracture.

Salter and Harris (1963) added two types of fracture to Poland's initial classification and produced the Salter–Harris classification, which remains the most widely used classification for epiphyseal fractures. This is detailed in Figure 1.10. The Salter–Harris type I fracture is a fracture through

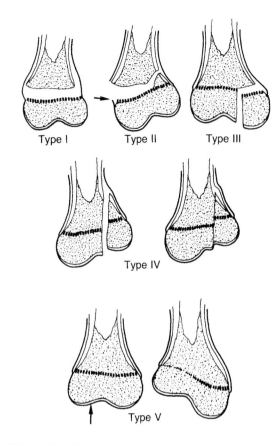

Figure 1.10   Salter–Harris classification of epiphyseal fractures

Type I: fracture through the physis. This tends to occur in younger children and is associated with birth injuries. The periosteal attachments may or may not remain intact

Type II: this is the most common type. The fracture line is mainly through the physis but a metaphyseal fragment of variable size remains attached to the epiphysis. This greatly aids reduction

Type III: the fracture line passes through the epiphysis to exit through the physis. A potentially unstable fracture

Type IV: the fracture line passes vertically through both metaphysis and epiphysis. The fracture tends to displace proximally

Type V: axial compressive force frequently causing partial or complete growth arrest

the physis without any evidence of metaphyseal or epiphyseal fracture. This type of fracture is more common in younger children and is especially associated with birth injuries. The type II fracture is more commonly seen. It consists of a fracture of the physis with an associated metaphyseal fracture. This configuration is most commonly seen in children over 10 years of age. The type III fracture passes through the physis and epiphysis and the type IV consists of a fracture through the metaphysis and epiphysis. Salter and Harris also described a fifth type of epiphyseal fracture, the compression fracture, this being associated with a higher incidence of growth arrest. It should be noted that in 1969 Rang described a sixth type of physeal injury. This is essentially a peripheral bruise to the perichondrial ring or its associated periosteum at the edge of the physis. There is little physeal damage, but the repair process may cause an osseous bridge to develop between the epiphysis and the metaphysis leading to angular deformity.

The two other classification systems that have been suggested are essentially variants of the Salter–Harris classification and will not therefore be reproduced here. Aitken (1965) described three types of epiphyseal fracture in which his type I lesion combined both the Salter–Harris type I and II fractures. His type II lesion was the equivalent of the Salter–Harris type III lesion and the Aitken type III lesion was the same as the Salter–Harris type IV lesion.

Weber (1980) also described a similar classification, dividing the physeal injuries into types A and B. This classification is based on AO principles, the type A fractures being extra-articular and the type B being intra-articular. Weber's type A1 is the same as the Salter–Harris type I. A type A2 fracture is the same as the Salter–Harris type II

fracture. Weber's B1 fracture is the same as the Salter–Harris type III fracture and Weber's B2 fracture is the same as the Salter–Harris type IV fracture.

Classification of comminution

Ellis (1958) and Nicoll (1964) both highlighted the importance of comminution of long-bone fractures as a prognostic indicator. Winquist and Hansen (1980) quantified comminution in the femoral shaft. This classification has been applied to the tibial diaphyseal fractures detailed in Chapter 2 and therefore will be detailed here. Winquist and Hansen separated their femoral fractures into four types dependent on the degree of comminution. Their classification system is detailed in Figure 1.11. There are four component types in the classification: in fractures with type I comminution, only a small piece of bone has broken away from the diaphyseal cortex; type II comminution exists when a larger butterfly fragment is broken away from the cortex, but the cortex is at least 50% intact – this facilitates control of rotation and bone length; in type III comminution there is a larger butterfly fragment, allowing less than 50% of cortical apposition which precludes the control of rotation and bone length; in type IV fractures there is major comminution allowing no cortical contact whatsoever.

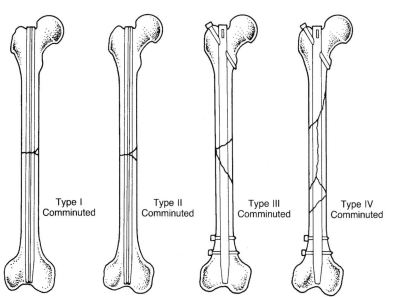

Type I　　　Type II　　　Type III　　　Type IV
Comminuted　Comminuted　Comminuted　Comminuted

Figure 1.11　Winquist–Hansen classification of comminution

Type I:　small bone fragment broken off the cortex
Type II:　larger butterfly fragment involving less than 50% of the cortex allowing control of rotation and length
Type III:　larger butterfly fragment involving more than 50% of the cortex. No control of rotation and/or length
Type IV:　no cortical abutment

Classification of soft tissue injury

Classification of soft tissue injury is much more difficult than classification of bone damage. The reason for this is obvious, as objective measurement of soft tissue damage is very difficult. The recent introduction of nuclear magnetic resonance imaging will help in the assessment of soft tissue injury as will the establishment of biochemical parameters for tissue damage. However, classifications based on these investigative modalities are not currently available and the classifications for soft tissue damage that are currently used are somewhat subjective and open to justifiable criticism. However, it is important that surgeons attempt to quantify soft tissue damage as it is the main prognostic determinant for fracture union, joint stiffness and eventual patient rehabilitation. Currently the classification of soft tissue damage takes two forms: the soft tissue lesion that accompanies open fractures has been categorized by a number of authorities, while more recently surgeons have become interested in the extent of soft tissue damage that accompanies closed fractures and attempts have been made to classify this type of injury.

Soft tissue damage associated with open fracture

Many surgeons, unfortunately, still merely differentiate between open and closed fractures and do not attempt to classify the degree of soft tissue damage that accompanies an open fracture. However, it is the severity of the soft tissue damage which governs the prognosis of open fractures and it is therefore important to divide open fractures according to the degree of damage. Cauchoix *et al.* (1965) based his classification on the size of the skin wound, but this may not directly relate to the extent of the underlying soft tissue and bone damage. Anderson (1971) divided open fractures into three types based on the size of the wound, the extent of the soft tissue damage and the degree of contamination.

Currently there are three classification systems that are used for open fractures. The most popular is that of Gustilo and Anderson (1976), modified later by Gustilo *et al.* (1984). This, like Anderson's earlier system, divides open fractures into three types based on the size of the wound, the extent of soft tissue damage and the degree of contamination. Gustilo's 1984 paper subdivided the type

Table 1.1   Gustilo classification of open fractures

Type I	Clean wound of less than 1 cm in length
Type II	Wound larger than 1 cm in length without extensive soft tissue damage
Type III	Wound associated with extensive soft tissue damage. Usually longer than 5 cm
	Open segmental fracture
	Traumatic amputation
	Gunshot injuries
	Farmyard injuries
	Fractures associated with vascular repair
	Fractures more than 8 hours old
Subtype IIIA	Type III wound with adequate periosteal cover
IIIB	Presence of significant periosteal stripping. Wound usually contaminated
IIIC	Vascular repair required to revascularize leg

III injury into three subtypes based on the extent of periosteal stripping and the presence of major vascular damage. Gustilo's complete classification is shown in Table 1.1. There has been recent criticism of the Gustilo classification (Brumback and Jones, 1995) because of lack of inter-observer reliability when classifying certain fractures. This criticism is probably justified but does not detract from the usefulness of this particular classification which is relatively easy to apply. With modern plastic surgery techniques the size of the skin wound is of little importance and it is the extent of the underlying soft tissue damage, particularly damage to the periosteum, which dictates the prognosis. The three Gustilo subtypes are therefore of considerable importance. Clinical usage of the Gustilo classification in Edinburgh has suggested that it is the transition from subtype IIIA to IIIB that most alters the eventual prognosis of the open fracture.

Oestern and Tscherne (1984) devised a similar open fracture classification to Gustilo's, but they included four types. Their types O1–O3 are very similar to Gustilo's types I–III. The major difference between the two classification systems is the former's inclusion of the O4 type, which the authors reserve for subtotal and total amputations.

The AO group (Muller *et al.*, 1991) have devised an open-integument classification with four groups. This is detailed in Table 1.2. They retain Allgöwer's (1971) earlier differentiation between inside-out and outside-in skin damage, although this has no real relevance to patient treatment. Like Gustilo they have taken a 5 cm length of wound as being of prognostic significance, but they have emphasized the importance of degloving, this

Table 1.2   The AO open integument classification designed for use with the long bone classification

IO1	Skin wound from inside out
IO2	Skin wound from outside in. Less than 5 cm in length. Contused edges
IO3	Skin wound greater than 5 cm in length. Increased contusion. Devitalized wound edges
IO4	Larger wounds. Full-thickness contusions. Extensive open degloving or skin loss

being ignored in the other classification systems for open fractures. Degloving injuries are of particular importance in the elderly.

Soft tissue damage associated with closed fractures

Tscherne (Oestern and Tscherne, 1984) has produced a classification system for closed fractures. This is based on the degree of soft tissue abrasion and contusion, the radiological features of the fracture, the presence of degloving, rupture of major blood vessels and the presence of a compartment syndrome. While skin abrasions and contusions are relatively easy to quantify, damage to underlying muscle is difficult to estimate in closed fractures. Tscherne's classification is detailed in Figure 1.12.

The AO group have also devised a closed integument classification, with five groups. This is somewhat easier to use, dealing as it does with skin abrasions, degloving and full-thickness necrosis (Table 1.3). They have also devised two further classifications for muscle tendon injury (Table 1.4) and neurovascular injury (Table 1.5). These latter classifications are for use in both open and closed fractures, although obviously it may be difficult to determine the extent of muscle damage in closed fractures.

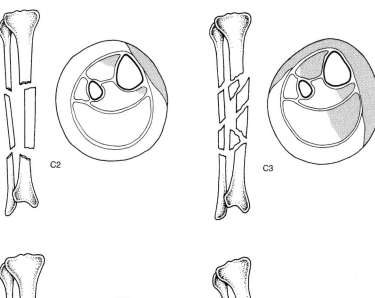

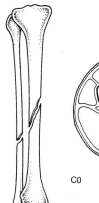
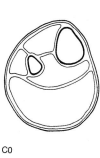

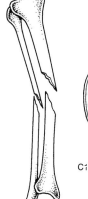
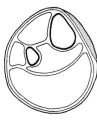

Figure 1.12   Tscherne classification of closed fractures

Type C0: simple fracture configuration with little or no soft tissue injury

Type C1: superficial abrasion. Mild to moderately severe fracture configuration

Type C2: deep contamination with local skin or muscle contusion. Moderately severe fracture configuration

Type C3: extensive contusion or crushing of skin or destruction of muscle. Severe fracture

Table 1.3   The AO closed integument classification

IC1	No skin lesion
IC2	No skin laceration but contusions present
IC3	Circumscribed degloving injury
IC4	Extensive closed degloving injury
IC5	Skin necrosis present

Table 1.4   The AO muscle/tendon injury classification

MT1	No muscle injury
MT2	Circumscribed muscle injury in one compartment
MT3	Muscle injury in two compartments
MT4	Muscle defect. Tendon laceration. Extensive muscle contusion
MT5	Compartment syndrome. Crush syndrome with wide injury zone

Table 1.5   AO neurovascular injury classification

NV1	No neurovascular injury
NV2	Isolated nerve injury
NV3	Localized vascular injury
NV4	Extensive segmental vascular injury
NV5	Combined neurovascular injury including subtotal or total amputation

It can be seen that the AO classification is all-embracing, and despite reservations about the ease of assessment of muscle tendon injury, it is the only currently available classification precisely to define a fracture. This makes fracture comparison easier and also allows for proper computerization and audit of results. As yet, however, the prognostic value of the AO classification systems has not been fully tested.

References

Aitken, A.P. (1965) Fractures of the epiphyses. *Clin. Orthop.*, **41**, 19–23

Allgöwer, M. (1971) Weichteilprobleme und infektrisiko der osteosynthese. *Langenbecks Arch. Chir.*, **329**, 1127

Anderson, L.D. (1971) Fractures. In *Campbell's Operative Orthopedics*, Mosby, St Louis

Ashurst, A.P.C. and Bromer, R.S. (1922) Classification and mechanism of fractures of the leg bones involving the ankle. *Arch. Surg.*, **4**, 51–129.

Bohler, L. (1936) *The Treatment of Fractures*, John Wright and Sons, Bristol.

Bradford, C.H., Kilfoyle, R.M., Kelleher, J.J., and Magill, H.K. (1950) Fractures of the lateral tibial condyle. *J. Bone Joint Surg.*, **32A**, 39–47

Brumback, R.J. and Jones, A.L. (1995) Interobserver agreement in the classification of open fractures of the tibia. *J. Bone Joint Surg.*, **77A**, 1291–2.

Carpenter, E.B., Dobbie, J.J. and Sewers, C.F. (1952) Fractures of the shaft of the tibia and fibula. Comparative end results from various types of treatment in a teaching hospital. *Arch. Surg.*, **64**, 433–56.

Cauchoix, J., Lagneau, P. and Boulez, P. (1965) Traitement des fracture ouvertes des jambe. Resultats de 234 cas observés entre le 1er Janvier 1955 et le 12 Juin 1964. *Ann. Chir.*, **19**, 1520.

Ellis, H. (1958) The speed of healing after fracture of the tibial shaft. *J. Bone Joint Surg.*, **40B**, 42–6

Gustilo, R.B. and Anderson, J.T. (1976) Prevention of infection in the treatment of 1,025 open fractures of long-bones: retrospective and prospective analysis. *J. Bone Joint Surg. (Am.)*, **58A**, 453–8

Gustilo, R.B., Mendoza, R.M. and Williams, D.N. (1984) Problems in the management of type III (severe) open fractures. A new classification of type III open fractures. *J. Trauma*, **24**, 742–6

Hohl, M. (1967) Tibial condylar fractures. *J. Bone Joint Surg.*, **49A**, 1455–67

Hohl, M. and Moore, T.M. (1983) Articular fractures of the proximal tibia. In *Surgery of the Musculo-Skeletal System* (ed. C.M. Evarts), Churchill Livingstone, New York.

Johner, R. and Wruhs, O. (1983) Classification of tibial shaft fractures and correlation with results after rigid internal fixation. *Clin Orthop.*, **178**, 7–25.

Kelikian, H. and Kelikian, A.S. (1985) *Disorders of the Ankle*, W.B. Saunders, Philadelphia

Lauge-Hansen, N. (1948) Fractures of the ankle. Analytic historic survey as basis of new experimental roentgenologic and clinical investigations. *Arch. Surg.*, **56**, 259–317

Lauge-Hansen, N. (1950) Fractures of the ankle II. Combined experimental-surgical and experimental-roentgenologic investigations. *Arch. Surg.*, **60**, 957–85

Lauge-Hansen, N. (1952) Fractures of the ankle IV. Clinical use of genetic reduction. *Arch. Surg.*, **64**, 488–500

Lauge-Hansen, N. (1953) Fractures of the ankle V. Pronation-dorsiflexion fracture. *Arch. Surg.*, **67**, 813–20

Lauge-Hansen, N. (1954) Fracture of the ankle III. Genetic roentgenologic diagnosis of fractures of the ankle. *Am. J. Roentgenol.*, **71**, 456–71

Maale, G. and Seligson, D. (1980) Fractures through the weight bearing surface of the distal tibia. *Orthopedics*, **3**, 517–21

Mast, J.W., Spiegel, P.G. and Pappas, J.N. (1986) Fractures of the tibial pilon. *Clin. Orthop.*, **230**, 68–81

Moore, T.M. (1981) Fracture-dislocation of the knee. *Clin. Orthop.*, **156**, 128–40

Müller, M.E., Nazarian, S., Koch, P. and Schatzker, J. (1987) *The Comprehensive Classification of Fractures of Long Bones.* Springer-Verlag, Berlin

Müller, M.E., Allgöwer, M., Schneider, R. and Willenegger, H. (1991) *Manual of Internal Fixation. Techniques Recommended by the AO–ASIF Group*, Springer-Verlag, Berlin

Nicoll, E.A. (1964) Fractures of the tibial shaft. A survey of 705 cases. *J. Bone Joint Surg.*, **46B**, 373–87

Oestern, H.-J. and Tscherne, H. Pathophysiology and classification of soft tissue injuries associated with fractures. In *Fractures with Soft Tissue Injuries* (eds H. Tscherne and L. Gotzen), Springer-Verlag, Berlin, pp. 1–9

Palmer, I. (1951) Fractures of the upper end of the tibia. *J. Bone Joint Surg.*, **33B**, 160–6

Poland, J. (1898) *Traumatic Separation of the Epiphyses*, Smith, Elder and Co, London

Rang, M. (1969) *The Growth Plate and Its Disorders*, Williams and Wilkins, Baltimore

Rüedi, T. and Allgöwer, M. (1973) Fractures of the lower end of the tibia into the ankle joint: results nine years after open reduction. *Injury*, **5**, 130–4

Salter, R.B. and Harris, W.R. (1963) Injuries involving the epiphyseal plate. *J. Bone Joint Surg.*, **45A**, 587–622

Schatzker, J., McBroom, R. and Bruce, D. (1979) The tibial plateau fracture. The Toronto experience 1968–1975. *Clin. Orthop.*, **138**, 94–104

Weber, B.G. (1980) *Treatment of Fractures in Children and adolescents* (ed. B.G. Weber), Springer Verlag, New York

Weissman, S.L., Herold, H.Z., and Engelberg, M. (1966) Fractures of the middle two-thirds of the tibial shaft. Results of treatment without internal fixation in 140 consecutive cases. *J. Bone Joint Surg.*, **48A**, 257–67

Winquist, R.A. and Hansen, S.T. (1980) Comminuted fractures of the femoral shaft treated by intramedullary nailing. *Orthop. Clin. North. Am.*, **11**, 633–48

2

Epidemiology of fractures of the tibia and fibula

C. Court-Brown

The epidemiology of the different fractures that occur in the tibia and fibula has been discussed by many authors over the years, although the data available in the literature are usually confined to one specific type of tibial fracture rather than to the entire tibia and fibula. It is surprisingly difficult to compare epidemiological data as surgeons usually examine selected groups of fractures and often use different classification systems. Thus some of the older data (Ellis, 1958; Nicoll, 1964) deal mainly with non-operatively managed fractures classified according to fairly rudimentary systems. More recent studies (Müller et al., 1987; Rommens and Schmit-Neuerberg, 1987) have tended to concentrate on operatively treated fractures and therefore have ignored some of the less severe tibial fractures. In addition in some countries there has been a tendency for subspecialization within the field of orthopaedic traumatology so that surgeons tend to deal either with fractures that occur following severe trauma or with less severe fractures. Thus surgeons working in a Level 1 trauma centre will rarely see tibial fractures occurring in the elderly after a simple fall and data derived from their experience will clearly be skewed towards the more severe end of the spectrum. To get detailed information about the epidemiology of fractures of the tibia and fibula in a community or area it is important to examine all fractures, particularly those that are treated on an outpatient basis.

This chapter contains an analysis of 2 450 consecutive fractures of the tibia and fibula treated by the Orthopaedic Trauma Unit of the Royal Infirmary of Edinburgh over a 3-year period between January 1988 and December 1990. All outpatient and in-patient fractures in patients over

12 years of age were included. The AO classification (Müller et al., 1987) was used to categorize the morphology of the fractures. Gustilo's classification (Gustilo and Anderson, 1976; Gustilo et al., 1984) was used to define the open fractures, although it is accepted that this classification is probably more appropriately used for diaphyseal, rather than metaphyseal, fractures. Closed diaphyseal fractures were graded by Oestern and Tscherne's (1984) classification and the degree of diaphyseal comminution was assessed using the Winquist–Hansen (1980) classification. Diaphyseal fractures were also separated into proximal, middle and distal tibial fractures, as well as those that extended across more than one-third of the bone.

Analysis of the literature suggests that causes of injury can reasonably be combined into a number of basic types. Simple falls, falls from a height, sports injuries and road traffic accidents account for the majority of injuries in most populations. Thus in this chapter the causes of injury have been separated into seven basic types dependent mainly on the kinetic energy involved, although sports injuries are grouped together and it is accepted that these may encompass a number of different types of injury. The categories for cause of accident used in this chapter are twisting injury, simple fall, fall down stairs (this includes outside steps, embankments and hillsides), fall from a height, sports injuries, direct blow or assaults (this includes work-related injuries not categorized in other sections) and road traffic accidents. The very few injuries caused by more severe accidents such as train accidents are included in the road traffic accident category. No gunshot injuries occurred in the 3 years of the study and it is recognized that the

Table 2.1 Incidence and average ages of the different fractures of the tibia and fibula

Type of fracture	Number	Incidence (%)	Average age (yr)
Plateau	225	9.2%	54.2
Diaphysis	523	21.3%	37.2
Pilon	66	2.7%	45.4
Ankle	1575	64.3%	44.4
Fibula	61	2.5%	43.2

data may therefore be different from those gained from equivalent populations in North America.

The Royal Infirmary of Edinburgh is the only Orthopaedic Trauma Centre for a catchment population of about 700 000 and it therefore handles all fractures of the tibia and fibula from minor ankle fractures to the Gustilo type IIIC open diaphyseal injuries. The types of fracture treated therefore mirror the spectrum of fractures in the population as a whole. In the 3-year period studied 2 450 patients with fractures of the tibia and fibula were treated in the Edinburgh Orthopaedic Trauma Unit. The mean age of the group was 43.4 years, with an age range of 12–98 years. The distribution of different fracture types is shown in Table 2.1. Ankle fractures were easily the most common fractures seen and pilon fractures and isolated fractures of the fibula without malleolar involvement were uncommon. The average age for pilon, malleolar and fibular fractures did not differ from the average age of the whole group, but in general tibial diaphyseal fractures occurred in a younger population and tibial plateau fractures in older patients.

Epidemiology of tibial plateau fractures

The distribution of tibial plateau fractures is shown in Table 2.2. The commonest type of tibial plateau fracture seen was AO type B, the partial articular fracture. This type of fracture tended to occur in the older population. Type A and type C fractures occurred with similar frequency. Fractures of the proximal tibial epiphysis in patients of 12 years and older are rare, accounting for only 1.3% of the overall group. A full breakdown of non-epiphyseal fractures according to the AO classification is shown in Table 2.3.

A review of the relative incidence of different tibial plateau fractures shows that a number of AO categories were not encountered. These were mainly extra-articular proximal tibial metaphyseal

fractures and it is quite possible that a number of these fractures have been included with the diaphyseal series of fractures as proximal third diaphyseal fractures. The most common type A lesion is unquestionably the A1.3 fracture, this being the cruciate avulsion fracture of the tibial eminence. The average age of patients who presented with the A1.3 fracture was 33.7 years, and of the 24 patients that made up this subgroup, only two had posterior cruciate avulsion fractures, the remainder all having anterior cruciate avulsion fractures. All other type A tibial plateau fractures were rare.

In the type B group the commonest fractures seen were the B1.1 lateral condylar split, the B2.1 lateral depression fracture, the B3.1 split depression fracture and the B2.2 central depression fracture. Type B medial condylar fractures (B1.2, B2.3 and B3.2) accounted for only 9.4% of the whole series, with medial condylar split fractures (B1.2) and medial condylar depression fractures (B2.3) being much more common, than the very rare medial condylar combined split depression fracture (B3.2). Oblique fractures involving the whole of a condyle including the tibial spines (B1.3 and B3.3) were also uncommon comprising 4.4% of the group. Type C fractures, despite a similar overall incidence to type A fractures, show a different spectrum when broken down into their subgroups. No C3.3 fracture was seen in the series although it is certainly a recognized fracture pattern. All Type C subgroups are rare, the commonest being

Table 2.2 Incidence and average ages of different types of tibial plateau fracture

Fracture type	Incidence (%)	Average age (yr)
AO type A	12.0	32.5
AO type B	73.3	57.1
AO type C	13.3	52.7
Epiphyseal	1.3	12.0

Table 2.3 The incidence of all the AO subgroups of tibial plateau fractures

Type A	Incidence (%)	Type B	Incidence (%)	Type C	Incidence (%)
1.1	0.4	1.1	18.0	1.1	1.8
1.2	0.4	1.2	4.5	1.2	2.7
1.3	10.8	1.3	3.1	1.3	0.9
2.1	—	2.1	16.6	2.1	1.3
2.2	0.4	2.2	9.9	2.2	3.1
2.3	—	2.3	4.5	2.3	1.3
3.1	—	3.1	15.3	3.1	1.8
3.2	—	3.2	0.4	3.2	0.4
3.3	—	3.3	1.3	3.3	—

the C2.2 fracture with simple articular involvement and a comminuted metaphysis. The C1.2 Y-shaped bicondylar split fracture with one displaced condyle was the next most frequent type C fracture, followed by the relatively undisplaced Y-shaped bicondylar fracture (C1.1) and the complete articular condylar fracture associated with a comminuted metaphysis (C3.1).

An analysis of the cause of tibial plateau fractures is shown in Table 2.4. This shows that tibial plateau fractures rarely occur following twisting injuries, falls down stairs or in sporting activities. The commonest causes of tibial plateau fractures are road traffic accidents and simple falls, with falls from a height producing the highest incidence of type C fractures. Predictably, tibial plateau fractures following road traffic accidents occur in a younger population. Tibial plateau fractures following a simple fall tend to occur in older people and usually take the form of partial articular fractures. In general the older the patient the more likelihood there will be of a depression fracture and comparison of the average ages of the three subgroups of B2 group shows that the B2.2 central depression fracture occurs in the very elderly. The average age for B2.1 lateral depression fractures is 58.7 years with the average age for the B2.3 median depression fracture being 57.1 years. This compares with the average age of the B2.2 central depression fracture which was 71.7 years. Table 2.4 also bears out the clinical impression that type A extra-articular fractures and type C complete articular fractures are unusual in the elderly population.

Tibial plateau fractures in younger patients are unusual. Analysis of the A1.3 subgroup with the anterior or posterior cruciate avulsion fracture showed an average age of 33.6 years. Contrary to the clinical impression, it is of interest that Table 2.4 shows that this injury only occurred during sporting activity in approximately a quarter of the patients. In fact a direct blow to the knee was the commonest cause of a tibial spine avulsion fracture.

Further analysis of the road traffic accident data shows that 62.8% of the plateau fractures associated with this mode of injury occurred in pedestrians with an average age of 51.2 years. A further 21.3% occurred in car drivers or passengers with an average age of 44.7 years and 16.0% occurred in motorcyclists or cyclists with an average age of 32.6 years.

Open fractures

Only 4 open fractures (1.8%) were seen in the tibial plateau group. No Gustilo type III fractures were encountered, there being one Gustilo type I and three Gustilo type II fractures. The average age of the open fracture group was 35.7 years and all open fractures occurred in road traffic accidents.

Epiphyseal fractures

Epiphyseal fractures of the tibial plateau in patients of 12 years or over are very unusual. There were only three fractures in this series (1.3%). One was a Salter–Harris (Salter and Harris, 1963) type II fracture and the other two were Salter–Harris type III fractures.

Comparison with previous epidemiological studies is difficult because of the relative complexity of the AO classification compared with earlier systems. The inclusion of extra-articular and tibial eminence fractures in the AO classification also alters the relative frequency of the different types of fractures. In addition, the revised Hohl classification (Hohl and Moore, 1983) allocated a separate category to undisplaced or minimally displaced fractures. Analysis of the literature suggests that between 18%–47.4% of tibial plateau fractures may be undisplaced or show insignificant displacement corresponding to Hohl's criteria (Roberts, 1968; Bakalim and Wilppula, 1973).

Table 2.4   Analysis of tibial plateau fractures by cause of accident

Cause of injury	Incidence (%)	Average age (yr)	AO type (%) A	B	C
Twist	1.8	34.2	25	75	—
Simple fall	31.1	67.7	6.6	88.3	5.0
Fall-stairs	3.1	64.1	14.3	71.4	14.3
Fall-height	8.4	48.9	5.2	52.6	42.1
Sport	3.1	39.0	28.6	71.4	—
Blow/assault	5.8	43.8	38.5	61.5	—
RTA	46.7	47.2	12.6	70.8	16.5

Hohl (1991) suggested that 22% of fractures were undisplaced or minimally displaced.

While it is possible to adjust the relative frequency of fractures in the different AO subgroups to take account of the presence of extra-articular fractures, it is impossible to allow for undisplaced or minimally displaced fractures when comparing this epidemiological study with previous ones.

The average age of patients with tibial plateau fractures is recorded as being between 44 and 55 years (Rasmussen, 1973; Brown and Sprague, 1976). The overall incidence of type C bicondylar fractures varies between 11% and 36% (Rasmussen, 1973; Hohl, 1991) although most investigators record their incidences being between 18% and 25% (Bakalim and Wilppula, 1973; Schatzker *et al.*, 1979; Duparc and Cavagna, 1987). If the Edinburgh figures are adjusted to remove the type A fractures, the relative incidence of type C bicondylar fractures is 16%.

It is impossible to adequately subdivide the unicondylar fractures of other classification systems into the different AO subgroups. The B1.1 fracture is, however, detailed in most classifications and is said to vary between 6% and 26.6% (Brown and Sprague, 1976; Schatzker *et al.*, 1979). Duparc and Cavagna (1987) combined B1.1, B2.1, B2.2 and B3.1 subgroups and showed a total incidence of 59.8%. Our equivalent total incidence for these subgroups after recalculation to remove the extra-articular fractures is 52.6%. Our data are also similar to those of Duparc and Cavagna for combined B1.2 and B3.2 fractures. They showed a 5.3% incidence, there being a 4.3% incidence in our study. Their series also had an identical incidence of epiphyseal injuries in the similar combined incidence of B1.3 and B3.3 fractures.

Other authors, however, have suggested a different distribution of fractures. Schatzker *et al.* (1979) had a 36% incidence of the central depression fracture (B2.2 subgroup), although Waddell *et al.* (1981) in the same town reported only a 26% incidence of the same fracture. Schatzker and his co-workers also recognized that the B2.2 fracture occurs in the elderly and the relative difference in frequency of this fracture in different studies may represent different patient populations. Schatzker *et al.* also reported a lower incidence of the split condylar fracture (B1.1) than other series.

The causes of tibial plateau fractures have been analysed by a number of authors. There is broad agreement about the incidence of fracture following road traffic accidents, most authorities quoting a figure between 40% and 60% (Roberts, 1968; Bakalim and Wilppula, 1973; Rasmussen, 1973;

Waddell *et al.*, 1981). The relative incidence of simple falls and twisting injuries varies greatly. Hohl (1991) documents a 12% incidence, but Bakalim and Wilppula (1973) and Brown and Sprague (1976) suggest that the incidence is over 40%. Sports injuries are universally reported as being rare, with Hohl (1991) quoting a 3% incidence.

Bengner (1987) has shown an increasing incidence of tibial plateau fractures in elderly women between the periods of 1950–1955 and 1980–1983 in Malmo, Sweden. They also recognize a slight increase in the incidence of more severe fractures between these two periods. Their results mirror the results of proximal femoral and proximal humeral fractures and illustrate that the incidence of tibial plateau fractures will in the population probably continue to increase.

Epidemiology of tibial diaphyseal fractures

Table 2.1 shows that tibial diaphyseal fractures were the second most common group of fractures of the tibia and fibula, with 523 being treated in the 3-year period. Table 2.5 shows the breakdown of these fractures into their AO groups. It is apparent that the average age rises almost linearly from type A to type C. The lower average age in the type A fractures probably reflects the increased incidence of type A fractures in sporting injuries. Table 2.6

Table 2.5 The relative incidence and average ages of the different AO types of tibial diaphyseal fractures

Fracture type	Incidence (%)	Average age (yr)
Type A	54.5	33.6
Type B	26.9	39.5
Type C	18.6	44.3

Table 2.6 The relative incidence of the AO subgroups of tibial diaphyseal fractures

Type A	Incidence (%)	Type B	Incidence (%)	Type C	Incidence (%)
1.1	3.7	1.1	1.2	1.1	1.9
1.2	8.3	1.2	2.9	1.2	0.8
1.3	4.8	1.3	1.9	1.3	—
2.1	2.9	2.1	1.9	2.1	1.5
2.2	2.7	2.2	1.7	2.2	4.8
2.3	7.7	2.3	6.4	2.3	0.2
3.1	11.0	3.1	1.2	3.1	3.1
3.2	1.5	3.2	1.7	3.2	2.5
3.3	11.4	3.3	8.9	3.3	3.5

Table 2.7   Average age and incidence of fracture types for the different causes of fracture

Cause of fracture	Incidence (%)	Average age (yr)	AO type (%) A	B	C
Twist	0	—	—	—	—
Fall	17.8	57.4	62.0	27.2	10.9
Fall-stairs	2.5	48.5	76.9	23.1	—
Fall-height	6.2	34.2	46.8	28.1	25.0
Sport	30.9	23.5	76.2	18.7	5.0
Blow/assault	4.5	29.5	69.6	21.7	8.7
RTA	47.5	39.8	30.9	34.0	35.0

shows an analysis of the incidence of the various AO subgroups. Only one subgroup was not found, this being the C1.3 complex spiral fracture with more than three intermediate segments. All other fracture types were seen, although some occurred in small numbers. Simple transverse fractures with the fibula and tibial fractures at different levels (A3.2) were unusual as was the spiral wedge fracture associated with an intact fibula (B1.1) and its comminuted variant, the B3.1 fracture. All type C complex spiral fractures were rare. Segmental fractures (group C2) accounted for 6.5% of the series, but the associated proximal or distal comminution meant that the majority were C2.2 fractures rather than the non-comminuted C2.1 fracture.

The commonest fractures occurred in the A3 group (23.9%), with the A3.1 fracture associated with an intact fibula and the A3.3 fracture with the tibia and fibula fracture at the same level displaying a very similar incidence. The A1.2 spiral fracture and the B2.3 bending wedge fracture were also commonly seen, as was its more severe variant associated with tibial comminution, the B3.3 fracture. Complex irregular fractures with complete cortical comminution were also quite commonly seen, the C3 group producing 9.1% of the fracture series.

An analysis of the causes of tibial diaphyseal fractures is shown in Table 2.7. It is obvious that the causes of fracture show a different spectrum from that of the tibial plateau fractures. Although road traffic accidents provide the largest number of diaphyseal fractures, sporting injuries account for almost one-third of all of the fractures. As with plateau fractures, simple falls are a relatively common cause of fractures in the older population but no diaphyseal fracture occurred after a twisting injury. Analysis of the types of fracture in the different causation groups shows that type C fractures most commonly occur following road traffic accidents and falls from a height. They are relatively unusual in sporting injuries, direct blows or simple falls.

Open fractures

Open fractures of the tibial diaphysis are more common than open fractures involving the other tibial segments. They occurred in 23.5% of the diaphyseal group, the patients having a mean age of 42.7 years. A breakdown of the open fractures according to the Gustilo types and subtypes is shown in Table 2.8. The majority of open tibial fractures fall into Gustilo's type III category, with types I and II fractures occurring with similar frequency. Breakdown of the type III fractures into the Gustilo subtypes IIIA, B and C shows that the majority of fractures are IIIB. Only 8.2% are Gustilo IIIC fractures requiring vascular reconstruction (Table 2.8). The average age for all the open fracture types and subtypes is very similar.

The review of the morphology of the open fractures (Table 2.8) shows that the Gustilo type I and II fractures have a similar pattern, although the type III fracture has a much higher incidence of AO type C morphology. The subtype analysis shows a similar pattern with decreasing type A and increasing type C characteristics from the IIIA to IIIC subtype.

Table 2.9 shows the percentage of open fractures in each causation group as well as the average age and incidence of Gustilo types. Simple falls, falls down stairs and sports fractures are not

Table 2.8   Incidences, average age and AO type of open fractures

Gustilo type	Age (yr)	Incidence (%) A	B	C
I	40.7	50	33.3	16.7
II	43.8	52.5	26.1	21.7
III	43.0	16.4	28.8	54.8
Subtypes				
IIIA	43.0	50	10	40
IIIB	42.3	4.2	38.3	57.5
IIIC	48.5	—	16.6	83.4

Table 2.9   Incidence of open fracture, average age and Gustilo type distribution for the different causes of fracture

Type of injury	Open fracture (%)	Average age (yr)	Gustilo type (%)		
			I	II	III
Simple fall	9.8	71.3	11.1	44.4	44.4
Fall – stairs	7.7	59.0	—	100	—
Fall – height	53.1	37.0	35.3	17.6	47.1
Sport	4.4	23.0	28.6	42.8	28.6
Direct blow	30.4	31.4	14.3	57.1	28.6
RTA	40.7	43.2	17.7	10.1	72.2

associated with a high incidence of open wounds but fractures following falls from a height, direct blows or road traffic accidents are. The average age for those patients who have open fractures following simple falls is significantly higher than the average for the whole open fracture group and it is of interest to note that the average age for those patients who had a Gustilo type III diaphyseal fracture following a simple fall is, in fact, 76.5 years. It is the elderly therefore that are responsible for the high incidence of Gustilo type III fractures after simple falls. The high incidence of such fractures after falls from a height or road traffic accidents is less surprising, these occurring mainly in younger people.

Closed fractures

The closed tibial fractures were analysed using Tscherne's classification. They comprised 76.5% of the diaphyseal group. The average age was lower than that of the open fractures at 35.6 years. Most fractures fell into the C1 and C2 categories,

with relatively few C0 and C3 fractures being seen. Table 2.10 shows the distribution, average age and morphology of the closed fracture group.

There is an obvious association between the Tscherne and AO classifications as fracture morphology is related to soft tissue injury. It is not surprising that all of the Tscherne C0 fractures were AO type A and virtually all of the Tscherne C3 fractures were AO type C. The distribution of closed fractures according to cause of fracture is shown in Table 2.11. As with the open fracture group (Table 2.9) closed tibial fractures occurring after simple falls tend to present in an older patient group, although younger than the equivalent open fracture group. With the exception of sports related fracture the closed fractures tended to occur at a younger age than the open fractures. Predictably, the highest incidence of C0 fractures was seen in sports fractures, with the lowest incidence occurring after falls down stairs, falls from a height or after road traffic accidents. As with open fractures, the most serious injuries tended to occur after falling from a height or a road traffic accident.

Table 2.10   Incidence, average age and AO distribution of the closed fracture group

Tscherne type	Incidence (%)	Average age (yr)	AO type (%)		
			A	B	C
C0	17.0	30.9	100	—	—
C1	53.6	33.6	82.9	15.2	1.9
C2	23.9	40.5	1.1	75.5	23.4
C3	5.6	45.2	—	4.5	95.5

Table 2.11   Incidence of closed fracture, average age and Tscherne type distribution for the different causes of fracture

Cause of injury	Closed fracture (%)	Average age (yr)	Tscherne types (%)			
			C0	C1	C2	C3
Fall	91.2	55.8	15.8	59.8	23.2	1.2
Fall – stairs	92.3	45.3	8.3	66.6	25.0	—
Fall – height	46.9	31.0	6.6	60.0	26.7	6.6
Sport	95.6	23.5	28.7	56.2	13.7	1.3
Direct blow	69.6	28.6	12.5	75.0	12.5	—
RTA	59.3	37.5	5.2	40.0	39.1	15.6

Table 2.12   Analysis of the characteristics of tibial fracture occurring at different locations

	Proximal	Middle	Distal	Others
Incidence (%)	6.9	44.0	37.8	11.3
Average age (yr)	49.8	31.3	40.4	42.4
AO type A (%)	47.2	63.5	60.5	—
AO type B (%)	36.1	28.9	28.7	7.2
AO type C (%)	16.6	7.4	10.8	92.8
Open fracture (%)	13.9	14.9	12.2	38.1
Tscherne 2 and 3 (%)	41.6	18.8	24.0	36.4
Winquist–Hansen 3 and 4 (%)	41.6	19.3	20.5	50.9
RTA (%)	80.6	36.4	20.4	70.9
Tibia only (%)	22.2	28.9	20.4	9.1

Location of tibial diaphyseal fractures

Traditionally surgeons have always separated the tibial diaphysis into thirds when classifying fractures. The popular belief for a long period was that distal third fractures carried the worst prognosis, probably because of the difficulty in managing them non-operatively. Nicoll (1964) disputed this, suggesting that middle third fractures were actually associated with a higher rate of non-union.

Tibial fractures can be divided into four groups dependent on the location of the fracture site. These comprise the proximal, middle and distal thirds of the bone with the fourth group containing those fractures which span more than one-third of the bone. For the purposes of this study spiral fractures occurring near the junction of the middle and distal thirds of the tibia were classified into the appropriate group depending on which third of the tibia contained the majority of the fracture. An analysis of the four different groups is shown in Table 2.12. This shows that the epidemiological characteristics of middle and distal third tibial fractures are very similar. The only difference relates to age and the incidence of fracture following road traffic accidents. In contrast, proximal diaphyseal tibial fractures show a significant difference from middle or distal third fractures and are much more comparable to those more complex fractures which span more than one third of the tibia. Proximal diaphyseal fractures occur in an older population and there is a higher incidence of AO type C, Tscherne types C2 and C3 and Winquist–Hansen grades 3 and 4 fractures. Most proximal diaphyseal fractures occur in road traffic accidents and 58.3% of the proximal diaphyseal fracture group occurred in pedestrians. It is obvious that the proximal tibial diaphyseal fracture is a high energy injury which occurs in an older population, usually as a result of a road traffic accident. From the data shown in Table 2.12 it would be reasonable to predict that these fractures would have a worse prognosis from those of the middle and distal thirds and this in fact is the case.

Isolated tibial diaphyseal fractures

There were 117 tibial fractures without an associated fibula fracture, giving an incidence of 22.4%. The average age of this group was 30.4 years. The AO classification lists isolated tibial fractures in each of the A and B groups, but fibula fractures are not included in the type C classification. This approach is vindicated by an analysis of the isolated tibial fractures shown in Table 2.13.

Isolated tibial fractures are usually type A fractures, with the transverse tibial fracture (A3.1) making up 62.6% of the isolated type A tibial fractures. The spiral variant (A1.1) occurred in 20.9% of this group, and the oblique type (A2.1) in 16.5% of the patients.

Type B isolated tibial fractures accounted for 18.8% of the series. In this group the isolated bending wedge fracture (B2.1) was the most common with 45.4%, followed equally by the spiral wedge (B1.1) and the fragmented wedge fracture (B3.1) with 27.3% each. Type C isolated tibial fractures are rare. Four were seen, three being associated with C1.1 complex spiral fractures and one with a C2.1 segmental fracture.

Table 2.13   Analysis of the isolated tibial fracture according to AO type and average age

AO type	Incidence (%)	Average age (yr)
A	77.8	29.6
B	18.8	33.8
C	3.4	28.2

Table 2.14   Cause of fracture, average age and AO distribution of isolated tibial fractures

Cause of fracture	Incidence (%)	Average age (yr)	AO type (%) A	B	C
Fall	14.5	57.5	82.3	11.8	5.9
Fall – stairs	2.6	46.0	100	—	—
Fall – height	2.6	38.6	33.3	66.7	—
Sport	56.4	21.4	84.8	13.6	1.5
Direct blow	2.6	24.0	100	—	—
RTA	21.4	33.8	56.0	36.0	8.0

An analysis of the cause of the isolated tibial fracture is shown in Table 2.14. As with the open and closed fracture groups, isolated tibial fractures occurring after a fall tend to occur in older patients. In contrast, the average age for isolated tibial fracture occurring after sporting activities was 21.4 years, the youngest average age seen in the analysis of all the data on diaphyseal fractures. As with a number of the other fracture groups, simple falls, sporting activities and road traffic accidents provided most isolated tibial fractures. Analysis of the cause of the rare AO type C isolated tibial fracture show that these occurred after simple falls in the elderly, sports injuries or road traffic accidents.

Sports-related tibial diaphyseal fractures

It is obvious that the epidemiology of sports-related tibial fractures will vary according to the popularity of different sports in different countries. In Scotland the sports of association football (soccer), rugby and skiing account for 93.7% of all tibial diaphyseal fractures, with soccer providing 80.1% of the series. The remaining 6.3% of tibial fractures occurred during karate, skate boarding and running, each occurring with an incidence of 1.2%. In addition, the sports of horse riding, ice hockey, motorcycle racing and windsurfing each accounted for 0.6% of the group. In view of the relative importance of soccer tibial fractures and the lack of epidemiological data currently available about them, data relating to the soccer group of tibial fractures are shown in Table 2.15. This shows that most soccer fractures are AO type A and that there are very few AO type C complex tibial fractures associated with soccer. Only 4.6% of the group were open fractures and of the six open fractures that occurred, three were Gustilo type I and only one open fracture was Gustilo type III in severity. A review of the Tscherne classification shows that only 10.8% were types C2 and C3, most of the fractures having relatively minor degrees of soft tissue injury. The Winquist–Hansen classification shows that only 5.4% of the group had significant comminution. Altogether 41.9% of the footballing tibial fractures were isolated fractures not associated with fractures of the fibula.

Tibial diaphyseal fractures in road traffic accidents

Table 2.7 shows that more tibial fractures occurred in road traffic accidents than from any other cause, accounting for 37.5% of the diaphyseal fracture group. Two victims of train accidents were placed in the road traffic accident group for the purpose of data analysis. If these fractures are removed from the road traffic accident group, further analysis shows that only two tibial fractures followed an accident involving a push bike. The remaining 194 fractures occurred in car drivers or passengers, motorcycle drivers or pillion passengers or in pedestrians. The epidemiological characteristics of these three groups of road traffic accident tibial fractures are shown in Table 2.16. When one bears in mind that recent legislation in the United Kingdom and other countries has been directed towards the wearing of seat belts and motorcycle helmets, it is interesting to note that almost 60% of the tibial fractures sustained in road traffic accidents, actually occurred in pedestrians. Table 2.16 shows that the average age of pedestrians involved in road traffic accidents is higher than that for car

Table 2.15   Analysis of the characteristics of tibial fracture caused by soccer

Average age (yr)	23.8
AO type A (%)	82.2
AO type B (%)	13.2
AO type C (%)	4.6
Open fracture (%)	4.6
Tscherne 2 and 3 (%)	10.8
Winquist–Hansen 3 and 4 (%)	5.4
Tibia only (%)	41.9

Table 2.16   Analysis of characteristics of tibial fracture occurring in road traffic accidents

	Pedestrian	Passenger/ driver	Motorcyclist
Incidence (%)	59.2	17.3	22.4
Average age (yr)	45.1	37.5	28.4
AO type A (%)	25.9	41.2	31.8
AO type B (%)	41.4	17.6	29.5
AO type C (%)	32.7	41.2	38.6
Open fracture (%)	32.7	35.3	63.6
Gustilo type III (%)	73.6	66.6	67.8
Tscherne types 2 and 3 (%)	69.8	47	59.1
Winquist–Hansen types 3 and 4 (%)	47.4	23.5	40.9

occupants or motorcyclists. In all groups at least one-third of the fractures showed an AO type C morphology.

Table 2.16 also shows that there is a very high incidence of open tibial fractures in motorcyclists. The overall incidence of Gustilo Type III fractures was similar throughout the three groups. Pedestrians and motorcyclists tended to show more soft tissue damage and comminution than did car occupants.

Considering the relative frequency of tibial shaft fractures and the considerable interest in the management of tibial diaphyseal fractures, it is remarkable how few studies there are of the epidemiology of these fractures. Most authors publish studies dealing with selected groups of tibial diaphyseal fractures and the studies of Ellis (1958) and Nicoll (1964) still remain the major epidemiological studies of tibial diaphyseal fractures. The AO group have analysed 2700 surgically treated diaphyseal fractures (Muller *et al.*, 1987), but as non-operative management is still a popular method of managing many tibial diaphyseal fractures, these data are not representative of the complete fracture spectrum.

The difficulties encountered in comparing the Edinburgh data on tibial plateau fractures with previous studies are minor compared with the analysis of the diaphyseal fractures. All previous classifications relied on fracture displacement as their main prognostic indicator (Ellis, 1958; Nicoll, 1964; Weissman *et al.*, 1966), and as the AO classification does not include displacement, comparison is virtually impossible. In addition, the early classification of open fractures was inadequate, as was the evaluation of outcome criteria. Thus, the only comparable parameters are location of fracture and cause of injury. Nicoll's distribution of fractures is similar to the Edinburgh results, with very few proximal diaphyseal fractures being seen.

In Nicoll's data 54.9% of fractures occurred in the middle third, compared with 44.0% in the Edinburgh study. Nicoll did not recognize the group of fractures extending over more than one-third of the bone.

The incidence of open fractures in Nicoll's series is 22.5% this being similar to the Edinburgh data. Interestingly, in two other series of consecutive tibial fractures the incidence of open fractures is 39% (Steen-Jensen *et al.*, 1977) and 55.7% (Rommens and Schmit-Neuerburg, 1987). In Sarmiento's large series (Sarmiento *et al.*, 1989) of braced tibial fractures 31% were open.

The difference in the incidence of open fractures is explained by analysis of the type of injury. In Germany, Rommes and Schmit-Neuerburg reported that 68.9% of their tibial fractures followed road traffic accidents. Steen-Jensen *et al.* (1977) in Denmark stated that 58.8% of the tibial fractures followed road traffic accidents. It is therefore obvious that the spectrum of tibial fractures encountered by surgeons varies directly with the cause of the fracture. Rommens and Schmit-Neuerburg reported only 7.9% sports fractures and Steen-Jensen *et al.* only 17.2% of these injuries, compared with the Edinburgh figure of 30.9%.

Despite different patient populations there is considerable agreement about the severity of tibial fracture in road traffic accidents. Burgess *et al.* (1987) documented the violence associated with pedestrian tibial injuries, and although the patient group was younger (30.2 years) than that seen in Edinburgh the results were not dissimilar. There was a high incidence of open fractures and complex fracture patterns. Zettas *et al.* (1979) have also noted the high incidence of open tibial fractures associated with the use of motorcycles.

Comparison of fracture morphology can only be made with the AO group (Müller *et al.*, 1987), and as stated previously, this differs from the Edinburgh data by being compiled from surgically treated fractures. There are some differences in the data. The AO group report a much higher incidence of type B tibial diaphyseal fractures (46%), but rather less type A and type C fractures at 45% and 9% respectively. The comparable Edinburgh data are shown in Table 2.6. Removal of the those type A fractures treated non-operatively from the Edinburgh data increases the relative incidence of type B and type C fractures, suggesting that the causes of tibial fracture in the Edinburgh and AO series may be different. The figures are, however, very similar for the numbers of type C complex spiral and segmental fractures. There are differences in the C3 group, where the AO group documented 2% tibial fractures, compared with the 9.1% seen in the Edinburgh population.

The Edinburgh data reflect the European experience in that there are no gunshot injuries in the series. Obviously this differs from the experience of trauma centres in urban North American hospitals, where gunshot wounds are not uncommon. Despite this, the literature regarding the epidemiology of tibial fractures associated with gun-shot wounds is scanty. Leffers and Chandler (1985) analysed 41 fractures caused by gunshot wounding. This number represented only 27% of the patients treated in a 41/2-year period and confirms the unreliability of this particular patient population. The low patient retrieval rate casts doubt upon the epidemiological data, but the results will be detailed as they do provide some interesting comparisons with the Edinburgh data.

In the Leffers and Chandler group 91% of all low energy wounds were Gustilo type I, all intermediate and high energy wounds being Gustilo types II and III in severity. A major difference from other studies of tibial fractures was the incidence of proximal tibial diaphyseal fractures. These are rare in non-gunshot injuries, but comprised 48.8% of Leffers and Chandler's series.

They described six types of fracture. Forty-eight per cent of the gunshot group had localized comminution, probably equivalent to a C3.1 or C3.2 fracture. A further 14.6% had unicortical fractures, this configuration being rare in healthy adult bone under other circumstances. Another 14% showed a 'drill hole' fracture of the metaphysis, a configuration that occurs almost exclusively with gunshot wounds. A further 14% showed an A1 type of long spiral fracture and 7% had a butterfly fragment. One patient in their series who had an oblique fracture of the tibia.

These results indicate that the spectrum of gunshot tibial diaphyseal fractures is quite different from that following other causes of diaphyseal fracture.

Epidemiology of tibial pilon fractures

Pilon fractures (bone segment 4.3) accounted for only 2.7% of the overall fracture population. The average age of the patients with pilon fractures was 45.4 years. The distribution of average ages for the different types of pilon fracture is shown in Table 2.17.

Unlike the other fractures of the tibia, the commonest type of pilon fracture encountered in this series was the type C complete articular fracture, the less severe type A and B fractures being less common. Interestingly the type B partial articular fracture tended to occur in younger people while the extra-articular metaphyseal type A fracture occurred in a much older group. The full breakdown of the pilon fractures is shown in Table 2.18. The commonest pilon fractures seen in this series were the simple articular fracture associated with a simple metaphyseal fracture extending proximally to the diaphysis (C1.3), the simple articular fracture associated with a comminuted metaphysis (C2.2), the transverse extra-articular fracture (A1.3) and the partial articular split fracture (B1.1), the majority of these latter fractures being isolated posterior malleolar fractures. The 'shattered' pilon fracture (C3.1–C3.3) was seen in 10.6% of the

Table 2.17 Distribution and average age of pilon fractures

AO type	Incidence (%)	Average age (yr)
A	28.8	60.0
B	25.7	32.5
C	45.4	43.1

Table 2.18 Relative incidences of the different AO subgroups of tibial pilon fractures

Type A	%	Type B	%	Type C	%
1.1	1.5	1.1	9.1	1.1	3.0
1.2	4.5	1.2	—	1.2	3.0
1.3	9.1	1.3	6.1	1.3	15.1
2.1	1.5	2.1	3.0	2.1	1.5
2.2	1.5	2.2	1.5	2.2	9.1
2.3	1.5	2.3	1.5	2.3	3.0
3.1	7.6	3.1	—	3.1	3.0
3.2	—	3.2	3.0	3.2	6.1
3.3	1.5	3.3	3.0	3.3	1.5

Table 2.19   Incidence, average age and AO distribution of the different causes of tibial pilon fracture

			AO type (%)		
Cause of fracture	Incidence(%)	Average age (yr)	A	B	C
Fall	27.2	57.6	33.3	33.3	33.3
Fall – stairs	6.1	64.6	50.0	25.0	25.0
Fall – height	50.0	37.9	15.1	27.3	57.6
Sport	4.5	22.0	66.6	—	33.3
Direct blow	1.5	62.0	—	—	100
RTA	10.6	52.6	57.1	14.3	28.6

cases. Three fracture types were not seen at all and eight fracture types were seen only once. As with the tibial plateau fracture, it is possible that some of the distal tibial diaphyseal fractures could be graded as type A pilon fractures. Analysis of the cause of the pilon fractures in relation to the average age and AO type is shown in Table 2.19.

The cause of pilon fractures is somewhat different from that of other tibial fractures. Unlike plateau and diaphyseal fractures, road traffic accidents are not a major cause. More than 80% of pilon fractures follow different types of fall: falls from a height account for half of the overall fractures, with simple falls causing pilon fractures in the older population. Pilon injuries following sporting activities and direct blows to the leg are very rare. The difficult type C pilon fracture is most commonly associated with falls from a height.

Open fractures

The incidence of open pilon fractures is low. Only 9.1% of the pilon fractures were open, but of these 83.3% were Gustilo type III and 80% were Gustilo IIIB. Eighty per cent of the open fractures followed a fall from a height and 20% occurred in road traffic accidents.

Pilon fractures in road traffic accidents

Analysis of the pilon fractures that occurred in road traffic accidents showed that in contrast to the tibial diaphyseal group, none occurred in motorcyclists. Fifty per cent of the fractures were seen in pedestrians, the remaining 50% occurring in car occupants.

Pilon fractures associated with sporting activities

Pilon fractures caused by sporting activities are very rare. Only three (4.5%) were seen and they all followed soccer injuries.

The comparative rarity of intra-articular pilon fractures has meant that there are comparatively few epidemiological studies relating to them. Rüedi and Allgöwer analysed 99 patients using their intra-articular classification. They found that 25% were type 1 without major disruption of the articular surface, 28% were type 2 with articular displacement, but without metaphyseal comminution. The remaining 47% were type 3 with both articular and metaphyseal comminution. The incidence of open fractures in their series was lower than that seen in Edinburgh, at 3%.

Epidemiology of ankle fractures

The largest group of fractures of the tibia and fibula involve the ankle (AO bone segment 4.4). A total of 1 575 malleolar fractures were admitted with an average age of 43.8 years. The distribution of the different types of malleolar fractures is shown in Table 2.20.

The type B trans-syndesmotic fracture accounts for about half of all ankle fractures with the infra-syndesmotic type A fracture occurring in 38.2% of the malleolar group. The supra-syndesmotic type C fracture is much rarer at 9.3% and the epiphyseal malleolar fracture in patients of 12 years and over accounts for only 2.2% of the group. The age distribution for the different groups is not remarkable.

A full breakdown of the AO type A, B and C fractures is shown in Table 2.21. A1.1 lesions were

Table 2.20   Incidence and average age of different types of malleolar fractures

AO type	Incidence (%)	Average age (yr)
A	38.2	42.5
B	50.3	47.9
C	9.3	38.7
Epiphyseal	2.2	12.8

Table 2.21 The distribution of the different AO subgroups of malleolar fracture

Type A	%	Type B	%	Type C	%
1.1	—	1.1	20.2	1.1	2.7
1.2	15.5	1.2	0.4	1.2	1.9
1.3	9.7	1.3	5.6	1.3	0.6
2.1	9.4	2.1	6.8	2.1	1.0
2.2	1.0	2.2	6.8	2.2	1.4
2.3	1.4	2.3	1.1	2.3	1.0
3.1	0.9	3.1	3.0	3.1	0.3
3.2	<0.1	3.2	0.3	3.2	0.4
3.3	0.3	3.3	6.1	3.3	<0.1

not considered in this study. They are isolated ruptures of the lateral collateral ligament without a co-existing fracture. All other AO types were seen in the series and the classification was relatively easy to apply although it is often difficult to distinguish between B1.1 and B1.2 fractures in the clinical situation.

The commonest fracture seen in the series was the trans-syndesmotic fibular (B1.1) fracture. This was followed by the avulsion fracture of the tip of the lateral malleolus (A1.2). When these two are combined with the isolated infra-syndesmotic lateral malleolar fracture (A1.3), the trans-syndesmotic fibular fracture with medial collateral ligament rupture (B2.1), the trans-syndesmotic fibular fracture (B1.3), it is apparent that 58.2% of all the ankle fractures in the series were isolated fractures of the lateral malleolus. In contrast, only 9.4% of the patients had isolated fractures of the medial malleolus. The two other relatively common type B fractures seen were the B2.2 bimalleolar fracture and the B3.3 trimalleolar fracture. The most common type C supra-syndesmotic fractures were the C1.1 and C2.1 lesions, these having a simple supra-syndesmotic fibular fracture with or without a medial malleolar fracture. Comminuted supra-syndesmotic fractures of the fibula (C2.1, C2.2 and C2.3) occurred in only 3.4% of ankle fractures and only 0.8% of the series had a high fibular fracture.

The least common ankle fractures encountered were the infra-syndesmotic lateral malleolar fracture with an associated posteromedial tibial fracture (A3.2) and the supra-syndesmotic equivalent (C3.3).

The cause of ankle fractures is analysed in Table 2.22. The same causative injuries are detailed as used for the other tibial fractures. However this is the only tibial fracture which is caused in significant numbers by a twisting type of injury. The AO type A fracture corresponds to the Lauge-Hansen supination–adduction injury and the type B fracture with the Lauge-Hansen supination–eversion injuries. The similarity of the incidence of these two types in the twist group suggests that inversion and external rotation twisting injuries are equally common. The type C fractures that follow a twisting injury occur in an older population (average age 58.3 years), with biomechanically weaker bones. Simple falls and falls down stairs show a similar fracture distribution with a high incidence of type B fractures. Sporting injuries and fractures following direct blows or assaults also show a similar distribution. The spectrum of ankle fractures associated with road traffic accidents is unusual in that the theoretically more benign type A fractures are the most common group and type C fractures account for a relatively small percentage. The epiphyseal fractures occurred mainly after falls from a height or in sporting activities.

A review of the epidemiology of the isolated lateral and medial malleolar fractures is shown in Table 2.23. The three main types of lateral malleolar fractures detailed in the AO classification (A1.2, A1.3, B1.1) show remarkable similarity in average age and cause of fracture. The less common B1.2 and B1.3 lateral malleolar fractures exhibit slight epidemiological differences but all five types of lateral malleolar fracture are very different from the A2.1 medial malleolar fracture. This occurs in younger people and is associated with more severe trauma. It occurs mainly in road

Table 2.22 Incidence, average age and types of fracture for each cause of fracture

| Cause of fracture | Incidence (%) | Average age (yr) | Type (%) | | | |
			A	B	C	Epiphyseal
Twist	25.8	47.4	44.3	52.5	1.5	1.7
Fall	30.3	53.3	25.5	64.2	9.0	0.8
Fall – stairs	8.2	48.6	28.7	58.9	8.5	3.9
Fall – height	6.1	34.6	41.7	31.6	19.0	7.6
Sport	16.2	25.0	40.1	40.1	13.5	6.4
Direct blow	5.3	36.1	36.9	45.2	15.5	2.4
RTA	7.8	41.7	56.4	25.0	16.9	1.6

Table 2.23   Epidemiology of isolated malleolar fractures showing the differences between lateral malleolar and medial malleolar fractures

Fracture type	Incidence (%)	Average age (yr)	Cause of fracture (%)						
			Twist	Fall	Stairs	Height	Sport	Blow	RTA
B1.1	20.2	46.2	40.2	27.3	6.0	2.5	17.9	5.3	0.6
A1.2	15.5	43.5	42.7	21.6	7.1	2.9	17.8	4.6	3.3
A1.3	9.7	42.5	40.8	20.1	7.3	4.9	9.8	2.4	7.3
B2.1	6.8	40.9	9.7	37.8	11.0	8.5	20.7	8.5	3.6
B1.3	5.6	52.1	54.7	29.3	2.6	1.3	2.6	2.6	6.6
B1.2	0.4	35.1	44.4	22.2	11.1	0	0	11.1	0
A2.1	9.4	33.3	7.6	12.5	2.8	13.2	29.4	9.0	25.0

traffic accidents and sports injuries and is very rarely associated with a simple twisting injury.

Open fractures

Open ankle fractures are relatively rare, accounting for only 1.6% of this series. The average age of the patients with open ankle fractures was 49.4 years. Analysis of the open ankle fracture shows that only 7.7% were type C, with 53.8% being type B and 38.5% being type A. Further analysis of the type B fracture showed that most fractures belonged to the B2 group, with 42.3% of all the open ankle fractures having a B2 morphology. The commonest Gustilo grading was the type II fracture, which accounted for 38.5% of the open fractures. A further 34.6% were type III and the remaining 26.9% were Gustilo type I open fractures.

Epidemiology of double tibial fractures

Of the 2450 tibiae in this series, 30 (1.2%) had double fractures, these being defined as two separate fractures occurring simultaneously in the tibia. Segmental tibial fractures were not included in this group. Analysis of these 30 patients showed that they had an average age of 43.6 years. There were three groups of double tibial fracture patients. Group 1 comprised of 4 patients (13.3%) who had fractures at each end of the tibia. Three of the patients had plateau and malleolar fractures with the fourth having a plateau and a pilon fracture. The rest of the double fracture group all had diaphyseal fractures, with either an associated proximal or distal intra-articular fracture. Group 2 comprised 12 patients (40.0%) who had diaphyseal and plateau fractures. Group 3 consisted of the

remaining 14 patients (46.7%), who had diaphyseal fractures and distal intra-articular fractures. Thirteen patients had malleolar fractures and one patient presented with a pilon fracture.

Analysis of the tibial diaphyseal component of the double fractures in groups 2 and 3 compared with the plateau and malleolar shows interesting differences. The diaphyseal fractures are more severe than the diaphyseal fractures that occurred without a second tibial fracture. Table 2.24 compares the descriptive criteria of the two groups of diaphyseal fractures.

The use of the AO classification confirms that in the double fracture group the diaphyseal fracture shows a more severe morphology. There is a higher incidence of open fractures, as well as a higher incidence of the more severe Tscherne and Winquist–Hansen groups. There is also a much lower incidence of tibial fractures associated with an intact fibula in the diaphyseal group associated with a double fracture.

A comparison of the plateau and malleolar fractures associated with double fractures does not show the same results as the diaphyseal fractures.

Table 2.24   Comparison of the tibial diaphyseal fractures associated with a double fracture with those occurring in isolation

	Diaphyseal fractures (%)	
	With double fracture	Without double fracture
AO type A	23.1	55.8
AO type B	46.1	25.8
AO type C	30.8	17.9
Open fracture	38.5	21.8
Tscherne groups 2 and 3	53.8	28.3
Winquist–Hansen groups 3 and 4	50.0	23.4
Tibia only	3.8	23.6

There is no evidence that the proximal and distal double fractures are more severe in type than the equivalent fractures not associated with a diaphyseal fracture.

Fibula fractures

These are uncommon, comprising only 2.5% of the whole group. Only 61 fibular fractures were seen that were not associated with malleolar fractures. The average age of this group was 43.2 years. Twenty-nine fractures (47.5%) occurred at the fibula neck with the remaining 32 (52.5%) being diaphyseal in location. Fractures of the fibular neck and diaphysis tended to have different causes with 58.6% of the fibular neck fractures being caused by road traffic accidents; the fractures usually being seen in pedestrians who had been struck by a car bumper. In contrast to this 50% of the fibular shaft fractures were seen in sporting accidents usually as a result of a direct kick. There were no open isolated fibular fractures.

References

Bakalim, G., and Wilppula, E. (1973) Fractures of the tibial condyles. *Acta Orthop. Scand.*, **44**, 311–22

Bengner U. *Age-related fractures*, Lund University, Malmo, Sweden

Brown, G.A. and Sprague, B.L. (1976) Cast-brace treatment of plateau and bicondylar fractures of the proximal tibia. *Clin. Orthop.*, **119**, 184–93

Burgess, A.R., Poka, A., Brumback, R.J. *et al.* (1987) Pedestrian tibial injuries. *J. Trauma*, **27**, 596–600

Duparc, J. and Cavagna, R. (1987) Resultats du traitement aperataine des plateaux tibiaux (a propos de II ocas). *Int. Orth.*, **11**, 205–13

Ellis, H. (1958) The speed of healing after fractures of the tibial shaft. *J. Bone Joint Surg.*, **40B**, 42–6

Gustilo, R.B. and Anderson, J.T. (1976) Prevention of infection in the treatment of 1,025 open fractures of long bones: retrospective and prospective analysis. *J. Bone Joint Surg.*, **58A**, 453–8

Gustilo, R.B., Mendoza, R.M. and Williams, D.N. (1984) Problems in the management of type III (severe) open fractures: a new classification of type III open fractures. *J. Trauma*, **24**, 742–6

Hohl, M. and Moore, T.M. (1983) Articular fractures of the proximal tibia. In *Surgery of the Musculo-Skeletal System* (ed. C.M. Evarts), Churchill Livingstone, New York

Hohl, M. (1991) Fractures of the proximal tibia and fibula. In *Fractures in Adults*, 3rd edn (eds C.A. Rockwood, D.P. Green and R.W. Bucholz), J.B. Lippincott, New York

Leffers, D. and Chandler, R.W. (1985) Tibial fractures associated with circular gunshot injuries. *J. Trauma*, **25**, 1059–65

Müller, M.E., Nazarian, S., Koch, P. and Schatzker, J. (1987) *The Comprehensive Classification of Fractures of the Long Bones*, Springer-Verlag, Berlin

Nicole E.A. (1964) Fractures of the tibial shaft. A survey of 705 cases. *J. Bone Joint Surg.*, **46B**, 373–87

Oestern, H-J. and Tscherne, H. (1984) Pathophysiology and classification of soft tissue injuries associated with fractures. In *Fractures with Soft Tissue Injuries* (eds H. Tscherne and L. Gotzon), Springer-Verlag, Berlin, pp. 1–9

Rasmussen, P.S. (1973) Tibial condylar fractures. *J. Bone Joint Surg.*, **55A**, 1331–50

Roberts, J.M. (1968) Fractures of the condyles of the tibia. *J. Bone Joint Surg.*, **50A**, 1505–21

Rommens, P. and Schmidt-Neuerberg, X. (1987) Ten years of experience with the operative management of tibial shaft fractures. *J. Trauma*, **27**, 917–27

Rüedi, T. and Allgöwer, M. (1973) Fractures of the lower end of the tibia into the ankle joint: results nine years after open reduction. *Injury*, **5**, 130–4

Salter, R.B. and Harris, W.R. (1963) Injuries involving the epiphyseal plate. *J. Bone Joint Surg.*, **45A**, 587–622

Sarmiento, A., Gersten, L.M., Sobol, P.A., Shjankwiler, J.A. and Vangsness, C.T. (1989) Tibial shaft fractures treated with functional braces. *J. Bone Joint Surg.*, **71B** 602–9

Schatzker, J., McBroom, R. and Bruce, D. (1979) The tibial plateau fracture. The Toronto experience 1968–1975. *Clin. Orthop.*, **138**, 94–104

Steen Jensen, J., Wang Hansen, S. and Johansen, J. (1977) Tibial shaft fractures: a comparison of conservative treatment and internal fixation with conventional plates or AO compression plates. *Acta Orthop. Scand.*, **48**, 204–12

Waddell, J.P., Johnston, D.W.C. and Neidre, A. (1981) Fractures of the tibial plateau: a review of 95 patients and comparison of treatment methods. *J. Trauma*, **21**, 376–80

Weissmann, S.C., Herold, H.Z. and Engelberg, M. (1966) Fractures of the middle two-thirds of the tibial shaft. Results of treatment without internal fixation in 140 conservative cases. *J. Bone Joint Surg.*, **48A**, 257–67

Winquist, R.A. and Hansen, S.T. (1980) Comminuted fractures of the femoral shaft treated by intramedullary nailing. *Orthop. Clin North Am.*, **11**, 633–48

Zettas, J.P., Zettas, P. and Thanasophon, B. (1979) Injury patterns in motorcycle accidents. *J. Trauma*, **19**, 833–6

3

Fractures of the tibial plateau

J. P. Waddell

Introduction

Few fractures generate so much debate regarding appropriate management as do fractures of the tibial plateau. There is an historical or literature precedent for virtually every possible treatment regime, no matter how conservative or how radical the treatment (Schatzker *et al.*, 1979; Waddell *et al.*, 1981; Angler and Healy, 1988; Duwelius and Connolly, 1988; Maheson and Colton, 1988; Delamarter and Hohl, 1989; Jensen *et al.*, 1990; Lachiewicz and Funcik, 1990; Stokel and Sadasivan, 1991; Benirschke *et al.*, 1992). This wide disparity and such strongly held views can be attributed to a lack of uniformity of fracture classification and lack of uniformity of assessing outcome following treatment.

It is now generally accepted that certain variables should be taken into account prior to decisions being made regarding treatment. These variables include age of the patient, age of the fracture, pre-existing knee pathology, presence or absence of osteoporosis, mechanism of injury, associated injuries (local and remote), pre-existing systemic health status and, finally, fracture type. Each of these variables must be considered prior to deciding upon definitive management. A fracture seen in an osteoporotic elderly female occurring as the result of a simple fall may require entirely different treatment than the same fracture type complicating multiple extremity fractures in a young male motorcyclist.

Therefore, treatment described for specific fracture types should be modified by reference to the variables described above.

Classification

A multitude of classifications have been proposed. In Chapter 1 a classification for these fractures has been outlined. All classifications of tibial plateau fractures should address the following:

1 Degree of articular surface depression.
2 Degree of articular surface damage.
3 Degree of metaphyseal widening.
4 Cortical disruption.
5 Metaphyseal/diaphyseal separation.

The classification used should be applicable to all fractures of the region, and *must* be useful in planning treatment and providing prognosis for the patient.

Assessment

History

The mechanism of injury is more important in tibial plateau fractures than many other fracture types. High velocity injury producing tibial plateau fracture is much more commonly associated with ligamentous disruption (Delamarter *et al.*, 1990), severe articular cartilage damage, associated fractures about the knee, and metaphyseal/diaphyseal separation. All of these factors have an adverse prognostic outcome and therefore mechanism of injury must be sought in the history. Similarly, a tibial plateau fracture which occurs as a consequence of a slip and fall accident is much more likely to have less displacement and be more stable than a fracture which has occurred as the result of a fall from a height (axial compression) or as the result of a blow to the weighted, extended knee (pedestrian/motor vehicle accident). Therefore despite similar radiographic appearance and perhaps similar fracture classification, the prognosis for these fractures is markedly different and may be determined by careful history.

A history of previous knee symptoms, particularly if it relates to instability or arthritis, is an important prognostic factor. Patients with pre-existing knee pathology frequently have a more difficult rehabilitation process and their symptoms from their pre-existing problem are frequently exaggerated as a result of injury.

Associated injury may have a significant prognostic effect as well as determining the priority of treatment. Patients with severe polytrauma or multiple fractures of the same limb may have their tibial plateau fracture surgery deferred; patients with femoral shaft fractures or tibial shaft fractures associated with tibial plateau fractures generally have a poorer prognosis for knee function than similar fractures of the tibial plateau occurring in isolation.

Physical examination

A careful physical examination is essential in all trauma patients. In patients with tibial plateau fractures the history of the mechanism of injury will frequently point to the need for careful physical examination of other areas of the musculoskeletal system or other organ systems. Associated injury in tibial plateau fractures is relatively common in high velocity injuries.

A careful inspection of the skin circumferentially about the knee to rule out an open fracture is essential. This is particularly true in those patients with other injuries where the limb has been splinted. Local associated injury includes laceration of patellar tendon, laceration of the quadriceps tendon, fractures of the patella, and fracture of the femoral condyles. Slightly more remote injuries include fractures of the tibial shaft or femoral shaft. In those patients who have fallen from a height careful attention to the foot and ankle, femoral neck, pelvis and lumbar spine is imperative. A significant number of patients with fractures of the tibial plateau will have associated major vascular and neurological lesions. Fractures of the tibial plateau extending to the diaphysis with significant displacement have a high incidence of associated vascular injuries (Schatzker *et al.*, 1979); displaced fractures of the tibial plateau often have associated peroneal nerve contusion with resulting symptoms.

Significant swelling of the soft tissues around the tibial plateau occurs as a consequence of the fractures. Because of the subcutaneous nature of the tibial plateau, compounding wounds are relatively common in fractures produced by direct blows (Benirschke *et al.*, 1992). With delay in treatment fracture blisters are common.

At the time of physical examination a careful assessment of knee stability may be appropriate. The deformity of the tibial plateau, if significant, will mimic ligamentous laxity on the contralateral side and therefore a true assessment of knee stability may not be possible. In the anaesthetized patient stress X-rays are frequently helpful to document ligamentous laxity (Delamarter *et al.*, 1990). These will often not be useful until after the fracture has been reduced. In fractures with intra-articular comminution, particularly around the tibial spines, anteroposterior laxity is frequently seen.

Imaging

Plain films are generally adequate for the assessment of many fractures of the proximal tibia. Anteroposterior and lateral films can be used effectively to measure increased width, joint depression and anterior or posterior displacement of articular fragments.

Oblique X-rays are mandatory to assess accurately the cortical fracture lines, particularly posteriorly, as well as to make an accurate assessment of joint depression.

Enhanced assessment of depression may be obtained by a 15° oblique AP film in which the X-ray beam parallels the tibial joint surface, thereby allowing the more accurate assessment of joint depression.

Tomography is frequently a valuable imaging technique to assess articular surface incongruity, comminution, shape and direction of posterior articular fragments and to assess significant cortical comminution. These studies are particularly helpful in central depression fractures, split depression with significant displacement, and bicondylar fractures.

Stress films are occasionally useful to assess the presence or absence of ligamentous instability in association with tibial plateau fractures. Clinical assessment of knee stability with the tibial plateau fracture unreduced is often impossible unless a stress X-ray is obtained to determine whether true ligamentous laxity exists or whether further fracture displacement is occurring as a consequence of valgus stress. In addition, stress films or fluoro-scopy can be used to assess fracture stability in the anaesthetized patient to assist in decisions with regard to approach and treatment.

Treatment

A final decision with regard to definitive manage-ment must be based on a careful analysis of all fractures influencing outcome.

Non-surgical treatment

Non-surgical treatment should be used in the fol-lowing circumstances:

1 Non-ambulatory patients.
2 Undisplaced fractures.
3 Anterior depression less than 5 mm.
4 Posterior depression less than 10 mm.
5 Fractures which defy open reduction and inter-nal fixation.

The type of non-surgical treatment is just as spe-cific as surgical treatment and should be tailored precisely to the patient's circumstances.

Non-ambulatory patients and patients with non-displaced or 'crack' fractures may be treated by simple knee immobilization until comfortable. Generally this requires 2–4 weeks in immobiliza-tion followed by appropriate physiotherapy.

Considerable argument exists with regard to appropriate management of fractures with minimal depression. Anterior articular surface depression is more functionally significant than posterior depres-sion since anterior depression may effect knee sta-bility in the stance phase of gait (Figure 3.1), while posterior depression alone has a minimal effect on stability. Therefore rather more posterior depres-sion (up to 10 mm) may be accepted as compared with anterior depression (up to 5 mm). It is rec-ommended that in patients with stable tibial plateau fractures with degrees of depression not exceeding those listed above, conservative treatment be utilized (Waddell *et al.*, 1981).

In patients who have minimally displaced tibial plateau fractures in which the knee is stable to clinical examination and the degree of depression falls within acceptable guidelines, cast-brace immobilization is an appropriate form of manage-ment. The cast-brace should be applied in a man-ner to unload the involved compartment of the knee. Thus a lateral tibial plateau fracture should have a cast-brace applied in such a way to main-

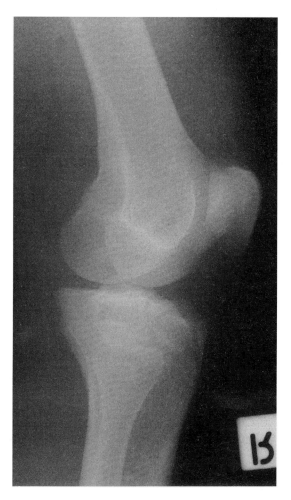

Figure 3.1   Oblique film demonstrating minimal anterior depression of the lateral tibial plateau

tain the knee in varus (Delamarter and Hohl, 1989). If the knee is particularly painful the cast-brace hinges should be locked to immobilize the knee completely; with resolution of effusion and decrease in pain active range of motion exercises can be started (Figure 3.2).

Weight bearing should be delayed for 2–4 weeks; progressive weight bearing is then permit-ted in the brace, which should be discontinued at approximately 8–10 weeks following fracture. At this time fracture healing should be well advanced, and when the patient is removed from the brace a good range of motion with excellent quadriceps bulk should be evident.

Occasionally patients are seen in whom open reduction and internal fixation is not advisable. Patients with severely compromised skin, patients

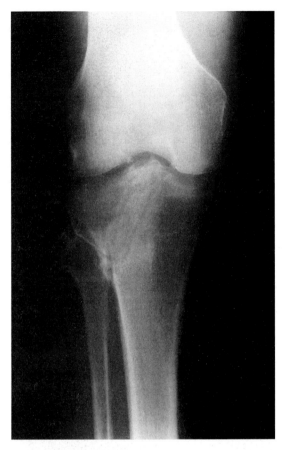

Figure 3.2 Minimally displaced tibial plateau fracture healed following cast-brace treatment

with frank skin loss, patients presenting late with secondary skin involvement and the occasional patient with extensive comminution precluding effective reconstruction all require some form of non-surgical management. Since virtually all of these patients will have significantly displaced and unstable fractures, simple immobilization is not adequate. These patients will require some form of traction.

External fixation may be used as a method of applying fixed traction across the joint. Anterior or lateral femoral pins and anteromedial tibial pins should be used and a frame of sufficient rigidity constructed that would permit correction of the deformity and also provide sufficient stability for secondary reconstructive procedures on the anterior soft tissues. This type of fixator frame precludes active knee motion and frequently the result of treatment is an unacceptable degree of knee stiffness or articular surface incongruity. This is a

small price to pay for satisfactory reconstruction of the soft tissue envelope of the knee; once the soft tissues have been satisfactorily reconstructed late reconstructive procedures for the articular surface might be contemplated.

The occasional patient may present with the fracture so extensively comminuted that effective fixation of the fracture would not be possible (Schatzker *et al.*, 1979). These patients may be treated effectively by skeletal traction. The skeletal traction should be applied in the tibia distal to the fracture site, but rather than using a transfixion pin for traction a small external fixator should be placed on the anteromedial surface of the tibia and traction attached to this frame. This prevents any interference with the anterior tibial musculature and avoids inadvertent injury to the anterior tibial neurovascular structures. Initially the traction can be applied with the patient placed in a Bohler Braun frame with the knee flexed approximately 45°. Once the acute swelling has subsided the limb may be transferred to a Thomas splint with a Pierson knee-piece and active range of motion exercises begun while in traction. A split bed of the Perkins type, if available, is also very helpful in the management of this type of traction.

Surgical treatment

Surgical treatment should be used in all patients who are not candidates for non-operative treatment. It is generally accepted that surgical treatment is required for those patients with unstable fractures, fractures that are associated with ligamentous disruption, bicondylar fractures, fractures with depression greater than 5 mm of the anterior tibia and fractures associated with other long-bone fractures in the same limb (Waddell *et al.*, 1981).

The surgical treatment for specific fracture types will be detailed under headings related to each type in the classification. It should not be forgotten, however, that many factors other than fracture type must be considered prior to a decision with regard to the appropriate approach to management for a particular patient.

Type I (Schatzker): AO 4.1 B1 (Figure 3.3)

This simple split fracture without significant depression most often occurs as the result of an indirect injury and is primarily seen in young people. Depression is infrequent, but significant widening of the tibial plateau is usually evident.

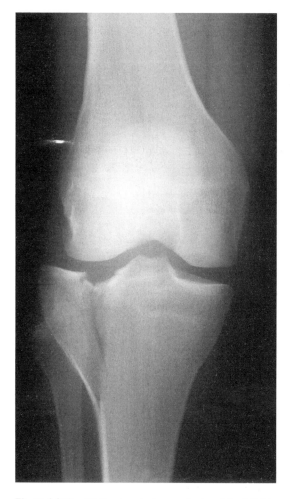

Figure 3.3(a)   AP film type I cleavage fracture lateral tibial plateau

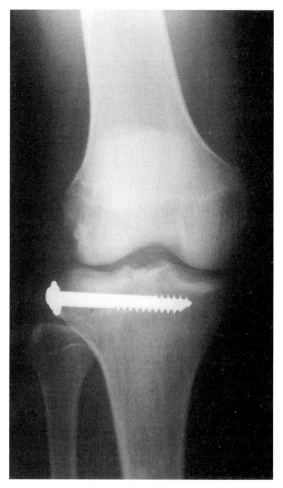

Figure 3.3(b)   Following successful treatment by open reduction, screw fixation

Widening of greater than 5 mm is an indication for surgical management. The fracture is rarely associated with other injuries.

Timing

Fracture management is not urgent, but should be carried out as soon as reasonably possible.

Exposure

A curvilinear incision is required, starting just proximal to the joint line at the posterior aspect of the femoral condyle and running parallel with the joint line to Gerdie's tubercle, then curving distally to parallel the patellar tendon. The anterior tibial musculature is carefully elevated from the under-

lying bone. The lateral meniscus is detached from the tibia in its anterior one-third and retracted proximally. This provides excellent visualization of the fracture and the joint surface.

After irrigating the knee thoroughly and removing the haematoma from the fracture site, reduction is accomplished by compression of the laterally displaced tibial plateau fragment. This can be accomplished by using a bone tenaculum or other large bone forceps. Elevation is not required.

Provisional fixation can be obtained with two parallel Kirschner wires. An intraoperative X-ray should then be obtained to ensure adequate reduction and appropriate placement of the Kirschner wires. Plain screws may then be inserted paralleling the wires; cannulated screws, if available, can be inserted directly over the wires. These should be lag screws and washers are required to prevent undue penetration of the screw head into the relatively soft lateral cortical bone.

A bone graft is not required.

Postoperatively the patient should be immobilized in a simple knee immobilizer and once soft tissue healing has occurred active range of motion is encouraged. Weight bearing should be restricted for 4 weeks and full weight bearing should be avoided for 8 weeks.

Type II (Schatzker): AO 4.1 B3 (Figure 3.4)

This is the commonest type of tibial plateau fracture. It is a combination of central depression of the tibial plateau as well as a lateral split; therefore the displaced fragment is generally depressed and laterally displaced. Varying degrees of articular surface comminution are associated with this fracture; associated fracture of the fibular neck is relatively common.

Timing

This fracture is not an urgent surgical procedure. Fracture management may be deferred until additional X-ray studies have been performed to permit accurate visualization of the articular surface comminution.

Exposure

Identical to the exposure for type I above. A curvilinear incision should be made starting just proximal to the joint line at the posterior aspect of the femoral condyle and running parallel with the joint line to Gerdie's tubercle, then curving distally to parallel the patellar tendon. The anterior tibial musculature is carefully elevated from the underlying bone. The lateral meniscus is detached from the tibia in its anterior one-third and retracted proximally. This provides excellent visualization of the fracture and the joint surface.

The skin incision should continue more distally on the tibia to provide full exposure of the lateral surface of the tibia for approximately 10 cm distal to the joint line.

Once the meniscus has been retracted proximally the interior of the joint can be carefully inspected. All blood clot should be irrigated from the knee to permit accurate visualization.

The periosteal hinge at the distal end of the split should be divided to permit the entire lateral cortex of the tibia to be swung away like opening the

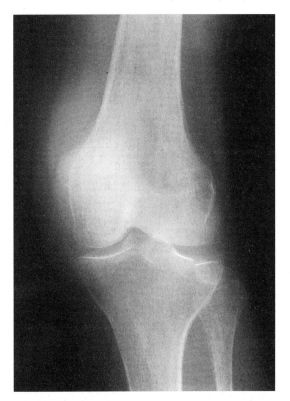

Figure 3.4 AP film Schatzker type II – a central depression plus lateral split

cover of a book. This permits excellent visualization of the fracture as well as the intra-articular portion of the fracture. Using an instrument such as a bone punch or a broad elevator the depressed central articular fracture fragments are elevated to their anatomical position. They may be held in position by a single Kirschner wire.

A bone graft should be placed under these fracture fragments in order to maintain their elevated position. The bone graft may be readily obtained by extending the proximal portion of the skin incision to the midpoint of the lateral femoral condyle from which a moderate amount of cancellous bone can be safely removed.

With this bone graft packed in place, the Kirschner wire holding the elevated fragments in position can be safely removed. The lateral tibial cortex is then swung back into position like closing the cover of a book and anatomical reduction of both the cortical and articular surface fracture lines is confirmed by direct inspection. Provisional fixation of this fragment is then obtained with one or more Kirschner wires and a check X-ray

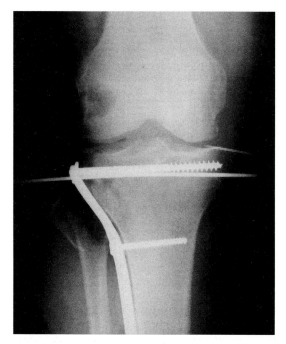

Figure 3.5(a)   With the fragment elevated and held with Kirschner wires, lag screw fixation of the fracture can be obtained

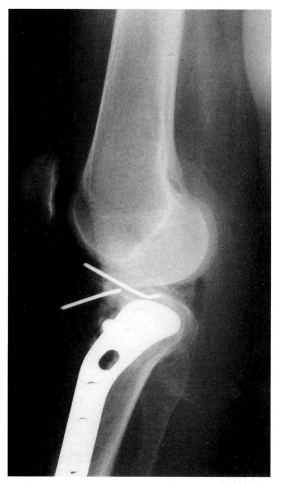

Figure 3.5(b)   Lateral view of same

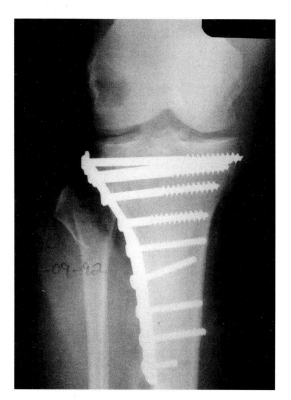

Figure 3.5(c)   Following check X-ray to show reduction plus provisional fixation with buttress plate, application is complete

obtained (Figure 3.5*a*, *b*). With this X-ray documenting the position of the wires and confirming satisfactory reduction of the fracture line, one or more lag screws should be used to ensure compression of the fracture fragment.

Because of the nature of the fracture some form of buttress plate is required to prevent collapse of the lateral fragment. Several such plates are available; the plate should be applied in such a way that it is closely contoured to the lateral surface of the bone and provides support for the vertical cortical fracture line. At least two screws should be in the proximal tibia providing additional compression across the fracture line and two or three screws should be in the distal tibial fragment. A final X-ray should be obtained once the plate has been applied (Figure 3.5*c*).

Postoperatively these patients should be on active knee motion as soon as pain and soft tissue healing permits. Weight bearing should be restricted for 6–8 weeks and full weight bearing discouraged for 12 weeks. The use of a supplemental fracture brace with the knee braced into varus may be of benefit, permitting earlier weight bearing, but is not used by the author.

Type III (Schatzker): AO 4.1 B2 (Figure 3.6)

This is the least common tibial plateau fracture. The central depression of the lateral tibial articular surface without associated cortical split or widening of the tibial plateau is rarely seen. It is infrequently associated with ligament injuries.

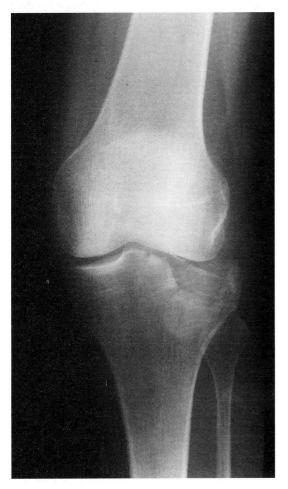

Figure 3.6　Schatzker type III AO 4.1 B2 central depression without lateral cortical fracture

Timing

This is not an urgent surgical procedure and reduction of this fracture might be delayed until supplemental imaging has confirmed the absence of a lateral fracture line.

Exposure

Exposure is identical to that for type I, consisting of a curvilinear incision starting just proximal to the joint line at the posterior aspect of the femoral condyle and running parallel with the joint line to Gerdie's tubercle and then curving distally to parallel the patellar tendon. Anterior tibial musculature is carefully elevated from the underlying bone. The lateral meniscus is detached from the tibia in its anterior one-third and retracted proximally. This provides excellent visualization of the fracture and the joint surface.

Once the lateral meniscal attachment has been severed and the meniscus retracted superiorly visualization of the depressed fracture is possible. There is often fissuring of the articular cartilage associated with the depression. Frank fracture lines are rarely seen.

A one-half inch or larger drill hole should be made in the lateral tibial cortex approximately 3–4 cm distal to the articular margin. Through this drill hole a large blunt bone punch should be inserted and the depressed articular surface of the tibia gently elevated by tapping on the punch. This can be observed directly by inspecting the joint surface as the articular fragment is being elevated. Over-reduction should be avoided. Once this procedure has been completed an X-ray should be obtained to document adequate reduction.

A bone graft is always required in these fractures. Adequate bone can usually be obtained from the lateral femoral condyle; if this is not possible or more bone is required, bone graft can be obtained from the iliac crest.

Internal fixation has little to offer in these patients, although one or two screws supporting the bone graft may be of benefit.

Postoperatively these patients can begin early active motion, but must be non-weight bearing for a mimimum of 8 weeks following surgery. Full weight bearing should not be permitted for at least 12 weeks.

Type IV (Schatzker): AO 4.1 B1 – medial (Figure 3.7)

Type IV are the rarest tibial plateau fractures. These fractures of the medial plateau are produced

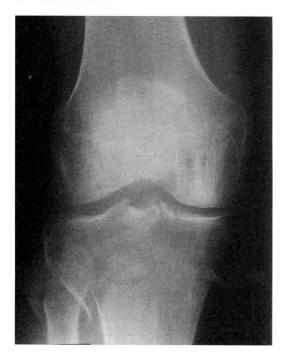

Figure 3.7(a)   AP film: open type IV with significant bone loss

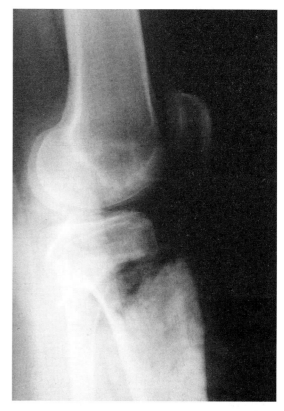

Figure 3.7(b)   Lateral film: open type IV with significant bone loss

by a varus stress upon the knee, and since this is an uncommon stress to be applied they are seen relatively infrequently. They are, however, always the product of high velocity injury and are commonly associated with injuries of the opposite knee because of the mechanism of production. They are also commonly associated with peroneal nerve injuries because of the amount of varus displacement at the time of fracture.

Timing

These are not urgent surgical problems in themselves, but frequently present with a constellation of other injuries that demand urgent treatment. These fractures may be fixed initially or delayed depending upon associated problems. They are rarely comminuted and additional preoperative imaging is rarely required.

Exposure

The fracture can be exposed through a medial parapatellar incision which is extended proximally and distally as required. The meniscus should be elevated by detaching its middle third through the coronary ligaments from the medial tibial margin; once elevated proximally, the interior of the joint can be clearly inspected. There is rarely significant compression or depression of the articular surface and most fractures tend to be cleavage injuries.

With the distal cortical fracture line exposed (this may occasionally require detachment of the portion of the pes anserinus) and the joint under direct vision, the knee should be irrigated and all clot removed. The medial fragment should then be elevated and compressed to provide an anatomical reduction. Provisional fixation should be obtained with K-wires. Once the Kirschner wires have been placed in a satisfactory position a check X-ray will confirm the adequacy of reduction as well as the placement of the wires. Solid or cannulated lag screws may be used to provide compression across the fracture line. Because of the very significant forces acting across the medial tibia, buttressing by additional plate fixation is always required. Plates specifically designed for the lateral tibial plateau frequently do not fit the medial tibia because the cortical border is much flatter; therefore a slightly modified straight plate may be more appropriate in terms of providing adequate fixation.

Postoperatively these patients should be kept on restricted weight bearing for a minimum of 8 weeks and should not be allowed full weight bearing until 12 weeks from the time of surgery.

Bone graft is rarely required since this tends to be a cleavage injury.

Type V (Schatzker): AO 4.1 C1–C3 (Figure 3.8)

Bicondylar fractures of the tibial plateau are the most serious tibial plateau injuries. They are invariably the result of high velocity injury and are therefore commonly associated with both systemic and other musculoskeletal injuries. In addition, since most are produced by direct blows to the anterior aspect of the knee or as a consequence of a fall from a height the incidence of open fractures is high (Benirschke *et al.*, 1992).

Timing

Because of the degree of instability of the knee, presence of associated injury and the possibility of skin compromise, a significant number of these fractures require urgent treatment. Since most of these fractures also have significant comminution treatment is occasionally undertaken without ideal additional imaging being available. This circumstance occasionally leads to real surgical difficulty.

Exposure

Exposure of these injuries is difficult. Three generally accepted surgical exposures to permit

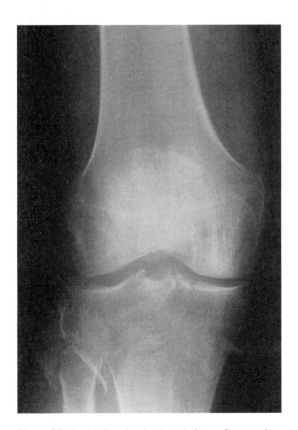

Figure 3.8(a)   AP film showing lateral plateau fracture plus possibility of medial plateau fracture

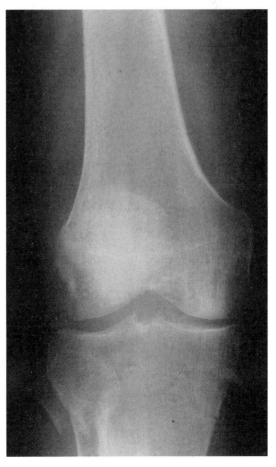

Figure 3.8(b)   Slightly more oblique projection confirming medial cortical fracture

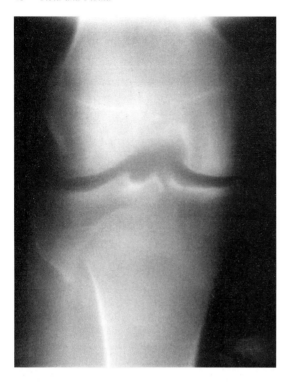

Figure 3.8(c)   Tomogram demonstrating intercondylar fracture in addition to confirming medial and lateral cortical disruption

visualization of both the medial and the lateral tibia as well as visualization of the joint surface have been described.

1 Reverse Mercedes   This approach, combining oblique medial and lateral incisions with a vertical distal incision, centred over the tibial tubercle, provides excellent exposure of the anterior medial and lateral tibia. It is, unfortunately, associated with significant skin healing problems at the junction of the three incision lines (Schatzker *et al.*, 1979). It should be used with great caution and should never be used in patients with vascular compromise of the anterior tibial skin.

2 Medial and lateral incisions   Separate medial and lateral incisions may be used to visualize the medial and lateral tibia and provide adequate visualization of the joint surface by bilateral submeniscal incisions. Unfortunately the skin bridge between the two incisions is often compromised by the injury and delayed healing of these incisions is possible. Furthermore, adequate visualization of the anterior tibia is difficult.

3 Anterior incision   The use of a long anterior incision, similar to that employed for total knee replacement, is gaining significant popularity. It is frequently necessary to osteotomize or reflect the fractured tibial tubercle laterally to permit good visualization (Fernandez, 1988). However, by using an anterior skin incision, medial parapatellar capsular incision and dislocating the patella laterally with or without reflection of the tibial tubercle excellent exposure to the anterior tibia and to the articular surface of the tibia is possible. Submeniscal exposure is not required since the articular surface visualization is generally adequate. The incision frequently must be extended distally down the tibia to provide adequate access.

The reduction of these fractures is extremely difficult. In general the medial side of the tibia has less comminution both of the cortical fracture line and of the articular surface. Therefore it is generally easier to approach the medial tibia first, and after appropriate exposure, irrigation and visualization obtain an anatomical reduction of the medial tibial plateau. This reduction should be held by provisional plate fixation utilizing short screws in the medial tibial fragment.

The lateral tibial plateau fragment, frequently with more comminution and significantly more depression of the articular surface as well as more comminution of the lateral cortical surface, is then reduced to the medial tibial plateau and to the lateral tibial cortex. This requires considerable time and patience in order to obtain an acceptable reduction. Once this reduction has been achieved, provisional fixation with Kirschner wires should be provided. X-ray examination of the knee should demonstrate anatomical reduction of both plateaus in relationship to one another as well as in relationship to the tibial shaft. Once the X-ray has confirmed this reduction lag screw fixation of the lateral tibial plateau to the medial tibial plateau should be secured. This can be done by exchanging the short screws in the medial tibial plate for full-length lag screws.

A buttress plate on the lateral side of the tibia is necessary to provide adequate stability (Vandenberghe *et al.*, 1990) There will therefore be a medial plate and a lateral plate with lag screws passing through both plates. Because of the triangular shape of the tibial diaphysis the distal screws in the two plates should not interfere with one another (Schatzker *et al.*, 1979).

Skin closure is frequently a problem in the acute situation. Every effort must be made to obtain soft tissue coverage of the joint and of the plates used to reconstruct the proximal tibia.

The use of bone graft should be encouraged. There will be many areas of comminution which will require buttressing with cancellous bone. This can be obtained from the distal femur or iliac crest.

These fractures are frequently complicated by a fracture of the posterior half of either the medial or the lateral tibial plateau (Figure 3.9). This fracture fragment is difficult to reduce and once reduced is difficult to maintain in the reduced position. However, if this fracture fragment is not reduced and stabilized, the end result will be poor because of persistent deformity of the proximal tibia. At the time of provisional fixation of the tibial plateau every effort should be made to ensure that the posterior fragment of the tibial plateau has been reduced to be congruent with the anterior fragment (Waddell *et al.*, 1981; Lachiewicz and Funcik, 1990; Stokel and Sadasivan, 1991). This can be secured by Kirschner wire fixation and single or parallel cannulated screws can then be passed over these wires to ensure adequate fixation and compression of this important fracture fragment.

In certain circumstances where skin compromise is felt to preclude safe exposure of both the medial and lateral tibia it has been suggested that isolated external fixation of the medial fracture fragment can be combined with open reduction and internal fixation of the lateral fracture fragment. Two fixator pins are placed percutaneously under image intensifier control in the medial tibial plateau fragment and two fixator pins are placed in the anterior-medial border of the tibia distal to the fracture site. An external fixator is applied to these pins and the plateau held in a reduced position. A single lateral incision is then used to reduce the lateral tibial plateau and fix it to the medial plateau with lag screws and to the lateral tibia with a buttress plate. This technique is particularly useful in the face of compromised anteromedial tibial skin.

Type VI (Schatzker): AO 4.1 C2 (Figure 3.10)

Fractures of both tibial plateaus with diaphyseal/metaphyseal discontinuity are relatively uncommon. They generally occur as a result of a fall from

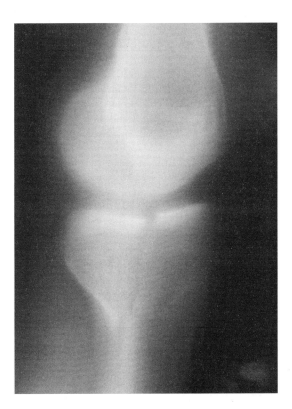

Figure 3.9 Lateral tomogram demonstrating posterior half of the lateral tibial plateau

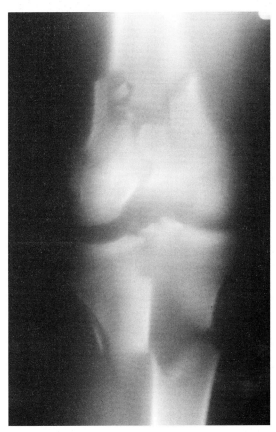

Figure 3.10 Tomogram to define fracture lines in Schatzker VI fracture type; note associated distal femoral fracture

a height or as a result of high velocity motor vehicle trauma. The problems associated with these fractures relate primarily to the high degree of instability plus the extensive comminution which frequently makes accurate restoration of the correct anatomical relationship of the bony plateaus to the diaphysis impossible. Cortical fractures are either extensively comminuted or buckled so that accurate fracture line matching is very difficult.

Timing

These are not emergency procedures, although because of the mechanism of injury they are often associated with other injuries because of high velocity trauma. Supplementary imaging is frequently useful, in particular to define the extent of intra-articular and central imminence comminution as well as to confirm the presence or absence of a separate posterior articular fragment.

Exposure

Exposure of these fractures is difficult since accurate reconstruction is dependent upon excellent visualization of medial and lateral surfaces of the tibia simultaneously; in addition, it is essential that both medial and lateral cortical surfaces are visualized in order to assist reduction. The best approach to accomplish these goals is an anterior approach with an anterior skin incision, medial parapatellar incision, and osteotomy of the tibial tubercle to permit superior reflection of the patellar tendon (Fernandez, 1988).

With this visualization submeniscal incisions are not necessary and the entire anterior surface of the proximal tibia can be readily visualized.

Reduction is difficult. Generally the medial tibial plateau has the least amount of comminution and the medial cortical fracture line is the least comminuted. There is a tendency, however, for the medial tibial cortex to buckle making exact fracture line matching difficult. It is recommended that provisional fixation of the medial tibial plateau be obtained utilizing a relatively short straight plate, contoured to the medial tibia, with full length screws in the distal fragment of the tibia and short screws in the medial tibial plateau fracture. With this in place an X-ray should be obtained to confirm reduction of the medial plateau. With the medial plateau reduced the lateral plateau can be reduced to the medial plateau and to the lateral tibial cortex. Provisional fixation of this lateral fragment should be secured with Kirschner wires and a second intraoperative X-ray obtained. At this time, additional posterior articular

fracture fragments must be reduced and held fixed with Kirschner wires. If the second intraoperative X-ray confirms satisfactory reduction lag screws may be placed parallel to or, if using cannulated screws, over the guidewires providing provisional fixation. A lateral buttress plate is usually required and the screws placed through the proximal holes of this plate should be lag screws to further enhance compression of the intra-articular portion of the fracture. The distal screws should be full length cortical screws. The osteotomized tibial tubercle should be fixed back into position with a single screw.

Bone graft is frequently required but generally only small volumes of bone are necessary. This can be readily obtained from the lateral femoral condyle.

Postoperatively the patient should be restricted to touch-down weight bearing for the first 6–8 weeks following surgery. Full weight bearing should be discouraged for 12–14 weeks, although active knee range of motion may be begun as soon as soft tissue healing permits.

In recent years there has been increased interest in the management of Schatzker VI or AO type C bicondylar tibial plateau fractures with external skeletal fixation. The popularization of the Ilizarov philosophy in the West has led to the increased use of hybrid frames utilizing small wires in the proximal tibial metaphysis and half pins in the diaphysis. Surgeons have been concerned about the amount of soft tissue stripping required to insert two plates into the proximal tibia and have adopted the policy of reconstructing the metaphysis with limited internal fixation, usually utilizing bone screws and then applying a small wire hybrid frame to secure the metaphysis to the diaphysis. Obviously bone grafting techniques are employed where appropriate, but in general the exposure is less and thus, in theory, there should be a lower incidence of infection and skin slough.

Stamer *et al.* (1994) treated 23 bicondylar tibial plateau fractures using this type of hybrid external fixator. Eight patients had limited open reduction and internal fixation and the remainder were treated with percutaneous cannulated screws to stabilize the articular surface. The average time to healing was 4.4 months and there were 16 excellent or good results. Similar results were obtained by Weiner *et al.* (1995), who treated 50 severe proximal tibial fractures of which 45 were bicondylar. In this series 82% of the patients had good results and there was a low incidence of complications.

Marsh *et al.* (1995) utilized the principle of external fixation but used a unilateral device which was placed on the lateral aspect of the leg. Half pins were used to immobilize the metaphyseal fragment after interfragmentary screws had been used to reconstruct it. Half pins were then placed in a conventional manner in the diaphysis and the external fixator secured. The main complication was pin track sepsis related to the proximal half pins. Two patients, however, developed septic arthritis that necessitated arthrotomy and debridement. The other patients did well and the authors showed using the SF-36 survey that most patients had function close to that of age-match controls.

Prospective randomized studies will be required to determine whether external fixation is superior to plating for the management of bicondylar fragments. In skilled hands both techniques will give good results but the technique of external fixation certainly remains a useful alternative to plating and orthopaedic traumatologists should be familiar with its use.

Associated diaphyseal and plateau fractures

Fractures of the tibial plateau associated with fractures of the tibial diaphysis are of significance primarily because of their effect on treatment of the tibial diaphyseal fracture. Co-existent tibial plateau fractures may preclude the use of intramedullary nails for tibial fractures, necessitating some other form of treatment. The presence of a tibial diaphyseal fracture should, however, not modify the treatment of the plateau fracture. An anatomical reduction of the tibial plateau is a prerequisite for satisfactory long-term knee function. Therefore the primary goal should be satisfactory reduction and fixation of the tibial plateau fracture and the tibial diaphyseal fracture should be treated by a method which will not compromise the tibial plateau. This is illustrated in Figure 3.11.

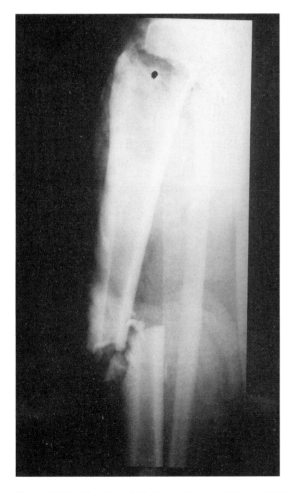
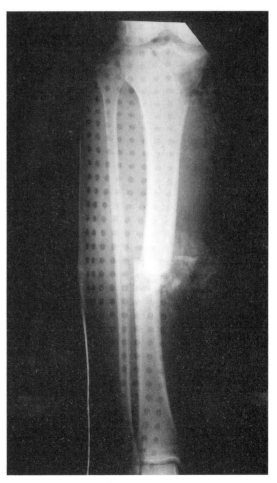

Figure 3.11(a, b) Open tibial plateau fracture with open tibial diaphyseal fracture

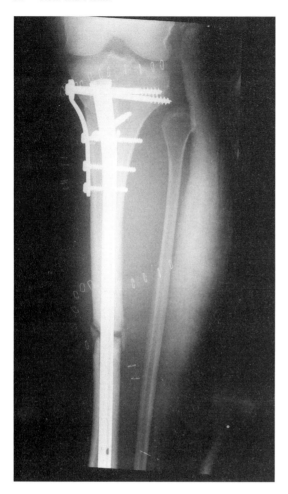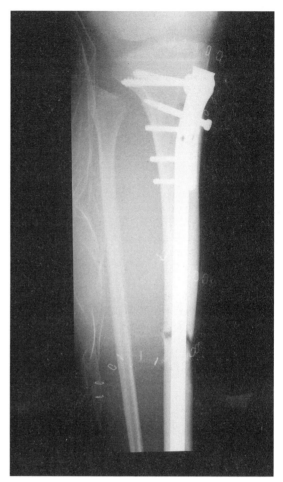

Figure 3.11(c, d) Postoperative appearance. Managed by plate and lag screw fixation of tibial plateau fracture and intramedullary nailing of the tibial diaphyseal fracture

Keating *et al.* (1994) examined the incidence and treatment of combined diaphyseal and plateau fractures. They performed a detailed audit of 523 diaphyseal fractures of the tibia which presented to the Edinburgh Orthopaedic Trauma Unit over a 3-year period and showed that 26 patients had 28 other fractures in the tibia. Eleven of these were tibial plateau fractures. Thus 2.1% of patients presenting with a tibial diaphyseal fracture also had a tibial plateau fracture. These patients tended to have more severe diaphyseal fractures, which usually showed AO type B or C morphology. In Keating's series of combined fractures there was a high incidence of open fractures with 36.3% of the open diaphyseal fractures being Gustilo grade III in severity. There was a high incidence of proximal tibial diaphyseal fractures in the series and the authors advocated the use of plates or external fixators for the management of the diaphyseal fractures.

Bone graft

Throughout this chapter reference has been made to bone graft. The author's personal preference is for autogenous bone from the femoral condyle or, rarely, from the ipsilateral iliac crest. In certain circumstances allograft bone may be used to augment autogenous bone but in the fracture situation allograft bone does not seem to possess the same osteogenic potential as does autogenous bone.

A number of bone graft substitutes have been

promoted for use in the region of the tibial plateau. Personal experience with these is very limited, but initial published reports have been relatively encouraging (Bucholz *et al.*, 1989). This is a development that may show promise with further clinical investigation.

Stability

Ligamentous injury associated with fractures of the tibial plateau has been variably reported as between 10 and 30% (Delamarter *et al.*, 1990). Avulsions of the cruciate ligament, usually with a small fragment of bone attached, are relatively common and can be diagnosed easily at the time of surgery (Schatzker *et al.*, 1979). These small avulsed bone fragments should be secured between the condyles in their anatomical position and can usually be held by simple compression across the major fracture line by lag screws.

Collateral ligament stability is much more difficult to assess. Generally assessment of knee stability is impossible in the emergency room and even under anaesthesia it is difficult to assess since depression of the lateral tibial plateau will allow excessive valgus deformity of the knee even in the presence of the intact medial collateral ligament. Therefore the usual tests for collateral stability are not useful. Stress X-rays may be useful in these circumstances, but also may be unreliable.

It is recommended that all patients with significant medial tenderness on clinical examination have stress testing of their medial collateral ligament following reduction and fixation of the tibial plateau fracture. With the fracture in the reduced position and securely fixed gentle testing of the medial collateral ligament will reveal any complete ruptures. These ruptures should be repaired at the time of surgery for the tibial plateau fracture, but of course must be done through a separate incision. If diagnosed preoperatively, the lateral tibial plateau fracture and the medial collateral ligament can both be addressed through an anterior knee incision.

Arthroscopy

There are a number of reports of arthroscopically assisted elevation and fixation of tibial plateau fractures. The author has no personal experience with this technique but recognizes its potential value in the following circumstances.

1 Simple split fractures in which the split can be visualized by the arthroscope, reduction obtained by simple compression of the fracture line with a tenaculum, and percutaneous cannulated screws inserted to compress the fracture line. This would require a combination of arthroscopy and fluoroscopy.
2 Simple depression fractures without cortical split. The arthroscope can be used to inspect the depressed articular surface and through a small skin incision the punch can be inserted through the drill hole in the lateral cortex and the articular surface observed directly as it is elevated with the punch. A bone graft can be inserted through the drill hole. Once again fluoroscopy would be an adjunct.
3 To assess the articular surface in those patients in whom extensive articular comminution may preclude satisfactory reduction and fixation by conventional methods.

Conclusion

Fractures of the tibial plateau continue to represent a significant therapeutic challenge. This challenge can be met, however, by a thorough understanding of fracture mechanics and fracture fixation and by careful assessment of the patient and the fracture. Careful preoperative planning, meticulous surgical technique and careful postoperative management should result in a satisfactory outcome in the majority of patients.

References

Anglen, J. and Healy, W.L. (1988) Tibial plateau fractures. *Orthopaedics*, **11**, 1527–34

Benirschke, S.K., Agnew, S.G., Mayo, K.A. *et al.* (1992): Immediate internal fixation of open complex tibial plateau fractures: treatment by a standard protocol. *J. Orthop. Trauma*, **6**, 78–86

Bucholz, R.W., Carlton, A. and Holmes, R. (1989) Interporous hydroxyapatite as a bone graft substitute in tibial plateau fractures. *Clin. Orthop. Rel. Res.*, **240**, 53–62

DeCoster, T.A., Nepola, J.V. and el-Khoury, G.Y. (1988) Cast-brace treatment of proximal tibial fractures. A ten-year follow-up study. *Clin. Orthop. Rel. Res.*, **231**, 196–204

Delamarter, R. and Hohl, M. (1989) The cast brace and tibial plateau fractures. *Clin. Orthop. Rel. Res.*, **242**, 26–31

Delamarter, R.B., Hohl, M. and Hopp, E. Jr (1990) Ligament injuries associated with tibial plateau fractures. *Clin. Orthop. Rel. Res.*, **250**, 226–33

Duwelius, P.J. and Connolly, J.F. (1988) Closed reduction of tibial plateau fractures. A comparison of functional and roentgenographic end results. *Clin. Orthop. Rel. Res.*, **230** 116–26

Fernandez, D.L. (1988) Anterior approach to the knee with osteotomy of the tibial tubercle for bicondylar tibial fractures. *J. Bone Joint Surg.*, **70A**, 208–19

Jensen, D.B., Rude, C., Duus, B. and Bjerg-Nielsen, A. (1990) Tibial plateau fractures. A comparison of conservative and surgical treatment. *J. Bone Joint Surg.*, **72B**, 49–52

Keating, J.F., Kuo, R.S. and Court-Brown, C.M. (1994) Bifocal fractures of the tibia and fibula. Incidence, classification and treatment. *J. Bone Joint Surg.*, **76B**, 395–400

Lachiewicz, P.F. and Funcik, T., (1990) Factors influencing the results of open reduction and internal fixation of tibial plateau fractures. *Clin. Orthop. Rel. Res.*, **259**, 210–15

Maheson, M. and Colton, C.L. (1988) Fractures of the tibial plateau in Nottingham. *Injury*, **19**, 324–8

Marsh, J.L., Smith, S.T. and Do, T.T. (1995) External fixation and limited internal fixation for complex fractures of the tibial plateau. *J. Bone Joint Surg.*, **77A**, 661–73

Schatzker, J., McBroom, R. and Bruce, D. (1979) *Clin. Orthop. Rel Res.*, **138**, 94–104

Stamer, D.T., Schenk, R., Staggers, B. *et al.* (1994). Bicondylar tibial plateau fractures treated with a hybrid ring external fixator: a preliminary study. *J. Orthop. Trauma*, **8**, 455–61

Stokel, E.A. and Sadasivan, K.K. (1991) Tibial plateau fractures: standardized evaluation of operative results. *Orthopaedics*, **14**, 263–70

Vandenberghe, D., Cuypers, L., Rombouts, L. *et al.* (1990) Internal fixation of tibial plateau fractures using the AO instrumentation. *Acta Orthop. Belg.*, **56**, 431–42

Waddell, J.P., Johnston, D.W.C. and Neidre, A. (1981) Fractures of the tibial plateau: a review of ninety-five patients and comparison of treatment methods. *J. Trauma*, **21**, 376–81

Weiner, L.S., Kelley, M., Yang, E. *et al.* (1995) The use of combination internal fixation and hybrid external fixation in severe proximal tibia fractures. *J. Orthop. Trauma*, **9**, 244–50

4

External casting of tibial diaphyseal fractures

C. Court-Brown

External splintage remains the most popular method of treating fractures of the tibial diaphysis throughout the world. In some more primitive cultures the use of wooden splints is still maintained, but usually either plaster of Paris or one of the more modern resin-based casting materials is used to immobilize the fracture. Many surgeons continue to use external casting for all closed tibial diaphyseal fractures, regardless of the type of fracture, the extent of bone comminution or the degree of soft tissue damage associated with the fracture. It is also widely used for the treatment of minor open fractures, although in recent years the trend has been towards the use of either internal or external skeletal fixation in severe open tibial fractures.

Calcaneal or distal tibial traction also remains in widespread use for the early management of severe closed tibial diaphyseal fractures associated with major soft tissue damage or comminution. The traction is either used prior to the application of a definitive external cast or before internal fixation. Traction is also sometimes used to stabilize open tibial diaphyseal fractures to allow examination of the soft tissues and occasionally to permit plastic surgery procedures to be performed.

Unfortunately, despite widespread use of external casting and traction, most of the literature dealing with the results and complications of these techniques is now at least 20 years old, being written before the advent of modern fracture classification systems and before it was appreciated by many surgeons that a successful outcome of fracture management depended not just on achieving bone union, but also on the time that the patient took to return to full function in the community. Thus it is probable that many of the older papers

dealing with casting methods overstate their usefulness. In the past 10–15 years, interest in the management of tibial diaphyseal fractures has mainly concentrated on the use of internal and external fixation. Recently, Sarmiento and his co-workers have provided the major in-depth analyses of the use of external casts in the management of tibial diaphyseal fractures (Sarmiento *et al.*, 1989).

The inevitable result of the recent interest in fixation techniques is that many younger orthopaedic surgeons know little of modern casting techniques and of their comparative qualities when compared with internal and external fixation methods.

History of external casting

The use of supportive dressings or splints stiffened with external agents, such as grease, honey and mud, goes back to the ancient Egyptian, Chinese and Indian civilizations. The Edwin-Smith papyrus written between 2800 and 3000 BC discusses the management of both closed and open fractures and highlights the futility of managing an open fracture at that time. Hippocrates (460–377 BC) introduced the use of roller bandages stiffened with cerate, an ointment consisting of lard or oil mixed with wax, resin or pitch. The bandages were renewed daily as the swelling subsided. Hippocrates also used a variety of different splints as well as mechanical aids to facilitate reduction of fractures or dislocations. Fractures were reduced at about seven days, after the initial swelling had settled, and the supportive dressing was then left for about three weeks.

Subsequent surgeons followed the Hippocratic method of using stiffened bandages, but Albucasis (936–1013) introduced the use of plasters or poultices as a method of managing lower limb fractures. These mixtures of mill-dust, egg white, clay and various plants were applied to the limb, left to harden and then left undisturbed for a long period.

In the thirteenth century, surgeons began to realize the importance of early fracture reduction. They employed techniques devised by both the Greek and Arabic surgical disciplines using bandages soaked in egg-white to support splints made of wood and other materials. During this period, the concept of balanced traction using a pulley and counter weights was developed by Guy de Chauliac in France.

In the following 500 years extraordinary progress was made in the understanding of anatomy and the management of open wounds and open fractures. However, although different types of splints and traction were devised, curiously little progress was made in the art of external cast immobilization. Patients continued to be treated by constant dressing changes and fracture manipulations. Peltier (1990) commented that by the beginning of the nineteenth century lower limb fractures were still treated by prolonged immobilization. Treatment was labour-intensive and expensive and presumably could only be afforded by the affluent few. The combination of the Napoleonic wars with its large number of casualties and the industrial revolution with its associated urbanization of the population meant that fracture management had to become easier, cheaper and more available to the general population. In addition, it was important that patients be mobile during their treatment. Larrey (1768–1842) and Seutin (1793–1865) both developed more effective bandage stiffeners allowing early mobilization, but it was Mathijsen (1805–78) and Pirogov (1810–81) who introduced the use of plaster of Paris impregnated bandages. These revolutionized fracture management as they dried quickly, conformed to the shape of the limb and could be windowed, bivalved and removed easily. The availability of an inexpensive effective casting material allowed surgeons to design different types of external cast and to introduce hinges to facilitate joint movement (Krause, 1891). Three areas of controversy soon emerged amongst surgeons treating tibial fractures. Discussion centred around the requirement for the knee to be included in the cast, whether or not the plaster should be skin-tight or adequately padded, and when weight bearing should be allowed. The first two points are

no longer of topical interest, but there is still debate as to the role of early or delayed weight bearing.

Inclusion of the knee joint into a long-leg cast facilitated the maintenance of fracture reduction and allowed early patient mobilization and weight bearing. The use of the long-leg cast, often following a period of traction, was extensively documented by Bohler (1885–1973) and Dehne (1905–83) and remains in use as a method of management of tibial diaphyseal fracture. However, long-leg casts are frequently awkward to wear and the immobilization of the knee joint for a prolonged period may lead to stiffness. This was recognized a hundred years ago by Reclus (1897) and later by Delbet (Tanton, 1916) who developed short weight bearing casts, the weight being borne by the proximal tibial flare. These are the forerunners of the modern patellar tendon-bearing cast and functional brace popularized by Sarmiento and now in widespread use.

The recent introduction of light, waterproof, radiolucent casting materials has certainly rendered external casts more 'user friendly', but basically the two different philosophies of Bohler (1958) and Sarmiento (1967, 1970) still persist when external cast treatment of tibial fractures is being considered.

Long-leg casts

Most externally casted tibial fractures are initially treated by the application of a long-leg cast from toes to groin (Figure 4.1). Bohler only treated 25% of his tibial diaphyseal fractures with an immediate long-leg cast and emphasized that if one was used it should be immediately split throughout its length and a definitive cast applied later. Usually he used a short period of traction through a calcaneal pin, the plaster being applied after the postoperative swelling had resolved. Once the long-leg plaster was applied a programme of early mobilization and weight bearing was encouraged. Dehne (1969) reviewed his experience with long-leg casts with and without preceding traction as well as his experience with internal fixation. He felt that the best results were gained from the use of a long-leg cast without preceding traction. He therefore instituted immediate weight bearing in a long-leg cast and reported good results in 349 consecutive, unselected tibial diaphyseal fractures. The mean time to union was 18 weeks and the main problem was shortening, with 33% showing tibial shortening of at least half an inch. He did not mention joint stiffness.

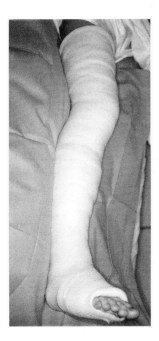

Figure 4.1 A long-leg cast. This is conventionally applied from the metatarsal heads to the proximal thigh with the knee in slight flexion and the foot in a plantigrade position

Dehne's technique was adopted by many surgeons in the United States. The Vietnam war had produced many open tibial fractures in addition to the more common sources of closed and open fractures. Brown and Urban (1969) and Burkhalter and Protzman (1975) analysed their results of the use of long-leg casts in two widely quoted papers. However, although reasonable results were clearly obtained, their papers illustrate some of the problems inherent in the literature of that time. Brown and Urban reviewed 63 open tibial fractures treated by long-leg casts and immediate mobilization wherever possible. The mean time to union was 19

weeks despite the presence of 'massive loss of skin and muscle' in many of their wounds. These were treated by split-skin grafting up to 4 weeks after the fracture. Fifty-seven patients had 'no disability', although many showed only 'good to normal' knee movement. Ten degrees of dorsiflexion of the ankle was considered adequate and subtalar function was not examined. Twenty-seven per cent had shortening of more than 1 cm, 60% showed a recurvatum deformity averaging 7°, 38% had a valgus deformity averaging 6° and 19% showed a varus deformity with an average of 5°. Infection was not thought to be a problem, although 15 fractures discharged for at least 27 weeks. Burkhalter and Protzman also documented a low infection rate at 3.8%, despite treating 159 open fractures with exposed bone without flap cover. Again time to union and the instance of delayed union are the only outcome criteria used by the authors.

Table 4.1 illustrates the results of the use of long-leg casts in recent years. Nicoll (1964) in a study of 674 cast-treated fractures including 144 open fractures, documented an average time to union of 15.9 weeks. As with other surgeons, he realized that there was an association between time to union and fracture severity, but because of the difficulty in adequately classifying the fractures he was unable to give average union times for different fracture types. He therefore arbitrarily defined normal union as being between 12 and 20 weeks and delayed union as being more than 20 weeks. He commented that 22% of the fractures took more than 20 weeks to unite and 5% had not united after one year. The cast-treated open fractures provided a particular problem, with a 15.3% infection rate and a 60% incidence of delayed or non-union. As Brown and Urban (1969) did later, Nicoll arbitrarily defined ranges of acceptable joint function, although they were somewhat more stringent than those of Brown and Urban. He stated that any loss

Table 4.1   The treatment of tibial fractures with long-leg casts

Series	No. of fractures	Open fractures (%)	Time to union (wk)	Malunion (%)	Joint stiffness (%)
Nicoll (1964)	674	22.5	15.9	8.6	25.0
Slatis and Rokkinen (1967)	198	33.3	19.8	?	?
Karahaju *et al.* (1979)	80	23.7	?	11.2*	27.5*
Steen Jensen *et al.* (1977)	102	?	?	21.0*	7.0*
Van der Linden and Larsen (1979)	50	12.0	17.0	50.0	24.0
Haines *et al.* (1984)	91	36.3	16.3	25.3	33.0
Kay *et al.* (1986)	79	22.8	19.1	9.1	?
Kyro *et al.* (1991)	165	21.0	13.7	30.0*	42.0*

*Indicates the value is a minimum figure. The true value is probably higher.

of knee extension and more than 10° loss of flexion was unacceptable. More than 25% loss of ankle dorsiflexion or plantar flexion or the same amount of subtalar inversion and eversion was also considered unacceptable. Using these criteria, 25% of his patients had residual stiffness in one or more joints, with 8% having disabling stiffness. There was a positive correlation between wound size and joint stiffness. In the absence of a wound, Nicoll found that the incidence of joint stiffness only increased by 20–25% as a result of prolonged immobilization secondary to delayed union. However, when there was a combination of a delayed union and severe soft tissue damage, the incidence of residual stiffness rose to 70%. He also documented an 8.6% incidence of residual deformity, taking 10° of angulatory or rotational deformity and 2 cm of shortening as being acceptable.

Slatis and Rokkanen (1967) prospectively analysed 198 adult tibial shaft fractures and commented that the mean time to union was 19.8 weeks. Forty-one per cent had united within 16 weeks and 69% within 20 weeks. Four cases (2%) remained ununited at one year. The authors examined the social consequences of the fracture by looking at the rate of return to walking with appropriate aids and the time taken to return to work. Fifty-five per cent of the group walked without a stick within 24 weeks and 38% had resumed work by that time.

Karaharju *et al.* (1979), Steen Jensen *et al.* (1977) and Van der Linden and Larsson (1979) all compared the use of long-leg casts with operative management. Karaharju *et al.* analysed a mixed group of intramedullary nails, AO plates and AO screws, whereas the other two groups compared cast management with plate fixation. Steen Jensen *et al.* used a number of different plates whereas Van der Linden and Larsson used only AO plates. Karaharju *et al.* followed up most of their patients for over one year and many for three years. Their treatment policy at that time was extremely conservative, the patients taking an average of 18 weeks to regain full weight bearing. The average period to return to work was 33 weeks, but there was no difference in the number or altered job status of the patients that returned to work between the cast and operatively managed group. They also showed no statistical difference between the operative and non-operative group as regards joint mobility, although they did demonstrate that joint mobility correlated well with the extent of fracture comminution, this being a reflection on the degree of soft tissue injury. They suggested that the commonest late complaint was loss of ankle and foot movement. Edwards (1965) outcome criteria were used, and no difference was found between the cast and operative groups. They felt that when operative fixation was required, intramedullary nailing was preferable to plating.

Steen Jensen *et al.* (1977) compared the use of a long-leg cast with AO, Eggers and Lane plates. They suggested that the advantage of plating was that union was faster than that associated with the use of a cast. However, they did admit that it was difficult to estimate bone union using AO plates and their conclusions about the relative times to fracture union are suspect. They did however point out that conservative management was associated with a high incidence of skin necrosis or superficial infection, with a 34% incidence of these complications in open fractures. In addition, 21% of the open fractures went on to non-union. Table 4.1 illustrates that they also had a high incidence of malunion, although their incidence of joint stiffness was low compared with other series. They concluded that at that time the use of AO plates could not be recommended for closed fractures but should be used for open fractures, because of the high incidence of complications associated with the use of casts.

Van der Linden and Larsson (1979) analysed 100 tibial fractures treated either by the use of a long-leg cast or by AO plate. All fractures were displaced and treatment was selected in a randomized fashion. The most striking result of their series was the high incidence of malalignment with conservative management. Their incidence of joint stiffness was comparable with other series and it is of interest that in addition to a 24% incidence of joint stiffness associated with cast management they had a 16% incidence of joint stiffness associated with plating. As with Steen Jensen *et al.*, they felt that the use of AO plates decreased the time to union, but unlike Steen Jensen's group their conclusions were that plating could not be recommended for open fractures but could be recommended for closed fractures.

Kay *et al.* (1986) studied 77 fractures over a five year period. They excluded all fractures with extensive soft tissue damage or bone loss. Their treatment was based on Bohler's original treatment with the application of a long-leg cast for the fractures in which the reduction could be easily maintained. Where this was not the case, they used os calcis traction for a period of 2–6 weeks. Table 4.1 shows that they had a relatively low incidence of malunion. They did not record joint stiffness. The use of traction greatly increased their patients' time in hospital, and it is interesting to note that of the 14 comminuted fractures, 9 required calcaneal traction for an average of 5.8 weeks. The authors made no conclusions, but did stress that the low malunion rate was only gained at the expense of doubling the hospital stay.

Haines *et al.* (1984) also adopted a very conservative policy with tibial fractures, again using os calcis traction for unstable and open fractures. They excluded undisplaced fractures from their series and analysed the results of treatment of 99 displaced adult fractures. Table 4.1 illustrates that they had a high incidence of malunion and joint stiffness. They stated that the lack of knee flexion deleteriously affected function and noted that the patients who had knee stiffness had been in plaster for an average of 4.6 weeks longer than those who had no stiffness. They did not document whether these fractures were more severe and might have had traction prior to the application of the cast. The inpatient stay averaged 14 days and of the patients who were employed at the time of fracture, the average time to restart their employment was 31 weeks. As with most other authors, Haines *et al.* took fracture union as their principle outcome criterion, and since all their fractures united with or without bone graft they felt that internal fixation was not only not indicated but might cause disaster.

Kyro *et al.* (1991) analysed the use of long-leg casts in 165 consecutive tibial fractures. In 23% of the group a calcaneal pin was incorporated into the plaster and in a number of severe open tibial fractures traction was used. Table 4.1 shows that they also had a high incidence of malunion and joint stiffness. The authors, however, examined the function of the patient in more detail than the other papers detailed in Table 4.1. They reported that 26% of their patients had limitation of knee flexion and 9% had impaired extension. Forty-two per cent had impaired ankle function and 37% had impaired toe movement. As far as functional handicap was concerned, they recorded that 25% of their patients had marked difficulty in squatting, with 23% having marked difficulty in walking and 38% having considerable difficulty in running. Only 27% of the overall group had no difficulty in running. Their conclusions differed markedly from those of Haines *et al.* Kyro *et al.* felt that satisfactory overall results will not be attained if all, or almost all, tibial fractures are conservatively treated. They felt that attempts to improve the final outcome should be based on appreciation of the

types of fracture, and that fracture management should be tailored towards the type of fracture being treated.

Short-leg casts

Sarmiento (1967) introduced the patellar tendon-bearing cast (Figure 4.2) in an effort to produce 'sufficient stabilisation of the fragments in the near physiological environment'. The cast enhanced rotational mobility, permitted knee flexion and extension and facilitated early weight bearing. Sarmiento suggested that a standard long-leg cast be applied until soft tissue swelling had largely resolved and felt that in most cases a one-week delay was desirable. In 1967 Sarmiento documented the use of the patellar tendon-bearing cast in 69 closed fractures which healed in an average of 13.6 weeks. He also used the cast in the treatment of 31 open fractures which healed in an average of 16.7 weeks. There were no cases of

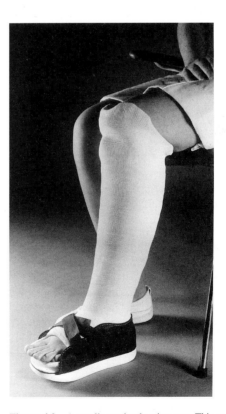

Figure 4.2 A patella tendon-bearing cast. This cast allows for free knee movement but the cast is so constructed proximally that in extension the cast grips the knee on each side of the patella, minimizing rotation

non-union or delayed union. Although the incidence of malalignment and joint stiffness was not detailed, the inference was that alignment was well maintained. Results of the use of patellar tendon-bearing casts are shown in Table 4.2.

The time of conversion from a long-leg cast to patellar tendon-bearing cast varies widely in the literature. Most authors wait for 4–6 weeks until a measure of bone stability has been achieved before applying the patellar tendon-bearing cast. Mollan and Bradley (1978) examined both early and late application of patellar tendon-bearing casts and showed improved time to union in the group treated by the Sarmiento technique of patellar tendon-bearing cast application within one week of fracture. They also stated that the union times were faster than an earlier group of patients treated with a long-leg cast. The groups were matched for age, sex and grade of injury, although the early patellar tendon-bearing group had significantly fewer open fractures. The average time to union for the early patellar tendon-bearing group was 10 weeks, with 15 weeks for the late patellar tendon-bearing group and 19 weeks for the earlier long-leg cast group. No mention was made of malalignment, joint stiffness or patient function.

Austin (1981) examined 132 patients treated with a Sarmiento patellar tendon-bearing cast. As with the other authors shown in Table 4.2, he had a high incidence of malunion and did not record the incidence of joint stiffness. He compared his results with those of Sarmiento and felt that the results were comparable, although he noted that his incidence of non-union was three times as high as that of Sarmiento. Austin also applied cumulative frequency curves to his results and to those of Ellis (1958), who used a long-leg plaster, and Burwell (1971), who used AO plates. Interestingly, his results are not as good as either of the other two authors. However, Austin felt that although the

method required care, the technique was useful and improved patient mobility and convenience.

Böstman and Hanninen (1982) examined an interesting group of 182 fractures of the adult tibial shaft caused by indirect violence. All of the fractures were located at the junction of the middle and distal thirds of the tibia. Cast management was used whenever an acceptable position of the fracture could be obtained by closed reduction, this occurring in 114 patients. The authors had a 2% infection rate for closed fractures treated with a cast and a 15% infection rate for cast-treated open fractures. They detailed the overall complication rate for conservative management as 18%. Sixty-eight patients in the series were managed by screw or plate fixation or by intramedullary nailing and the authors list the overall complication rates for these techniques as 22% for screw fixation, 28% for plate fixation and 12% for intramedullary nailing.

Puno et al. (1986) retrospectively compared 60 patients with tibial fractures treated by reamed nailing with 141 patients who were treated by closed reduction and casting. In their group a long-leg cast was applied for 4–6 weeks and then changed to a patella tendon-bearing cast. They analysed their fracture population according to the fracture configuration, the mechanism of injury and the degree of fracture displacement and showed the two fracture populations were very similar. A comparison of the results for the two groups showed that there was a 9.9% incidence of delayed or non-union in the cast-managed group in addition to a 1.4% incidence of infection and a 4.3% incidence of malunion. Nineteen of the patients had secondary surgery because of inadequate reduction or loss of fracture position. In the intramedullary nailing group there was a 1.7% incidence of non-union, 3.3% incidence of infection and there were no cases with malunion. The

Table 4.2   The treatment of tibial fractures with patellar tendon-bearing casts

Series	No. of fractures	Open fractures (%)	Time to union (wk)	Malunion (%)	Joint stiffness (%)
Sarmiento (1967)	69	0	13.6	?	?
Mollan and Bradley (1978)	106	38.3	10.0	?	?
Austin (1981)	132	11.4	16.7	39.0	?
Böstman and Hanninen (1982)	114	16.0	15.3	40.0	?
Puno et al. (1986)	141	17.0	16.7	4.4	?
Oni et al. (1988)	100	0	?	21.0*	43.0
Wu and Shih (1990)	145	0	19.9	29.0	?
Hooper et al. (1991)	33	21.0	18.3	27.3	15.0

*Indicates the value is a minimum figure. The true value is probably higher.

authors showed that the average time to union for the closed fractures treated with intramedullary nailing was 9.1 weeks compared with 15.3 weeks for the closed fractures treated with a cast. They did not subdivide their open fractures according to the degree of soft tissue injury but they did show the mean time to union for the open fractures treated with intramedullary nails as 15.2 weeks compared with 23.5 weeks for the open fractures treated with a cast.

The average time interval between the injury and restarting work was 22 weeks for the intramedullary nailing group and 26 weeks for the cast group. This was a retrospective study and it is interesting to compare it with the results of Hooper *et al.* (1991) who undertook a similar study on a prospective basis.

Oni *et al.* (1988) examined the use of patellar tendon-bearing casts in the management of 100 consecutive closed fractures of adult tibiae. They took fracture union as their principal outcome criterion and showed that 81% of the fractures were united at 20 weeks. They continued with conservative management beyond this time, a further 15% healing without further intervention. Based on these results they believed that few closed tibial diaphyseal fractures required operative intervention. They stated there were no complications worthy of note, although 43% of their patients had objective or subjective restriction of ankle or subtalar movement and at least 21% had significant malunion. Patient function was not examined. Wu and Shih (1990) used a similar technique to Oni *et al.* and examined 182 closed tibial fractures treated by a patellar tendon-bearing cast applied after 6 weeks. They recorded a 28.3% incidence of delayed or non-union and a 29% incidence of malunion.

Hooper *et al.* (1991) undertook a prospective randomized trial comparing the use of a patellar tendon-bearing cast applied 4 weeks after fracture with the use of an interlocking intramedullary nail in 62 tibial diaphyseal fractures. In the cast managed group, 27% of the patients had significant varus or valgus malalignment, 9% showed antecurvatum or recurvatum and 46% had significant shortening. They found the mean time to union was significantly shorter in the nail group, as was the mean delay before return to work. Malunion, shortening and time in hospital also showed better results than the nail group. Interestingly, although movement at the knee, ankle and hindfoot was regained earlier in the nailed group, at the end of the treatment period, both groups had similar ranges. The only difference was that moderate hindfoot stiffness was apparent in 15% of the cast managed group, as against 3.4% of the nailed group. The authors went as far as to say that they considered it unethical to continue cast management of displaced tibial shaft fractures. Obviously this view is at variance with the views of Sarmiento and other workers.

Functional bracing

In 1970 Sarmiento published a report on 135 tibial fractures treated by a total contact functional brace which allowed both knee and ankle movements. The brace was initially made of plaster of Paris, but subsequently a thermoplastic material was used (Figure 4.3). Rotation was controlled by a patellar tendon bearing top to the cast and ankle movement was facilitated by the use of a cable ankle joint. He reported an average time to union of 15.5 weeks with no cases of non-union. The average shortening in this series was 6.4 mm, with the maximum shortening being 1.9 cm. Angular deformity and joint motion were not adequately discussed. The results of this study and others

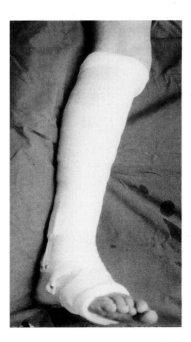

Figure 4.3 A functional brace. Nowadays this type of brace is usually made of plastic and theoretically it allows for free movement of knee and ankle joints. The fact that the heel is usually supported by medial and lateral hinges obviously minimizes subtalar movements

Table 4.3   The treatment of tibial fractures with functional braces

Series	No. of fractures	Open fractures (%)	Time to union (wk)	Malunion (%)	Joint stiffness (%)
Sarmiento (1970)	135	24.4	15.5	?	?
Sarmiento *et al.* (1989)	780	31.0	18.7	13.7	?
Suman (1982)	82	36.6	14.7	?	9.7
Digby *et al.* (1983)	82	20.7	17.4	9.0*	45.0
Den Outer *et al.* (1990)	94	11.7	?	40.0	?
Pun *et al.* (1991)	97	7.2	17.1	23.7*	28.9*
Alho *et al.* (1992)	35	31.4	17.0	8.6*	26.0*

*Indicates the value is a minimum figure. The true value is probably higher.

concerned with functional bracing are detailed in Table 4.3.

Sarmiento *et al.* (1989) subsequently analysed 780 patients treated with a functional brace. At that time they stated that their indications for the use of bracing included most closed and many open fractures with minimal soft tissue damage. They only used the technique on ambulatory patients. Contraindications to bracing included fractures with excessive initial shortening and fractures which showed increasing angular deformity in the initial cast. In addition, they excluded patients with significant neurovascular damage, segmental bone loss and those requiring soft tissue flaps. Gustilo type III open fractures were treated by external fixation, but if the fractures were stable and the soft tissues healed, a functional brace was frequently applied 6 weeks after the fracture.

The average time to application of the function brace after injury was 3.8 weeks for closed fractures and 5.2 weeks for the open group. The mean time to bone union was 18.7 weeks, with the closed fractures healing in an average of 17.4 weeks and the open fractures in 21.7 weeks. They found that the fractures that were braced within the first 6 weeks healed more quickly than those braced later. Non-union was defined as a failure to unite by one year and this occurred in 2.5% of the series. Varus angulation of >5° occurred in 13.7% of the group with varus angulation of >5° occurring in 2.3%. Anterior angulation occurred in 4.3% and posterior angulation in 10.5% of the group. Ten per cent of the patients healed with shortening of >1 cm.

The authors feel that functional bracing is an appropriate treatment for closed and Gustilo type I open fractures, but emphasize that if success is to be achieved, rigid adherence to technical details is important. They also emphasize the importance of an understanding of the degree of soft tissue injury and they suggest that few Gustilo type III fractures are suitable for functional bracing.

Suman (1982) reported the results of 82 tibial shaft fractures treated with an orthoplast functional brace. Unlike Sarmiento and his co-workers, Suman did not report the incidence of malunion, but he did document a functional assessment of the patient. He reported a full range of knee movements was achieved in all patients, but that 7.3% of patients complained of ankle stiffness and 9.7% had mild subtalar stiffness. Some patients developed troublesome oedema of the ankle and foot and a number of patients also had to have the use of the brace discontinued because of severe sweat rashes.

Digby *et al.* (1983) reviewed 103 adult tibial diaphyseal fractures treated with a functional brace. They reported an average time to union of 16.7 weeks for the closed fractures and 19.9 weeks for open fractures. They also found full knee movement, but reported that only 89% of their group regained normal ankle movements. Interestingly, only 55% had normal subtalar function at final follow-up. Those patients who had commenced weight bearing at an early stage showed a significantly better range of ankle and subtalar movement. Nine patients had shortening of >2 cm, but only one patient had significant angulation. Those patients in employment took an average of 16 weeks to return to their jobs, and many were able to resume full employment while still wearing the brace, while 49.5% of the patients returned to sport in an average time of 21.5 weeks. However, 21.3% of the patients could not run at final follow-up. These were obviously the patients with more severe soft tissue injuries as the average time to healing in this group was 20.8 weeks, compared with 14.8 weeks for those who could run.

Pun *et al.* (1991) undertook a comprehensive examination of the use of functional bracing in the management of tibial fractures and analysed 93 patients treated initially with a long-leg cast but changed to a functional brace between 2–6 weeks after fracture. They assessed patient mobility and joint function after brace removal with an average follow-up of 1.6 years. Fifty-three patients had a longer follow-up, averaging 2.83 years. They found that at an average of 1.86 years, 68.4% of patients had normal ankle motion and 60% had normal inversion and eversion. By 2.83 years these figures had risen to 75.5% and 71.1% respectively. After 1.86 years all patients could fully extend their knees, although 13.2% had some restriction of knee flexion. This persisted at the later follow-up date. The authors found that 15.8% of the group had shortening of greater than 4 mm, 23.7% had varus or valgus angulation of more than 5°, and 20.6% had anteroposterior angulation of more than 5°.

Den Outer *et al.* (1990) and Alho *et al.* (1992) both conducted retrospective studies comparing the use of functional braces with other methods of tibial diaphyseal treatment. Den Outer *et al.* (1990) compared a number of different types of cast with different types of internal fixation. However, 63% of their cast-managed fractures were treated in a functional brace. They only selected relatively straightforward AO type A fractures, excluding polytraumatized patients, second- and third-degree open fractures and those patients with more than one fracture of the lower extremity. Despite these somewhat stringent criteria, they still had a 40% malunion rate in their cast-managed group and 32% of the group took more than 20 weeks to unite. However, they stated that they only had a 3.2% incidence of complications in the cast-managed group compared with 11.8% incidence in the operatively treated group. They did not document their incidence of joint stiffness, but they did comment that there was no significant difference in either knee or ankle function between the two groups. They also commented that there was no evidence that the patients with malalignment had any associated sequelae. They concluded that functional bracing was the preferred method of management for AO type A closed or grade I open tibial diaphyseal fracture.

Alho *et al.* (1992) compared functional bracing with locked intramedullary nailing. However, 14.3% of their brace managed group were initially treated with external skeletal fixation. They commented that the incidence of joint stiffness and complications was less with intramedullary nailing than with the use of functional bracing. They also

reported that a higher proportion of nailed patients had excellent and good results, compared with braced patients.

Disability following cast immobilization

Considering the number of papers written about tibial fractures, it is surprising just how little is understood about them or how little work has been done to examine patients' function and disability after tibial fracture. The main outcome criteria employed by authors are the time to fracture union and the incidence of non-union after an arbitrary time limit. The latter measure has arisen because of a virtually uniform failure adequately to classify fractures. Despite many authors commenting on the importance of the associated soft tissue injury, there has been little recognition that some fractures may take a considerable time to unite and if they are immobilized in a cast for the complete treatment period joint stiffness is almost inevitable. The other problem associated with cast or brace immobilization is malalignment and subsequent malunion, although it must be stated that a positive relationship between tibial malalignment and subsequent post-traumatic osteoarthritis has yet to be proved (Kristensen *et al.*, 1989; Netz *et al.*, 1991).

Tables 4.1–4.3 illustrate the high incidence of both joint stiffness and malalignment that occurs after cast or brace treatment. Most of the joint stiffness detailed in the various papers in Table 4.1 is in the hindfoot. Knee stiffness does not appear to be a particular problem, even after prolonged immobilization. It is perhaps not surprising that the incidence of joint stiffness and malalignment is very similar between long-leg casts and patellar tendon-bearing casts (Table 4.2), but it is more surprising that the joint stiffness and malunion rates after functional bracing are comparable (Table 4.3).

Hindfoot disability was examined by McMaster (1976). He looked at 100 patients with heel tibial diaphyseal fractures following the use of a long-leg cast. All were unilateral and 15% had required further surgery in the form of grafting for non-union. Forty-three per cent of the patients experienced trouble in walking over rough ground, although only 12% had symptoms severe enough to interfere with recreational activities or work.

He divided the patients into four groups, consisting of normal function, in addition to mild, moderate and severe stiffness. Interestingly, the patients with normal hindfoot function had been immobilized for an average of 15.4 weeks, whereas the patients with severe stiffness had been in a cast for an average of 24.5 weeks. However, the normal group were much younger and contained a higher proportion of less severe injuries than the moderate or severe disability groups.

Horne *et al.* (1990) investigated residual disability following tibial shaft fracture in a group of 97 patients. Seventy-five per cent of the patients had been treated by either a long-leg cast for the whole of their treatment period or by the sequential use of a long-leg cast followed by a below-knee cast. Twenty-five per cent of the group had had some form of internal fixation.

It is interesting to note that 79% of the patients felt subjectively that they had symptoms in their legs. Of this group, 31% stated that the symptoms were severe, although only 19% had constant symptoms. Forty per cent of the patients stated that they were asymptomatic and could participate in all activities. In the remaining 60%, the most frequent complaints related to walking over rough ground, walking up hills or running. In addition, 24% of the patients had had to modify their work activities because of their tibial fracture and 37% had had to downgrade their level of sporting activity.

Physical examination of the patients showed asymmetrical shoe wear in 42% of the patients, overt tibial deformity in 60% of the cases and clawing of the toes in 5% of the patients. Examination of the range of ankle movement showed that dorsiflexion was normal in only 48% of the patients and subtalar motion was normal in only 28% of the group. The authors concluded that there was no correlation between the loss of subtalar motion and subsequent symptoms, but they did feel that there was a direct relationship between ankle stiffness and the presence of pain and they concluded that treatment of tibial fractures should be directed at preventing ankle stiffness.

Netz *et al.* (1991) also investigated a group of tibial fractures treated by closed reduction and plaster fixation. They analysed subjective and objective criteria, concluding that 52% of the patients reported some kind of problem following the fracture at an average of 7 years and 8 months after the injury. Muscle force analysis was performed which showed that despite the long follow-up period, all muscle force parameters were significantly stronger in the non-fractured leg, the differences being accentuated in those patients who had subjective complaints and in those who had high energy trauma. Netz *et al.* also found that the most common functional problem was reduced dorsiflexion of the ankle, which affected squatting and stride length.

Kyro *et al.* (1991) questioned 137 patients who had had a tibial fracture treated with a long-leg cast. Only 47% considered the healing to be excellent or good. It is interesting to note that 54% of the patients complained of pain in the lower leg, while 49% complained of pain in the ankle and 34% of pain in the foot. Unlike other studies, Kyro *et al.* found a considerable problem with knee stiffness, 9% of the group complaining of limited extension and 26% complaining of limited flexion. In addition, 42% complained of limited ankle movement and 27% of limited toe movement. Only 47% of the group could squat without symptoms, while only 40% could walk and 27% run without any problems. The authors took the view that their data suggested that satisfactory overall results would not be obtained if casting was used to treat all tibial fractures.

Merchant and Deitz (1989) analysed 37 patients at an average of 29 years after surgery. They looked at knee and ankle function, concluding that the outcome was good or excellent in 78% of the ankles and excellent in 92% of the knees. They felt that the clinical and radiological outcomes were not affected by the degree of tibial malalignment or by the length of fracture immobilization.

One of the striking features about the literature concerning functional bracing is how little discussion of patient function there actually is. The incidence of joint stiffness is high despite the theoretical ability to move the ankle and subtalar joints as well as the knee. The results of Pun *et al.* (1991) have been detailed. They have drawn attention to the fairly high incidence of stiffness in the ankle and subtalar joints over 2.5 years after fracture. They also demonstrated that the ankle and subtalar joint stiffness was associated with an abnormal walking pattern.

Combined external casting and supplementary fracture fixation

A literature review shows that orthopaedic surgeons have found it difficult to maintain the reduced position of an unstable fracture of the tibia and fibula by the use of an external cast. It is this difficulty which has given rise to the attempted definition of what constitutes an acceptable reduction. In an effort to facilitate the maintenance of fracture reduction, surgeons have either incorporated metal pins into a cast or have used minimal internal fixation as an ancillary fixation method. Bohler (1958) stated that he used a pins and plaster technique between 1929 and 1933 on 65 closed and 36 open fractures. The pins were conventionally placed in the proximal and distal tibial metaphyses and a cast applied around them. However, he reported 15 cases of proximal pin site infection, with 3 patients requiring sequestrectomy, and abandoned the technique. He felt that it offered no advantage over properly supervised continuous traction in the management of unstable fractures and merely added the danger of infection. Despite Bohler's early pessimism, the technique of pins and plaster continued to be used. It was popularized in the United States of America initially by Moore (1960) and later by Anderson *et al.* (1974). Anderson and his co-workers documented the use of pins and plaster in 208 selected patients. They emphasized that the technique should be used in unstable comminuted and open fractures and reported that 95.2% of the fractures healed without grafting and that 88% of the patients had good results in that shortening was less than half an inch, varus or valgus deformity was less than 5 ° and anteroposterior deformity was less than 10 °. The range of joint movement was not assessed, although they stated that almost all patients regained satisfactory joint motion. This apparently occurred despite the average cast time for the united fractures being 24 weeks, with 42 weeks for the group that had union problems. They reported only 5 patients with pin tract sepsis. Anderson *et al.* (1974) used a long-leg cast and delayed weight bearing for an average of 3 months. However, Scudese *et al.* (1970) allowed early weight bearing in a short-leg cast, but used four transfixion pins. One was placed proximally at the level of the tuberosity, one was transcalcaneal and two were adjacent to the fracture site. The mean time to union for 60 closed and 15 open fractures was 18.5 weeks. There was no shortening and only two unacceptable angulatory deformities. Only two pin tract infections were noted. As in other series, joint movement and patient function were not assessed.

Kay (1970) described the use of a long-leg cast with two transfixion pins, one placed just below the tibial tuberosity and the second through the calcaneus. The absence of traction from the management of comminuted fractures brought the average hospital stay down to 4 days for closed fractures and 10 days for minor open fractures. The mean time to union was 14 weeks for closed fractures

and 17.5 weeks for the open fracture group. Despite a calcaneal pin and a prolonged period in plaster, apparently only 12% had hind foot stiffness. Six per cent showed evidence of pin tract sepsis.

Scheck (1965) extended the use of the pins and plaster technique by inserting a proximal tibial and a transcalcaneal pin. If intermediate bone fragments remained unreduced, he opened the fracture and used one or more bone screws to reattach the fragments. He still reported malalignment problems as many of the fractures were comminuted and screw fixation did not immobilize all the fragments. He reported no pin tract or wound infection. Kushner (1970) used a similar technique substituting a thin wire for the bone screws. He treated 28 patients and reported five complications, of which two were infective.

Watson-Jones (1976) advocated screw fixation and a subsequent long-leg cast for unstable, oblique and spiral tibial fractures. He stressed that in comminuted spiral fractures a plate might be required. White *et al.* (1953) described 66 cases of screw fixation with the subsequent use of a standard long-leg cast. They suggested careful assessment of the fracture as their poor results were often associated with comminution or fracture distraction. More recently Dent and Hadden (1987) analysed 54 patients treated with interfragmentary screws and showed that despite an initial excellent reduction, 32% healed with a degree of malunion. They also had a 12.9% incidence of union problems and they concluded that superior techniques were available and suggested that the technique of infragmentary screws with a supplementary cast should not be used.

Cerclage wiring

Open wiring of the tibia was one of the six internal fixation methods described by Berenger-Feraud in 1870. It was widely used by many early orthopaedic surgeons such as Putti, Parham and Arbuthnott-Lane. However, it was accompanied by a high complication rate and was particularly associated with non-union and infection (Bohler, 1974). Goetze (1933) published a method of percutaneous extra-periosteal wire cerclage, and despite initial reservations, the method continues to be used in parts of Europe. Ahrer *et al.* (1966) reported on 188 patients treated with percutaneous cerclage and recorded only a 0.17% incidence of infection and a 2.65% incidence of delayed union.

Habernek *et al.* (1989) documented the results of percutaneous cerclage in 186 patients. They used the Johner and Wruhs (1983) forerunner of the AO classification. In their fracture population there were 59% B1 fractures, 22% A1 fractures and 11% C1 fractures. Complications included 13 cases of secondary malalignment, six superficial infections, five cases of peroneal nerve palsy and eight cases of delayed union. Joint mobility and patient function was not reported.

Traction

Traction remains a popular method of treating both closed and open tibial diaphyseal fractures associated with comminution of soft tissue damage. Traction can either be applied through the distal tibia, or more commonly through the calcaneus. It is interesting that calcaneal fixation is still in relatively widespread use, as it has gained a poor reputation over the years. White and Young (1966) reported a 50% incidence of infection and other complications, including lateral popliteal nerve palsy, hallux flexus and calcaneo-cavus deformity.

Calcaneal traction is an ostensibly easy technique, but is in fact associated with disadvantages other than those detailed by White and Young. Haines *et al.* (1984) and Kay *et al.* (1986) have illustrated the length of time for which traction must be applied before a long-leg cast can be applied without significant risk of fracture displacement. Haines *et al.* (1984) used traction for between two and three weeks but Kay *et al.* (1986) kept their oblique fractures in traction for 5.1 weeks, the transverse fractures for 4.6 weeks and the comminuted fractures for 5.8 weeks. The enforced bed rest that is associated with this method of management is associated with a considerable number of problems such as deep venous thrombosis, muscle wasting and joint stiffness in the young, with many other potentially more serious problems in the elderly.

Watson-Jones and Coltart (1943) recognized that skeletal traction was associated with delayed union in tibial fractures. Watson-Jones (1976) did, however, find the method useful for preventing loss of reduction in open tibial fractures. He emphasized that the traction weight should merely steady the leg and not exceed 5 lb. Bohler (1958) agreed that traction could cause enormous damage if incorrectly used. He proposed strict guidelines to govern the use of traction, suggesting that at most 3 kg should be used. He stressed the traction was only used to maintain alignment and should be combined with correct patient positioning to achieve its goals. He also stated that some overlap of fracture site was acceptable when applying traction to the tibia. Nicoll (1964) disagreed about the consequences of traction. He noted that there was a higher incidence of delayed union in his tibial fracture cases treated by traction. These fractures were associated with 31% incidence of delayed union compared with 19% in the fracture group treated without traction, but he attributed this to the type of fracture treated by traction rather than to the traction itself. Shakespeare and Henderson (1982) studied the effects of calcaneal traction on the compartmental pressures in the legs of five patients with tibial fractures. They used a slit catheter technique (Rorabeck *et al.*, 1981) to measure the pressure in the deep posterior compartment and in the anterior compartment. They found that the mean resting pressures without traction were 31.9 mmHg for the deep posterior compartment and 27.0 mmHg for the anterior compartment. For each kilogramme weight of traction applied, deep posterior pressure rose by an average of 5.2% of the resting value and the anterior pressure by 1.6%. They concluded that excessive traction was likely to increase the risk of compartmental ischaemia. The association of fracture non-union with increased compartmental pressure was shown by Court-Brown and McQueen (1987) and it seems likely that the increased compartment pressure following ill-judged calcaneal traction will cause delayed or non-union.

Isolated fractures of the tibia

A number of authors have examined the prognosis for tibial fractures without an associated fibula fracture. Much interest has centred around whether isolated tibial fractures heal more quickly or more slowly than fractures which involve both bones. Most of the literature now points to a shorter time to union in the isolated tibial fracture and this is not surprising when one considers that most isolated tibial fractures are low velocity injuries and are not associated with significant soft tissue damage. The other point that is commented on by many authors is the tendency of isolated tibial fractures to go into varus malalignment. Table 4.4 illustrates that the overall incidence of malalignment following isolated tibial fractures differs little from fractures of both the tibia and fibula treated by different types of plasters and braces. Interestingly, none of

Table 4.4   The treatment of isolated fractures of the tibial diaphysis

Series	Type of cast	No. of fractures	Open fractures (%)	Time to union (wk)	Malunion (%)	Joint stiffness (%)
Teitz *et al.* (1980)	Mixed	68	13.2	9.4	26.5	?
Hooper *et al.* (1981)	Long-leg	106	18.9	?	40.0	?
Wu and Shih (1990)	PTB	40	0	19.9	29.0	?
O'Dwyer *et al.* (1992)	Long-leg	48	10.4	16.5	?	?

the papers quoted in Table 4.4 talks about patient function following isolated tibial fractures. It seems reasonable to conclude from analysis of Table 4.4 that the isolated tibial fracture should be treated in the same way as fractures of both the tibia and fibula. The isolated tibial fracture is discussed further in Chapter 15.

Comments

1 Generally speaking, all authors dealing with the use of casts to treat tibia and fibula fractures have failed to classify fracture morphology or the degree of soft tissue damage associated with the fracture. Comparison of results between publications is therefore difficult.
2 In recent years many authors have reserved cast management for simpler tibial fractures, using operative techniques to manage more difficult fractures. Again, this makes comparison between different series difficult and also tends to accentuate the usefulness of cast management as the simpler tibial fractures are associated with a better prognosis.
3 Patient function has been virtually ignored by most authors. A number of recent papers have dealt with some aspects of patient function, but these have been retrospective studies and there are no studies dealing prospectively with the reestablishment of patient function after fracture. Most authors have merely used the rate and time of fracture union as the criteria of success.
4 The incidence of malalignment is frequently measured, but there is debate as to what constitutes malalignment. The literature suggests that malalignment <10° is not associated with significant long-term sequelae. This statement, however, must be subject to the proviso that recent series have shown much greater morbidity than earlier series. It may yet be shown that the increased mobility is at least in part related to malalignment.
5 Joint stiffness, particularly of the ankle and sub-

talar joints, is clearly the major problem associated with the use of casts or braces. As with malalignment, earlier authors suggested that hindfoot stiffness was not associated with significant morbidity. However, later authors clearly dispute this and there seems little doubt that ankle stiffness in particular is associated with significant morbidity and is a common problem following the use of casts or braces.
6 The use of subjective rather than objective criteria to assess patient disability is suspect. Patients tend to accommodate to their disability and often make light of it. This, however, does not lessen the effect of the disability and if questioned most patients would prefer not to have any disability. An example of this is commonly seen in patients who have lost ankle dorsiflexion and cannot adequately squat. They frequently get down to the ground by abducting the affected hip, flexing the knee and supporting themselves on their knee, rather than the foot. Most patients when questioned about this say that they would prefer to be able to squat, but have got used to this trick motion.
7 Long-term follow-up studies are of dubious relevance. An assessment of a patient 20 or 25 years after fracture provides little information as to what happened over the intervening years. It is likely that the patient has accommodated to any disability. It is also perfectly possible that the patient has relatively few symptoms even 5 years after fracture, but had significant medical, functional and social problems for a year or two after injury.
8 Isolated tibial fractures have a similar prognosis to tibia and fibula fractures of equivalent severity.
9 Functional braces may be lighter to wear, but otherwise appear to confer little benefit to the patient. What little literature there is suggests that the incidence of malalignment and joint stiffness following the use of functional bracing is much the same as that seen following patellar tendon-bearing plasters and even following long-leg casts, although recent works suggest

that the incidence of knee stiffness following use of a long-leg cast is higher than was previously thought. It appears that merely keeping the ankle free from a supportive cast does not ensure that the patient actually uses it.

Recommendations

1 The choice of the method of management for a tibial fracture should be directed towards reducing morbidity, particularly the complication of hindfoot stiffness.
2 In view of the fact that hindfoot stiffness appears to be increased in high energy injuries and by the prolonged use of a supportive cast, it is suggested that cast management of tibial fractures is confined to low energy injuries in which the surgeon can be reasonably sure of being able to remove the cast within 12–16 weeks of the injury.
3 High energy tibial fractures should be treated by operative means to facilitate joint movement.
4 Prolonged calcaneal traction should not be used. It is a difficult technique and, if badly managed, associated with a considerable morbidity. If the surgeon is considering calcaneal traction, external skeletal fixation should be used instead. Not only is this a more controllable technique, but it confers greater stability to the fracture.
5 The technique of pins and plaster should not be used. Again external skeletal fixation provides a better method of managing tibial fractures using transfixion pins. Cast materials are biomechanically poor pin clamps and the fractures are not rigidly held. In addition, the use of plaster obscures open wounds and denies examination of the soft tissue.
6 Interfragmentary screw fixation supplemented by an external cast should not be used. It combines the twin disadvantages of open surgery and further soft tissue stripping with inadequate fracture fixation.
7 All Gustilo types II and III open fractures should be treated operatively. The use of a plaster cast with this type of fracture not only hides the wound, but provides inadequate fracture stabilization. Internal or external fixation should be used for these fractures.

References

Ahrer, E., Philadelphy, G. and Vogl, W. (1966) Erfahrungen mit den percutanen draht-osteosynthese bei unterschenkeld rehbruchen. *Hefte Unfallheilk.*, **89**, 107

Alho, A., Benterud, J.G., Hogevold, H.E., Ekeland, A. and Stromsoe, K. (1992) Comparison of functional bracing and locked intramedullary nailing in the treatment of displaced tibial shaft fractures. *Clin. Orthop.*, **277**, 243–50

Anderson, L.D., Hutchins, W.C., Wright, P.E., and Disney, J.M. (1974) Fractures of the tibia and fibula treated by casts and transfixing pins. *Clin. Orthop.*, **105**, 179–91

Austin, R.T. (1981) The Sarmiento tibial plaster: a prospective study of 145 fractures. *Injury*, **13**, 12–22

Berenger-Feraud, L.J.B. (1870) *Traite de l'immobilisation directe des fragments ossieux dans les fractures*, Adiene Delahaye, Paris

Bohler, L. (1958) *The Treatment of Fractures*, Grune and Stratton, New York

Bohler, J. (1974) Percutaneous cerclage of tibial fractures. *Clin. Orthop.*, **105**, 276–82

Böstman, O. and Hanninen, A. (1982) Tibial shaft fractures caused by indirect violence. *Acta Orthop. Scand.*, **53**, 981–90

Brown, P.W. and Urban, J.G. (1969) Early weight bearing treatment of open fractures of the tibia. *J. Bone Joint Surg.*, **51A**, 59–75

Burkhalter, W.E. and Protzman, R. (1975) The tibial shaft fracture. *J. Trauma*, **15**, 785–94

Burwell, H.N. (1971) Plate fixation of tibial shaft fractures. *J. Bone Joint Surg.*, **53B**, 258–71

Court-Brown, C.M. and McQueen, M.M. (1987) Compartment syndrome delays tibial union. *Acta Orthop. Scand.*, **58**, 249–52

Dehne, E. (1969) Treatment of fractures of the tibial shaft. *Clin. Orthop.*, **66**, 159–73

Den Outer, A.J., Meeuwis, J.D., Hermans, J. and Zwaveling A. (1990) Conservative versus operative treatment of displaced non-comminuted tibial shaft fractures. *Clin. Orthop.*, **252**, 231–7

Dent, J.A., and Hadden, W.A. (1987) Interfragmentary screw fixation of fractures of the tibial shaft. *Injury*, **18**, 28–32

Digby, J.M., Holloway, J.M.N and Webb, J.K. (1983) A study of function after tibial cast bracing. *Injury*, **14**, 432–9

Edwards, P. (1965) Fractures of the shaft of tibia: 492 consecutive cases in adults. *Acta Orthop. Scand.*, Suppl. 76

Ellis, H. (1958) The speed of healing after fractures of the tibial shaft. *J. Bone Joint Surg.*, **40B**, 42–6

Goetze, O. (1933) Subcutane drahtnaht bel tibia schragfrakturen. *Arch. Klin. Chir*, **177**, 445–9

Habernek, H., Walch, G. and Dengg, C. (1989) Cerclage for torsional fractures of the tibia. *J. Bone Joint Surg.*, **71B**, 311–13

Haines, J.F., Williams, E.A., Hargadon, E.J. and Davies, D.R.A. (1984) Is conservative treatment of displaced tibial shaft fractures justified? *J. Bone Joint Surg.*, **66B**, 84–8

Hooper, G., Buxton, R.A. and Gillespie, W.J. (1981) Isolated fractures of the shaft of the tibia. *Injury*, **12**, 283–7

Hooper, G.J., Keddell, R.G. and Penny, I.D. (1991) Conservative management or closed nailing for tibial shaft fractures. *J. Bone Joint Surg.*, **73B**, 83–5

Horne, G., Iceton, J., Twist, J. and Malony, R. (1990) Disability following fractures of the tibial shaft. *Orthopedics*, **13**, 423–7

Johner, R. and Wruhs, O. (1983) Classification of tibial shaft fractures and correlation with results after rigid internal fixation. *Clin. Orthop.*, **178**, 7–25

Kay, N.R.M. (1970) The treatment of unstable fractures of the tibia by the double pin technique. *Injury*, **2**, 55–60

Kay, L. Hansen, B.A. and Raaschou, H.O. (1986) Fracture of the tibial shaft conservatively treated. *Injury*, **17**, 5–11

Karaharju, E.O., Alho, A. and Nieminen, J. (1979) The results of operative and non-operative management of tibial fractures. *Injury*, **7**, 49–52

Krause, F. (1891) Beitrage zur behanglung der knochenbrucke der unteren gliedmaassen im umhergehen. *Dtsch. Med. Wochenschr.*, **17**, 457–60

Kristensen, K.D., Kiaer, T. and Blicher, J. (1989) No arthrosis of the ankle 20 years after malaligned tibial shaft fractures. *Acta Orthop. Scand.*, **60**, 208–9

Kushner, A. (1970) Treatment of open tibial fractures by cross-fracture pin fixation. *Clin. Orthop.*, **73**, 136–45

Kyro, A., Tunturi, I. and Soukka, A. (1991) Conservative management of tibial fractures. *Ann. Chir. Gynaecol.*, **80**, 294–300

McMaster, M. (1976) Disability of the hindfoot after fractures of the tibial shaft. *J. Bone Joint Surg.*, **58B**, 90–3

Merchant, T.C. and Deitz, F.R. (1989) Long term follow-up after fracture of the tibial and fibular shafts. *J. Bone Joint Surg.*, **71A**, 599–606

Mollan, R.A.B. and Bradley, B. (1978) Fractures of the tibial shaft treated in a patellar tendon-bearing cast. *Injury*, **10**, 124–7

Moore, J.R. (1960) The closed fracture of the long bones. *J. Bone Joint Surg.*, **42A**, 869–74

Netz, P., Olsson, E., Ringertz, H. and Stark, A. (1991) Functional restitution after lower leg fractures. *Arch. Orthop. Trauma Surg.*, **110**, 238–41

Nicoll, E.A. (1964) Fractures of the tibial shaft. A survey of 705 cases. *J. Bone Joint Surg.*, **46B**, 373–87

O'Dwyer, K.J., De Vriese, L., Feys, H. Vercruysse, L. and Jameson-Evans, D.C. (1992) The intact fibula. *Injury*, **23**, 314–16

Oni, O.O.A., Hui, A. and Gregg, P.J. (1988) The healing of closed tibial shaft fractures. *J. Bone Joint Surg.*, **70B**, 787–90

Peltier, L.F. (1990) *Fractures: a History and Iconography of Their Treatment*, Norman Publishing, San Francisco

Pun, W.K., Chow, S.P., Fang, D. *et al.* (1991) A study of function and residual joint stiffness after functional bracing of tibial shaft fractures. *Clin. Orthop.*, **267**, 157–63

Puno, R.M., Teynor, J.T., Nagano, J. and Gustilo, R.B. (1986) Critical analysis of results of treatment of 201 tibial shaft fractures. *Clin. Orthop.*, **212**, 113–21

Reclus, P. (1897) *Bulletins et memoires de la societe de chirurgie de Paris*, **23**, 267

Rorabeck, C.H., Castle, G.S.P., Hardie, R. and Logan, J. (1981) Compartmental pressure measurements: an experimental investigation using a split catheter. *J. Trauma*, **21**, 446–9

Sarmiento, A. (1967) A functional below-the-knee cast for tibial fractures. *J. Bone Joint Surg.*, **49A**, 855–75

Sarmiento, A. (1970) A functional below-the-knee brace for tibial fractures. *J. Bone Joint Surg.*, **52A**, 295–311

Sarmiento, A., Gersten, L.M., Sobol, P.A., Shankwiler, J.A. and Vangsness, C.T. (1989) Tibial fractures treated with functional braces. *J. Bone Joint Surg.*, **71B**, 602–9

Scudese, V.A., Birotte, A. and Gialanella, J. (1970) Tibial shaft fractures: percutaneous multiple pin fixation, short-leg cast and immediate weight bearing. *Clin. Orthop.*, **72**, 271–82

Shakespeare, D.T. and Henderson, N.J. (1982) Compartmental pressure changes during calcaneal traction in tibial fractures. *J. Bone Joint Surg.*, **64B**, 498–9

Sheck, M. (1965) Treatment of comminuted distal tibial fractures by combined dual pin fixation and limited open reduction. *J. Bone Joint Surg.*, **47A**, 1537–53

Slatis, P. and Rokkanen, P. (1967) Conservative treatment of tibial shaft fractures. *Acta Chir. Scand.*, **134**, 41–7

Steen Jensen, J., Wang Hansen, S. and Hoansen, J. (1977) Tibial shaft fractures: a comparison of conservative treatment and internal fixation with conventional plates or AO compression plates. *Acta Orthop. Scand.*, **48**, 204–12

Suman, R.K. (1982) Orthoplast brace for the treatment of tibial shaft fractures. *Injury*, **13**, 133–8

Tanton, J. (1916) Fractures du membre inferieur. In *Noveau traite de chirurgie* (eds A. Le Dentu and P. Delbet), Ballière et fils, Paris

Teitz, C., Carter, D. and Frankel, V. (1980) Tibial fractures with intact fibulae. *J. Bone Joint Surg.*, **62A**, 770–6

Van der Linden, W. and Larsson, K. (1979) Plate fixation versus conservative treatment of tibial shaft fractures. *J. Bone Joint Surg.*, **61A**, 873–8

Watson-Jones, R. and Coltart, W.D. (1943) Critical review. Slow union of fractures with a study of 804 fractures of the shafts of the tibia and femur. *Br. J. Surg.*, **30**, 260–76

Watson-Jones, R. (1976) *Fractures and Joint Injuries* (ed. J.N. Wilson), 5th edn, Churchill Livingstone, Edinburgh

White, E.M., Radley, T.J. and Earley, N.N. (1953) Screw stabilisation in fractures of the tibial shaft. *J. Bone Joint Surg.*, **35A**, 749–55

White, E.H., Radley, T.J. and Earley, N.N. (1966) Screw stabilisation in fractures of the tibial shaft. *J. Bone Joint Surg.*, **48A**, 257–67

White, J. and Young, A.B. (1966) The complications of skeletal traction through the calcaneum. *Brit. J. Surg.*, **53**, 348–50

Wu, C.C. and Shih, C.H. (1990) Tibial fracture with or without fibular fracture – clinical studies. *Chang Gung Med. J.*, **13**, 191–8

5

Plating of tibial diaphyseal fractures

D. Pennig

Introduction

Tibial shaft fractures are caused by direct injury, penetrating trauma or indirect forces such as those experienced in shearing and rotational injuries. The exposed subcutaneous location of the tibia offers little protection against these forces and in displaced fractures the surgeon must be aware of the additional problem of soft tissue injuries (Billroth, 1866).

Plating is one of the original methods of treating displaced tibial shaft fractures. This method attracted the interest of surgeons because of the ease with which they could control fracture reduction. The first surgeon to use a plate for stabilization of a tibial fracture was Hansmann from Hamburg in 1886. The Hansmann plate is shown in Figure 5.1. Sir William Arbuthnot-Lane (1893a, b, 1897, 1914) of Scotland and Albin Lambotte

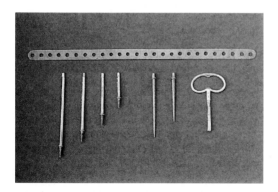

Figure 5.1 The Hansmann plate (Hamburg 1886). Photograph from the archives of Aesculap, Tuttlingen, Germany

(1907) of Belgium established this method of internal fixation and promoted its use. Lane's book was published in 1905 and Lambotte's in 1907. By that time both surgeons had tested their techniques over some years. The plates were made of metal and were fixed to the bone by means of metallic screws driven through the cortex.

Stimulated by the work of Lambotte, Robert Danis of Belgium described several internal fixation techniques, including plate fixation, in his textbook published in 1947. Danis coined the term 'soudure autogène' which later became known as 'primary bone healing' (Danis, 1979). Until the 1960s scientific reports dealing with plating of acute fractures were scarce and the complications associated with plating were frequently severe (Anderson, 1965; Karlström and Olerud, 1974). The 'Arbeitsgemeinschaft für Osteosynthesefragen' in Switzerland (AO) played an important role in metallurgical research, the improvement of plate design and in the biomechanical studies of fracture plating (Allgöwer *et al.*, 1973; Allgöwer and Spiegel, 1979; Hutzschenreuter and Brummer, 1980; Müller *et al.*, 1990; Pennig, 1994). They defined plate fixation as aiming at accurate anatomical reduction and direct bone healing with no visible callus (Anderson, 1965). In the 1970s the technique of bone plating was very popular (Burwell, 1971; Olerud and Karlström, 1972; Smith 1974; Thunold *et al.*, 1975; Rüedi *et al.*, 1976; Laros and Spiegel, 1979; Allgöwer and Perren, 1982) but the enthusiasm for the technique has faded over the last 10–15 years (Johner and Wruhs, 1983; Rommens and Schmitt-Neuerberg, 1987a; Hegelmaier *et al.*, 1990) with other techniques showing better results (Bach and Hansen, 1990).

A literature search for the period January 1990 until August 1994 revealed 152 publications dealing with tibial shaft fractures. It is interesting to observe that only 7.9% of these publications dealt with plating whereas 37.5% of the publications concerned external fixation and 54.6% dealt with intramedullary nailings.

Lag screw

A simple way to compress two fragments of bone together is with the use of a lag screw (Schatzker, 1974; Schatzker *et al.*, 1975a; Müller *et al.*, 1990). The lag screw exerts intrafragmental compression. Lag screws have to be inserted into the centre of bone fragments and at right-angles to the plane of the fracture. Since one single lag screw is generally not strong enough to achieve stable fixation in the diaphysis a minimum of two screws is required.

Accurate reduction is important prior to insertion of the screws. The first hole to be drilled is the gliding hole in the proximal fragment. This has to have the same size as the outer diameter of the screw thread. The gliding hole is drilled through the proximal cortex only and subsequently a drill guide is inserted into the gliding hole. An appropriately smaller drill is then inserted through the drill guide to drill the distal cortex. The screw is then inserted and tightening of the screw causes the fragments to be compressed (Figure 5.2).

Screws may be either self-tapping or non-self-tapping. The original belief was that self-tapping screws provided a poorer hold in bone because they created more damage during insertion (Hutzschenreuter and Brummer, 1980). This however has now been shown to be incorrect (Schatzker *et al.*, 1975a, b). Non-self tapping screws have an advantage where the screws have to be passed obliquely through a thick cortex. In these cases non-self-tapping screws are easier to insert (Schatzker *et al.*, 1975a).

The biomechanics of compression plate fixation

The introduction of compression plating improved postoperative stability (Anderson, 1965; Allgöwer *et al.*, 1973; Schatzker, 1974; Müller *et al.*, 1990). Stability was not only achieved by the rigidity of the implant but also by impaction of the fragments. This reduces the stresses borne by the implant thereby protecting it (Figures 5.3, 5.4).

In the areas of bone contact fracture healing occurs as a result of osteons crossing the fracture lines. The osteons grow parallel to the long axis of the bone in Haversian systems. A persistent gap after rigid internal fixation hinders the osteons ability to cross the fracture line with a consequent delay in union (Uhthoff and Finnegan, 1983; Pennig, 1994; Uhthoff *et al.*, 1994). The aim of compression plate osteosynthesis is accurate reduction of the fracture fragments and secure permanent fixation

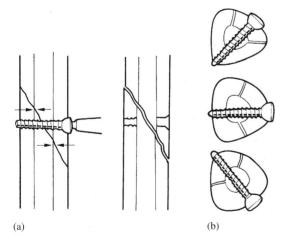

(a)   (b)

Figure 5.2 (a) Lag screw fixation: the hole next to the screw head is larger than the thread diameter to allow gliding. The hole in the opposite cortex is the thread hole (gliding hole 4.5 mm drill bit, thread hole 3.2 mm drill bit). (b) Orientation of the screw in lag screw fixation: the screw is inserted into the centre of the fragments. The fracture plane is crossed at right-angles

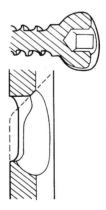

Figure 5.3 Dynamic compression plates allow the application of the spherical gliding principle. The screw hole is designed as an inclined half-cylinder for self-compression or self-loading with a slope of the hole corresponding to the spherical screw head. (After Müller *et al.*, 1990)

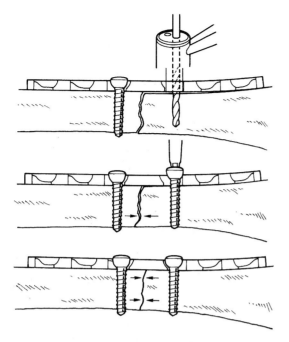

Figure 5.4 With the dynamic compression plate and eccentric drilling of the gliding hole on the right hand side tightening of the screw results in a movement of screw and bone towards the fracture line. This causes axial compression. (After Allgöwer *et al.*, 1973)

(Figures 5.5, 5.6). Initially the philosophy of plating involved the reduction of the fracture such that the entire fracture surface was brought into contact and compressed by the plate (Rüedi *et al.*, 1984; Müller *et al.*, 1990) and lag screws. Recently however this concept has been altered to allow for more indirect control of the smaller fragments with modified reduction techniques (Mast *et al.*; Hegelmaier *et al.*, 1990). The current philosophy is that a bone plate will anchor the main fragments leaving the comminuted fragments as little disturbed as possible. Using these indirect plating techniques periosteal callus formation is frequently visible.

The biomechanical principles of compression plating consist of plate positioning and contouring, screw placement and interfragmentary compression (Müller *et al.*, 1990). With regard to the positioning of the plate it should be placed in such a way that muscle forces acting across the fracture tend to close it (Figure 5.7). This generally means that the plate should be placed on the convex side of the bone, a location which does not exist in the tibia. In addition during normal gait the loading pattern of the tibia varies from compression to tension (Chao and Aro, 1994).

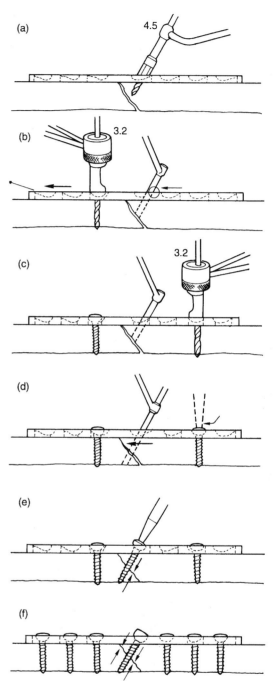

Figure 5.5 Application of a dynamic compression plate and a lag screw for interfragmentary compression. (a) Selection and contouring of the plate. The cortex under the plate is drilled for insertion of a lag screw. (b) Fixation of the plate with one screw drilled in the neutral position. (c) Second screw drilled in the eccentric load position. Tightening of the screw results in axial compression. (d) Drilling of the thread hole for the lag screw (3.2 drill bit). (f) Insertion of the remaining screws in the neutral position. (After Müller *et al.*, 1990)

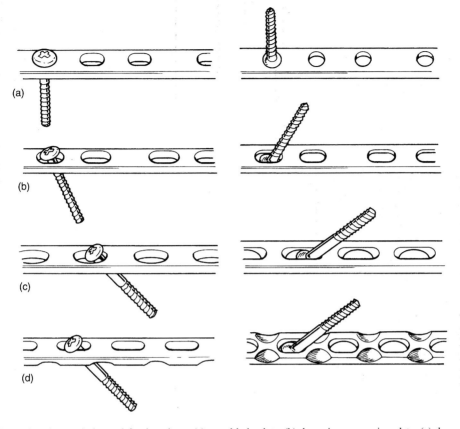

Figure 5.6 Design changes in internal fixation plates: (a) round hole plate: (b) dynamic compression plate; (c) dynamic compression unit; (d) limited contact dynamic compression plate (LC-DCP). (After Müller *et al.*, 1990)

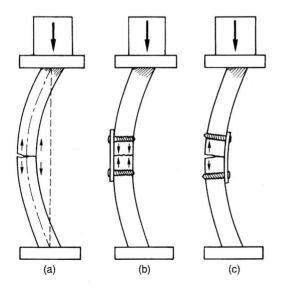

Figure 5.7 The plate acts as a tension bend in eccentric loading of long bones. It is important to know which side of the bone is under tension. (b) Plate applied on the convex side to neutralize all tension forces. (c) Application on the concave side resulting in inadequate fixation and bending of the implant. (After M.E. Müller *et al.*, New York, 1970)

Screws are used to hold the implant onto the bone and it is important to place the screws close to the fracture site. Some screws may act as lag screws in that they are designed to compress a fracture surface. Lag screws may also be inserted independent of the plate to facilitate fracture reduction. It should be remembered that these screws require 4.5 mm holes which cause defects in the cortex which persist after screw removal. It should also be remembered that although interfragmentary compression is a biomechanical prerequisite for increased rigidity of the plate bone construct the interfragmentary compression is not constant since bone resorption at the fracture may considerably reduce the compressive forces (Schatzker *et al.*, 1975b; Hutzschenreuter and Brummer, 1980; Chao and Aro, 1994).

Contouring of the plate is performed to create more uniform compressive contact stresses at the fracture site (Figure 5.8). If a plate fits the bone surface exactly there is less eccentric compression when it is screwed onto the bone. If the plate is not contoured the cortex under the plate is compressed whereas the opposite cortex tends to open as the screws are tightened (Frankle *et al.*, 1994). In addition experimental studies examining plated bones after 16–32 weeks observed that the removal torques of the screws were low. This indicates the plates tend to loosen after a relatively short period

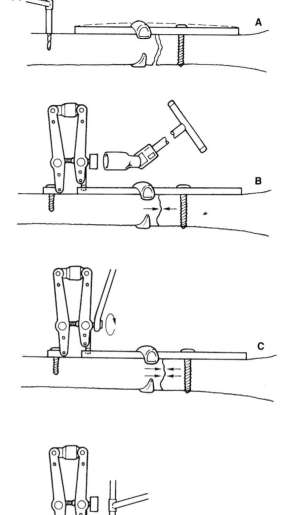

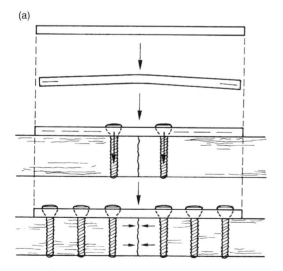

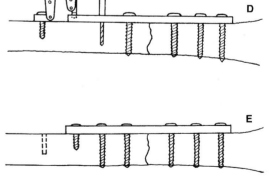

Figure 5.8 (a) Application of a contoured plate. The inner screws have to be placed first. Insertion of the outer screws first would result in a persistent gap under the plate. (b) The tension device to apply compression. **A**, reduction of the fracture is followed by application of the plate and insertion of the screw in one fragment. Holding of the plate with a bone clamp. Drilling of an additional hole for fixation of the tension device. **B**, Compression of the fracture by loading of the tension device. The bone clamp may have to be loosened temporarily. **C**, Insertion of two further screws in one fragment. **D, E**, Insertion of remaining screws. (After Müller *et al.*, 1990)

(Hutzschenreuter and Brummer, 1980; Chao and Aro, 1994).

The axial stiffness of a rigid stainless steel plate is several times that of intact bone. A consequence of this is that the bone is frequently osteopenic after union and refractures not infrequently occur after plate removal. Although this can theoretically be linked to the stiffness of the implant (Uhthoff and Finnegan, 1983; Uhthoff *et al.*, 1994), lowering the axial stiffness of plates has not thus far had any effect on the incidence of refracture (Tayton and Bradley, 1983; Woo *et al.*, 1984). Ideal plate technology has to provide immediate maximum rigidity to replace the lost structural integrity of the bone but at the same time this rigidity should not be spread over the whole length of the bone. In the later phases of bone union and remodelling the axial stiffness of the plate should be reduced so that the underlying bone can absorb a higher proportion of the physiological loading, this being necessary for bone healing and remodelling. This mechanical dilemma has not as yet been solved (Pennig, 1990).

Open reduction is a prerequisite of adequate plate fixation. However open reduction disturbs the periosteal blood supply as does the presence of the plate on top of the periosteum (Pennig, 1990; Uhthoff *et al.*, 1994). The primary cell source for the formation of external (periosteal) callus is the cambium cell layer (Pennig, 1990). In an attempt to reduce the vascular problems associated with plates limited contact plates have been designed which are thought to maintain a greater degree of periosteal integrity than conventional plates (Perren, 1991). However experiments in dogs have shown that both conventional plates and limited contact plates cause similar amounts of cortical necrosis and osteoporosis and thus far there is no evidence that limited contact plates are superior to conventional plates (Uhthoff *et al.*, 1994).

Operative technique in tibial shaft fractures

Timing of surgery

In tibial plating the exact timing of surgery is extremely important and will have a major influence on the eventual outcome (Rüedi *et al.*, 1984). Ideally early surgery is preferable but may be associated with significant complications if there is significant damage to the skin or other soft tissues. As with the management of all fractures factors such as the severity of coexisting injuries in the multiply injured patient and the general medical state of the patient should be taken into account when making a decision about the type of fixation to be used.

Local factors that the surgeon should be aware of include the elapsed time since injury, the state of the soft tissues and the type of surgical intervention planned. If the patient is assessed shortly after the injury the operation should ideally be carried out within 6 hours of the injury. However if there is the slightest doubt regarding the state of the soft tissues the procedure should be delayed. The advantage of early surgery is that fracture reduction is easier since no shortening of the soft tissues has occurred (Rüedi *et al.*, 1984). Not infrequently the operation has to be delayed for between 6 and 10 days because of general or local factors. During this period any bone shortening associated with fracture instability should be avoided by means of traction.

The standard approach to the tibia is anterolateral (Figure 5.9) (Rüedi *et al.*, 1984; Mast *et al.*, 1989). An incision is made 1 cm lateral to the subcutaneous anterior border over the anterior compartment muscle mass. The advantages of this approach include the ability to expose the entire tibia from the knee to ankle if this is required. The incision chosen should be long enough to avoid forceful handling of the soft tissue envelope. At

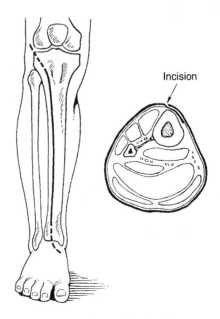

Figure 5.9   Anterolateral approach to the tibia

the distal end of the tibia in the region of the tibialis anterior tendon the incision should curve
medial to the tendon. The surgeon should avoid
opening the tendon sheath and if this manoeuvre
is required the sheath should be resutured. The
surgeon should also be careful to elevate the skin
and subcutaneous tissues together and to avoid
thinning of the skin edges by unnecessary dissection as this may result in skin necrosis. Once
the incision has been made the fracture is carefully
exposed while protecting the periosteum. Periosteal stripping should be avoided.

The surgeon should always be aware of other
possible surgical approaches. Some patients will
have other incisions on the leg and if at all possible a previous incision should be used. Where
there is a pre-existing skin flap the surgeon should
be careful not to devascularize the flap and if there
is any doubt about this a plastic surgeon should be
consulted.

If decompression of the posterior compartment
of the leg is required a posteromedial incision
1 cm posterior to the medial border of the tibia can
be used (Figure 5.10). Open reduction can be performed along the posterior surface of the tibia
(Rüedi *et al.*, 1984; Rommens and Schmitt-
Neuerburg, 1987b; Mast *et al.*, 1989).

A posterolateral approach can be used when the
anterior portion of the soft tissue envelope is
severely damaged (Figure 5.11) (Rüedi *et al.*,
1984; Mast *et al.*, 1989; Heitemeyer *et al.*, 1990).
This approach is also very useful for secondary

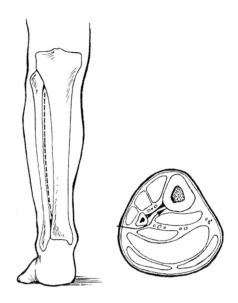

Figure 5.11 Posterolateral approach to the tibia

bone grafting and the fibular may be incorporated
in the grafting procedure.

Implant selection

Preoperative planning is important if bone plating
is to be undertaken correctly. Preoperative draw-
ings should be carried out using translucent or
transparent paper or plastic over the X-rays. The
most frequently used plate is a standard dynamic
compression plate with 4.5 mm cortical screws
(Müller *et al.*, 1990). The plate can be placed on
the anteromedial or lateral surfaces of the tibia. At
the distal end of the tibia the anteromedial location is the only possible option. When selecting the
correct implant the surgeon should remember that
satisfactory plating involves fixation of 6 cortices
above and below the fracture (Müller *et al.*, 1990).
Any less than this is mechanically inappropriate.

The plate should be pre-bent to allow more uniform compression of the fracture site (Figure 5.12).
As originally detailed the early philosophy of plating required that even the smallest fragments were
identified, reduced and fixed by screws. Recently
however there has been an acceptance of a more
indirect reduction techniques. This can be assisted
by the use of a fracture distractor (see Chapter 7).
If an indirect reduction technique is used the plate
is essentially a neutralization device which bridges
the comminuted area in an attempt to minimize
vascular damage to the smaller fragments (Rüedi
et al., 1984).

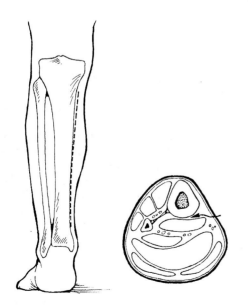

Figure 5.10 Posteromedial approach to the tibia

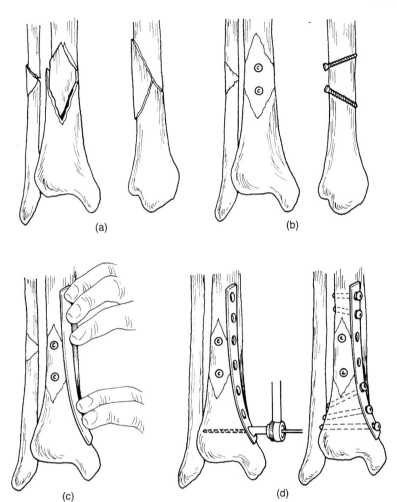

Figure 5.12 Plate application in a distal tibial fracture with a third fragment. (a) Fracture reduction. (b) Stabilization with two lag screws. (c) Contouring of the plate with a malleable plate. (d) Screw placement starting at the distal end of the tibia

(a)

(b)

(c)

(d)

It is advisable to start with the smaller main fragment and to place one or two screws in this fragment (Figure 5.13). The reduction is then completed with the use of a Verbrugge bone reduction clamp to hold the part of the plate not yet secured to the bone (Figure 5.14).

It should be remembered that the stiffer the implant the greater the precision of plate contouring must be. Even small inconsistencies between the contour of the bone and the plate will result in angulation or opening of the fracture. Repeated application of the plate may therefore be necessary to contour it exactly.

At this point the fracture reduction should be checked radiographically in both anteroposterior and lateral planes. The position is then secured by two screws in the other fragment and a further check is carried out after tightening these screws.

It is usually necessary to use one or two reduction forceps until the last screws are inserted.

Contouring of the plate is more difficult in the distal tibia where the plate acts as an anti-glide plate (Mast *et al.*, 1989). Pre-contoured plates exist but even with these some fine tuning is necessary. Plate fixation in this area relies on adequate bone stock and if the bone is osteoporotic the purchase of the screws in the bone may be inadequate. Other methods of treatment should be employed if this is the case.

Bone grafting

In closed fractures bone grafting may be required if there is extensive comminution. The indication for bone grafting has to be established during surgery and should be performed during the procedure.

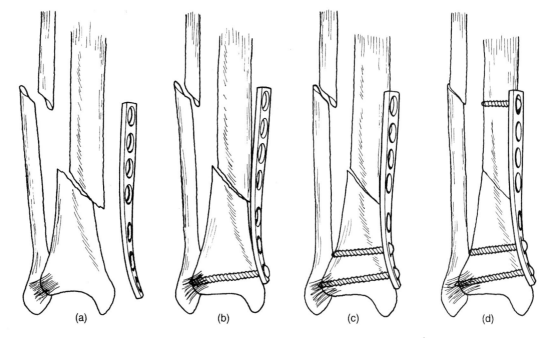

Figure 5.13 Plate application in a distal tibial fracture with the dynamic compression plate. (a) Exposure of the fracture, selection of the implant (7–10 hole plate). Contouring of the distal part of the plate by twisting and bending. (b) Fixation of the plate to the distal fragment just above the medial malleolus. Joint penetration has to be avoided. The screw is not definitively tightened at this point. (c) Reduction of the fracture and insertion of the second distal screw. (d) Anatomical reduction of the fracture and insertion of the most proximal screw. Radiographic check at this point and placement of the remaining screws depending on the direction of the fracture line. A loading screw may be inserted

Cancellous bone and corticocancellous chips are best used and should be packed in the area of comminution. In open fractures primary bone grafting is not advisable because of the risk of infection (Müller *et al.*, 1990).

Open fractures

Despite good initial results with the use of plates in open fractures (Rittmann *et al.*, 1979; Heitemeyer *et al.*, 1990) the enthusiasm for this technique has decreased in recent years. The requirement for a large skin incision and further soft tissue dissection in an area where there is already soft tissue injury in addition to a large implant surface in a potentially contaminated area has led to unacceptably high infection rates (Johner and Wruhs, 1983; Hegelmaier *et al.*, 1990). The use of plates in open tibial shaft fractures cannot be recommended.

Complications

Intraoperative complications include arterial and nerve damage from drilling. This can be avoided with careful technique. Over-stressing of the screws may lead to stripping of the thread and the screw will then need to be resited. Poor implant selection or incorrect plate contouring leads to inadequate reduction which has to be corrected (Frankle *et al.*, 1994).

When closing the skin the surgeon should ensure that there is no tension. Inability to gain skin cover over the plate constitutes a major intraoperative problem (Hegelmaier *et al.*, 1990). On one hand it is necessary to cover the plate to avoid infection but on the other hand tension on the skin will lead to skin necrosis and subsequent infection. Scarification of the skin has been carried out to reduce the tension on the main incision. However this leads to impaired skin circulation and cannot be recommended. If the plate and bone cannot be covered one must consider removal of the implant and a change of fixation method to either external fixation or intramedullary nailing. Alternatively the

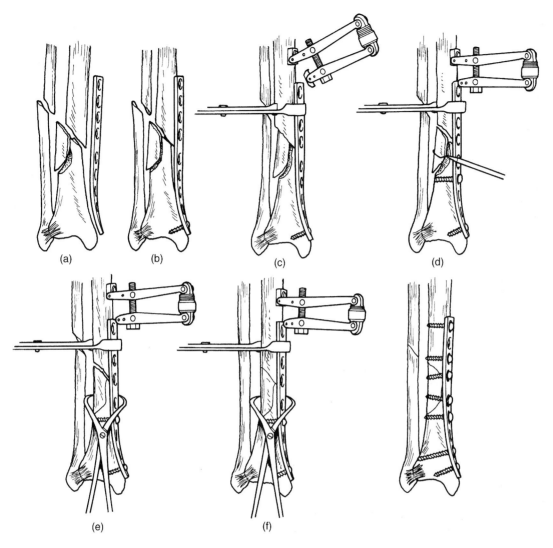

Figure 5.14 Use of plate fixation in a comminuted distal tibial fracture and application of the tensioner. (a) Contouring of the plate. (b) Fixation of the plate to the distal fragment with one screw. (c) Use of a Verbrugge bone clamp. (d) After insertion of a further screw into the distal fragment the tension device is used for distraction, the plate is allowed to slide under the Verbrugge clamp. The third fragment may reduce. Due to the soft tissue attachments this requires careful manipulation and fixation with a pointed reduction forceps (e). (f) Compression is applied with the tension device. (g) Insertion of the remaining screws. The two central screws are used as lag screws to stabilize the third fragment

soft tissue defect can be covered by a flap, this usually being a fasciocutaneous or muscle flap.

Postoperative complications include skin necrosis and wound infection (Johner and Wruhs, 1983). If the condition of the soft tissue is poor a supportive plaster cast is recommended to aid soft tissue stabilization (Figure 5.15). If soft tissue necrosis develops early plate removal and a change to external fixation is advisable (Figure 5.16). If bone is left

exposed for more than 24 hours the risk of infection is considerable. Under these circumstances the help of a plastic surgeon must be sought and flap cover undertaken as soon as possible. The worst prognosis is in those cases where infection occurs and is ignored for a long period (Figure 5.17).

Another problem associated with plating is that union is often slow and sometimes difficult to detect on the X-rays. If no radiological progress is

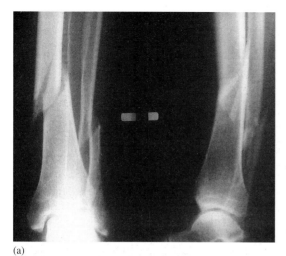

(a)

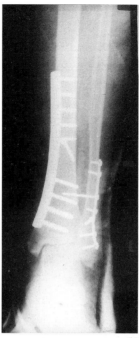

(b)

Figure 5.15 (a) Fracture of the distal tibia with soft tissue damage in a 28-year-old male. The fibular fracture extends distally to the level of the syndesmosis. (b) Stabilization of the tibia with a dynamic compression plate. Stabilization of the fibula with a one-third tubular plate. The repair of the syndesmosis is secured with a fibulo-tibial screw. Plaster application to protect the soft tissues

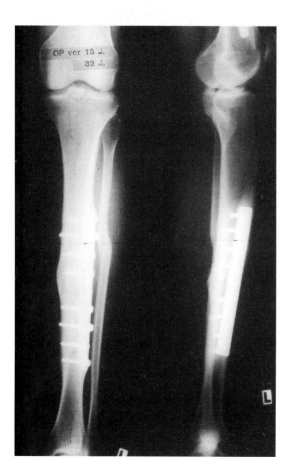

Figure 5.16 Lateral plate fixation in a 32-year-old male. The plate has been in place for 13 years. Notice the dense bone with visible remodelling

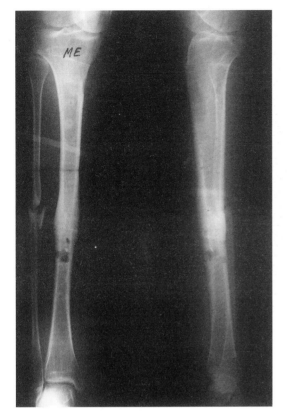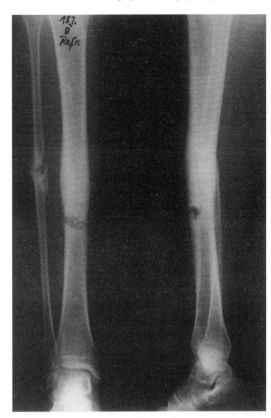

Figure 5.17 (a) Situation after removal of an internal fixation plate with two lag screws resulting in a large cortical defect (18-year-old female). (b) Unprotected loading resulted in a fatigue fracture of the medial cortex

visible early posterolateral bone grafting is advisable to avoid a fatigue fracture of the plate. If this occurs in the presence of delayed union or non-union a change to intramedullary stabilization is recommended (Perren, 1979). This should be carried out by a surgeon experienced in the technique.

Implant removal

It is recommended that plates be removed after 12–24 months (Müller *et al.*, 1990). The plate should of course only be removed when union is confirmed clinically and radiologically. When removing a long plate we routinely protect the soft tissue with a plaster backslab until wound healing is established. Strenuous activities are prohibited for 3 months and in the presence of one or more gliding holes for lag screw fixation the protective brace is used for 6–8 weeks (Figure 5.18).

Postoperative management

Postoperative management starts with an intra-operative assessment of the fracture stability. If the surgeon considers that the stability is excellent then early mobilization of the extremity may be undertaken. Postoperatively the leg is elevated with the ankle splinted at 95° of dorsiflexion. The splint is removed to initiate physiotherapy on the sixth post-operative day. Until then a daily inspection of the soft tissues is advisable. The splint is reapplied after exercise and at night until the patient has adequate active control of dorsiflexion. If this is not done the patient is at risk of developing an equinus deformity which is difficult to control and will invariably cause disability. Two to three weeks after injury the patient can discard his splint completely and 10 kg of weight bearing is allowed after the soft tissues have healed. If the patient is uncooperative a cast or cast brace must be retained until fracture union is established otherwise implant failure and other problems may occur. It is recommended

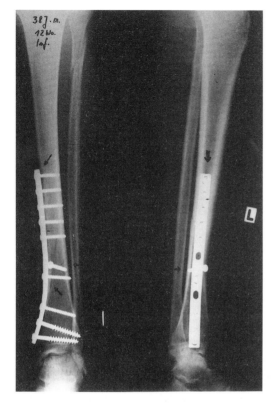

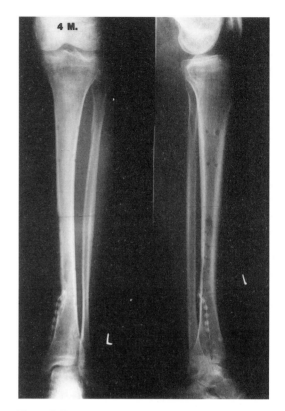

Figure 5.18   (a) Plate fixation in a tibial fracture (38-year-old male). Twelve weeks after surgery an infection with wound breakdown developed. Fracture lines still visible

Figure 5.18   (c) Healing 4 months after fixator application. Note the cortical defect on the medial side

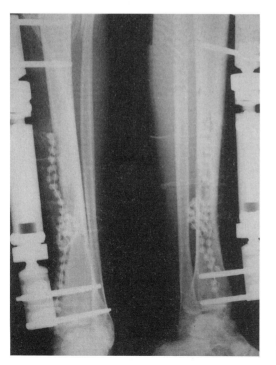

Figure 5.18   (b) Removal of the plate, removal of avital bone, gentamycin beads and stabilization with an external fixator

that X-rays be carried out on the first postoperative day and again after 3 weeks, 6 weeks and 4 months. After 4 months it should be apparent that union is proceeding and weight bearing may then be increased. Until this time only partial weight bearing can be allowed.

Results

The initial series published by Rüedi *et al.* (1976) reported 97% excellent and good results in 323 closed tibial fractures treated with dynamic compression plates. The infection rate was less than 1%. However these results could not be reproduced by other authors. Johner and Wruhs (1983) reported significant complications in 9.5% of their simple fractures, this rising to 18.1% in their complex fractures and 48.3% in the comminuted fractures. Osteitis in their different groups ranged from 2.1% to 10.3%. Where there was more comminution the complication rate was significantly raised.

Most authors now view tibial shaft fractures associated with displaced intra-articular fractures of the knee as one of the few remaining indications for compression plate and screw fixation. Other indications include a displaced tibial fracture below a total knee procedure.

Careful preoperative planning, assessment of the soft tissue injury and a good technical understanding of implant and instrumentation are the key factors for an acceptable outcome with this technique. Plate fixation is not a forgiving technique and even small mistakes may result in serious complications (Johner and Wruhs, 1983).

Conclusion

The tibial diaphysis has the disadvantage of having a poor soft tissue envelope on the subcutaneous anteromedial border. The vascular supply to this area is often suspect and arterial and venous disorders are known to lead to chronic ulceration which can occur either spontaneously or after minimal trauma. Significant trauma to the soft tissue envelope associated with a displaced tibial shaft fracture often involves considerable damage to this area and any incision placed through the damaged soft tissue in front of the tibia may add insult to injury.

Plate fixation aims at an accurate anatomical reduction of the bone fracture and under ideal circumstances direct bone healing should occur without visible callus formation. However healing without callus produces a weak union which relies on the implant for supplementary stabilization. The rigidity of the implant does not allow the bone to respond with normal periosteal callus formation. Since plating is essentially non-physiological its use in diaphyseal fractures of the tibia should be viewed with extreme caution and, if undertaken by a surgeon, meticulous adherence to technique should be employed. In periarticular fractures plating may have a more important role but here again the plate has to compete with other forms of stabilization. One of the few remaining indications for plating a displaced tibial diaphyseal fracture is where a total knee replacement has been implanted prior to the fracture. In virtually all other situations, no matter whether the fracture be closed or open, alternative methods such as cast bracing, intramedullary nailing and external fixation are to be recommended.

References

Allgöwer, M., Matter, P., Perren, S.M. *et al.* (1973) *The Dynamic Compression Plate (DCP)*, Springer-Verlag, New York–Berlin–Heidelberg

Allgöwer, M. and Perren, S.M. (1982) Voraussetzungen und Indikationen der operativen Behandlung von Tibiafrakturen. *Akt. Chir.*, **1**, 1

Allgöwer, M. and Spiegel, P.G. (1979) Internal fixation of fractures: evolution of concepts. *Clin. Orthop. Rel. Res.*, **138**, 26

Anderson, L.D. (1965) Compression plate fixation and the effect of different types of internal fixation on fracture healing. *J. Bone Joint Surg.*, **47A**, 191

Bach, A.W. and Hansen, T. Jr (1989) Plates versus external fixation in severe open tibial shaft fractures. *Clin. Orthop. Rel. Res.*, **241**, 89

Billroth, T. (1866) *Die allgemeine chirurgische Pathologie und Therapie in 50 Vorlesungen*, Verlag Georg Reimer, Berlin

Burwell, H.N. (1971) Plate fixation of tibial shaft fractures: a survey of 181 injuries. *J. Bone Joint Surg.*, **53B**, 258

Chao, E.Y.S. and Aro, H.T. (1994) Biomechanics of fracture repair and fracture fixation. In *Current Practice of Fracture Treatment* (ed. P.C. Leung), Springer-Verlag, Berlin

Danis, R. (1947) *Theorie et pratique de l'osteosynthèse*, Masson, Paris

Danis, R. (1979) The classic: the aims of internal fixation. *Clin. Orthop.*, **138**, 23

Frankle, M.A., Crodey, J., Frankle, M.D. *et al.* (1994) A retrospective analysis of plate contouring in the tibia using the conventional 4.5 (narrow) dynamic compression plate. *J. Orthop. Trauma*, **8**, 59

Hegelmaier, C., Bierwirth, P. and Schulz, S. (1990) Sind Komplikationen nach Plattenosteosynthese am diaphysären Unterschenkelschaft unvermeidlich? *Unfallchirurg*, **93**, 544

Heitemeyer, U., Bohm, H.J. and Hierholzer, G. (1990) Die dorsale Plattenosteosynthese am Tibiaschaft. Ergebnisse einer Sammelstudie der Deutschen Sektion der AO-International. *Unfallchirurg.*, **93**, 391

Hutzschenreuter, P. and Brummer, H. (1980) Screw design and stability. In *Current Concepts of Internal Fixation of Fractures*, (ed. H.K. Uthoff), Springer-Verlag, Berlin

Johner, R. and Wruhs, O. (1983) Classification of tibial shaft fractures and correlation with results after rigid internal fixation. *Clin. Orthop.*, **178**, 7

Karlström, G. and Olerud, S. (1974) Fractures of the tibial shaft: a critical evaluation of treatment alternatives. *Clin. Orthop.*, **105**, 82

Lambotte, A. (1907) *Le traitement des fractures*, Masson, Paris

Lane, W.A. (1893a) A method of treating simple oblique fractures of the tibia and fibula more efficient than those in common use. *Trans. Clin. Soc. Lond.*, **72**, 167

Lane, W.A. (1893b) On the advantage of the steel screw in the treatment of ununited fractures. *Lancet*, **i**, 1500

Lane, W.A. (1897) Treatment of simple fractures by operation. *Clin. J.*, **10**, 161

Lane, W.A. (1905) *Operative Treatment of Fractures*, London Medical Publishing Co.

Lane, A.W. (1914) *The Operative Treatment of Fractures*, 2nd edn, London Medical Publishing Co.

Laros, G.S. and Spiegel, P.G. (1979) Rigid internal fixation of fractures. *Clin. Orthop. Rel. Res.*, **138**, 2

Mast, J., Jakob, R. and Ganz, R. (1989) *Planning and Reduction Technique in Fracture Surgery*, Springer-Verlag, Berlin

Müller, M.E., Allgöwer, M. and Willenegger, H. (1970) *Manual of Internal Fixation*, Springer-Verlag, New York

Müller, M.E., Allgöwer, M., Schneider, R. *et al.* (1990) *Manual of Internal Fixation*: *Techniques Recommended by the AO–ASIF*, 3rd edn, Springer-Verlag, Berlin

Olerud, S. and Karlström, G. (1972) Tibial fractures treated by AO compression osteosynthesis: experiences from a five year material. *Acta Orthop. Scand. (Suppl.)*, **140**, 1

Pennig, D. (1990) Zur Biologie des Knochens und der Knochenbruchheilung. *Unfallchirurg*, **93**, 488

Pennig, D. (1994) Current use of the intramedullary nail. In *Current Practice of Fracture Treatment* (ed. P.C. Leung), Springer-Verlag, Berlin, p. 119

Perren, S.M. (1979) Physical and biological aspects of fracture healing with special reference to internal fixation. *Clin. Orthop. Rel. Res.*, **138**, 175

Perren, S.M. (1991) The concepts of biological plating using the limited contact-dynamic compression plate (LC-DCP). *Injury*, **22** (Supplement 1), 1

Rittmann, W.W., Schibli, M., Matter, P. *et al.* (1979) Open fractures: long-term results in 200 consecutive cases. *Clin. Orthop. Rel. Res.*, **138**, 132

Rommens, P. and Schmitt-Neuerberg, K.P. (1987a) Ten years of experience with the operative management of tibial shaft fractures. *J. Trauma*, **27**, 917

Rommens, P. and Schmitt-Neuerburg, K.P. (1987b) Indikation und Ergebnisse der dorsalen Plattenosteosynthese am Tibiaschaft. *Unfallchirurg.*, **90**, 309

Rüedi, T., von Hostetter, A.H.C. and Schlumpf, R. (1984) *Surgical Approaches for Internal Fixation*, Springer-Verlag, Berlin

Rüedi, T., Webb, J.K. and Allgöwer, M. (1976) Experience with the dynamic compression plate (DCP) in 418 recent fractures of the tibial shaft. *Injury*, **7**, 252

Schatzker, J. (1974) Compression in surgical treatment of fractures of the tibia. *Clin. Orthop.*, **105**, 220

Schatzker, J., Horne, J.G. and Summer-Smith, G. (1975a) The holding power of orthopaedic screws in vivo. *Clin. Orthop.*, **108**, 115

Schatzker, J., Horne, J.G. and Summer-Smith, G. (1975b) The effects of movement on the holding power of screws in bone. *Clin. Orthop.*, **111**, 257

Siebert, Ch., Rinke, F., Lehrbass-Sokeland, K.P. *et al.* (1993) Sekundare Versorgung von Tibiafrakturen mittels Plattenosteosynthese. *Akt. Traumatol.*, **23**, 307

Smith, J.E.M. (1974) Results of early and delayed internal fixation for tibial shaft fractures: a review of 470 fractures. *J. Bone Joint Surg.*, **56B**, 469

Tayton, K. and Bradley, J. (1983) How stiff should semi-rigid fixation of the human tibia be? A clue to the answer. *J. Bone Joint Surg.*, **65B**, 312

Thunold, J., Varhaug, J.E. and Bjerkeset, T. (1975) Tibial shaft fractures treated by rigid internal fixation: the early results in a 4-year series. *Injury*, **7**, 125

Uhthoff, H.K., Boisvert, M.S.C., Finnegan, M. *et al.* (1994) Cortical porosis under plates. *J. Bone Joint Surg.*, **76A**, 1507

Uhthoff, H.K. and Finnegan, M. (1983) The effects of metal plates on posttraumatic remodeling and bone mass. *J. Bone Joint Surg.*, **65B**, 66

Wolter, D. (ed.) (1992) Historische Entwicklungen in der operativen Frakturbehandlung (von Hansmann bis Ilisarov). In *Schriftenreihe Unfallmedizinische Tagungen der Landesverbände der gewerblichen Berufsgenossenschaften*, Heft 79, 21

Woo, S.L.-Y. *et al.* (1984) Less rigid internal fixation plates: historical perspectives and new concepts. *J. Orthop. Res.*, **1**, 431

6

Intramedullary nailing of the tibia

C. Court-Brown

There are two principal techniques for nailing tibial diaphyseal fractures. The most widely used is the introduction of a single large diameter nail into the intramedullary canal. In recent years these nails have been of the interlocking type such that proximal and distal screws can be inserted to stabilize the fracture. These nails may be inserted with or without prior intramedullary reaming and currently there is debate as to which is the better technique. An example of the use of a large diameter reamed nail is shown in Figure 6.1.

The alternative technique is to use flexible small diameter intramedullary nails without prior reaming. With the introduction of interlocking tibial nailing the use of small diameter flexible tibial nails has declined but the technique will be described at the end of the chapter as it still remains in use for less severe tibial fractures. Figure 6.2 shows an example of a tibial diaphyseal fracture stabilized using Rush pins.

Tibial nailing using a single large diameter nail

Intramedullary nailing of the tibia has enjoyed a considerable resurgence in the past ten years to the extent that many surgeons have forgotten that the technique has a relatively long pedigree and their current interest merely represents an example of the cyclical nature of orthopaedic surgery. Interest in tibial nailing was initiated by the invention of the Kuntscher–Herzog nail, this being an unlocked open section nail with a proximal bend to facilitate its placement in the tibia. Despite the fact that Kuntscher strongly advocated reamed intramedullary

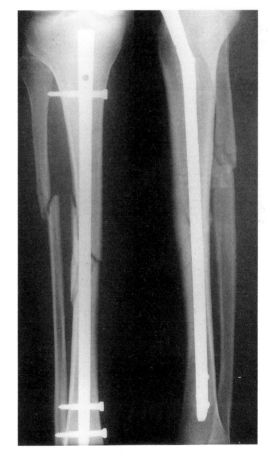

Figure 6.1 A statically locked reamed Grosse–Kempf nail used to stabilize a closed tibial diaphyseal fracture. Union was secured in 17 weeks and full joint mobility was achieved

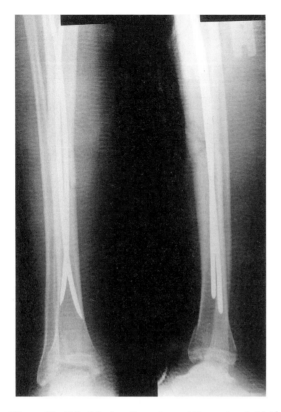

Figure 6.2   Paired Rush nails used to stabilize a closed tibial diaphyseal fracture. Note the use of three point fixation but also the cast necessary to ensure maintenance of fracture position

nailing, the Kuntscher–Herzog tibial nail was used in both reamed and unreamed forms. Although considerable success was achieved with this nail (Kempf *et al.*, 1969; Zucman and Maurer, 1970; Merle d'Aubigne *et al.*, 1974), the technique was not without its problems.

The problems encountered using an unlocked tibial nail mainly related to the difficulty in securing good fixation in inherently unstable tibial fractures without the use of locking screws. As many tibial fractures are located in the distal third or are spiral or comminuted in type, it is obvious that stable fixation cannot always be achieved. Early workers such as Merle d'Aubigne (1974) advocated the use of postoperative casts, but this combined method of treating fractures had obvious disadvantages and improved fixation techniques were sought. Lottes (1952) attempted to improve on the original Kuntscher design by developing a flexible unreamed nail. However he still needed to use postoperative casts because of the inherent instability of many of the tibial fractures that he treated.

The AO group (Müller *et al.*, 1965) solved the problem of postoperative instability by advocating the use of open plating for many tibial fractures, but this technique also had a number of complications and the invention of interlocking intramedullary tibial nails by Klemm and Schellman (1972) and Grosse and Kempf (Kempf *et al.*, 1978) allowed surgeons to combine the advantages of the closed technique of tibial nailing with the avoidance of postoperative casts. It quickly became clear to many surgeons that the tibia was much easier to nail than the femur and the technique of interlocking tibial nailing became rapidly accepted.

The relative success of tibial nailing is demonstrated by reviewing the results of a number of the surgeons who used unlocked nails. Despite the disadvantage of having to use postoperative casts, the authors were absolutely clear that the technique of closed tibial nailing represented a major advance over non-operative closed tibial fracture treatment. Zucman and Maurer (1970) used unreamed Kuntscher nails in 356 fractures. In 207 closed fractures they had 200 good results with no infection. They had a 2.1% incidence of non-union and 0.5% incidence of malunion. In 136 open fractures there was an 8.1% infection rate with a 0.7% incidence of aseptic non-union and no malunions. However, the proportion of distal third and comminuted fractures was low and only 15% of the open fractures were severe. Merle d'Aubigne and his co-workers (1974) documented the use of unreamed Kuntscher nailing in 640 tibial fractures. They also had a lower infection rate, with 0.7% infection in 384 closed fractures and a 6.6% incidence in 256 open fractures. The union rates were high and they reported only a 1.04% incidence of non-union in the closed fractures, with 2.4% in the open fractures. Unlike Zucman and Maurer they did encounter malunion, stressing that this occurred in proximal and distal fractures and rarely in the mid-diaphyseal areas. They compared their results with the use of plaster, traction and plating and reported lower complication rates and reoperation rates using nailing. They advocated the use of plaster for undisplaced or stable fractures or for very comminuted fractures.

Lottes (1974), using his unreamed nail, also reported relatively low complication rates in both closed and open tibial fractures. He analysed the results of tibial nailing, reporting 0.9% infection in 330 closed single fractures and no infection in closed segmental fractures. There was a 7.3% infection rate in the open single fractures and 6.3% in the open segmental fractures. There were only two cases of non-union in the closed group and 8 non-unions were seen out of 251 open fractures. As with the other early workers, Lottes felt that intramedullary tibial nailing was an excellent technique.

Later researchers have also confirmed the usefulness of both reamed and unreamed unlocked tibial nailing. Weller *et al.* (1979) documented the Swiss experience with the early AO nail. This had the facility of using antirotation wires to stabilize some fractures and therefore represented a form of interlocking nailing. In 1882 open and closed tibial fractures they documented an infection rate of 3.2%, a malunion incidence of 2.4% and good recovery of joint and patient function. Similar results using the AO nail were reported by Puno *et al.* (1986) who found a 3.3% infection rate and a 1.7% incidence of malunion in a mixed group of open and closed tibial fractures. Donald and Seligson (1983) also reported reasonable results using a Kuntscher nail modified to facilitate the use of antirotation wires.

Locked intramedullary nailing

The introduction of the Klemm–Schellmann and Grosse–Kempf nails which substituted proximal and distal cross screws for the antirotation wires of the earlier nails permitted adequate stabilization of virtually all tibial diaphyseal fractures. Both these nails were designed to be used as reamed nails but interest in the unreamed concept continued and improvement in metallurgy and nail design allowed the introduction of unreamed interlocking intramedullary nails which also used proximal and distal locking screws to gain stability. Examples of this type of unreamed nail include the Russell-Taylor nail (Whittle *et al.*, 1992) and AO nail (Haas *et al.*, 1993; Oedekoven *et al.*, 1993; Renner *et al.*, 1993).

Reamed interlocking tibial nailing

The first results of the use of reamed interlocking tibial nails in a large group of patients came from Klemm (Klemm and Borner, 1986). He examined the results of 401 closed and Gustilo type I open tibial fractures treated with the Klemm-Schellmann nail. Table 6.1 shows his basic results, indicating low infection and non-union rates. He defined function according to his own criteria, with excellent function (full knee and ankle motion, no muscle atrophy and normal radiological alignment) occurring in 62.5% of patients. A good result (slight loss of knee or ankle motion, less than 2 cm of muscle atrophy or angular deformity of less than 5°) occurred in 31.8% of patients and a fair or poor result in the remaining 5.7%. He concluded that interlocking intramedullary nailing was the treatment of choice for closed tibial fractures in the skeletally mature individual and that delayed interlocking nailing could be used in grade I open fractures. He reserved external skeletal fixation for type II and III open fractures.

One of the problems about most of the literature relating to nailing of tibial fractures is patient selection. Most surgeons apply a bias to their inclusion criteria using nailing for a predetermined group of patients without any objective evidence that it is appropriate for that particular group. In an attempt to explore the usefulness of nailing in all closed and type I open tibial fractures Court-Brown *et al.* (1990a) adopted a policy of nailing all tibial fractures that required an anaesthetic in their treatment. Thus minor undisplaced fractures were treated non-operatively but all other fractures were treated by primary reamed intramedullary nailing using the Grosse–Kempf nail. One hundred and twenty-five patients were followed prospectively for one year after nailing. The basic results of the trial are shown in Table 6.1. Overall the

Table 6.1   Results of use of interlocking intramedullary nailing in the management of closed and open tibial diaphyseal fractures

	No.	Type	Union (wk)	Infection (%)	Non-union (%)	Malunion (%)	Joint stiffness (%)	Compartment syndrome (%)
Klemm and Borner (1986)	267	Closed Open (G1)	?	2.2	1.1	?	?	0.4
Henley (1989)	24	Closed Open (GI,II)	24	0	0	4.2	?	0
Court-Brown *et al.* (1990a)	125	Closed Open (G1)	16.7	1.6	1.6	2.4	7.2	1.6
Alho *et al.* (1990)	93	Closed Open (GI,II)	15	3.2	3.2	10.7	9.7	3.2
Hooper *et al.* (1991)	29	Closed Open (GI)	15.7	0	0	3.4	13.7	3.4
Habernek *et al.* (1992)	109	Closed Open (GI,II)	?	1.8	6.4	12.8	?	1.8

G = Gustilo type.

complication rate was low, with no specific fracture grade or type showing an increased complication rate. All the closed fractures were classified according to Tscherne's classification and the mean union time shown in Table 6.1 merely represents the figure based on the relative number of the different Tscherne types. A breakdown of the time to union according to Tscherne's classification is shown in Table 6.2. This illustrates that the relationship between the mean time to union and the Tscherne fracture grade is virtually linear and indicates the importance of adequately classifying closed fractures. Most fracture series combine all their closed fractures and Table 6.2 illustrates that this is inappropriate. It is obvious that the union time for a C3 fracture is almost twice that of a C0 fracture and the mean time to union for most series will therefore depend on the proportion of each type of fracture within the fracture population.

Court-Brown *et al.* found the functional results following nailing were better than those reported for other treatment methods. They found that the mean time to resumption of full activities except sports in those patients who did not have multiple injuries was 14.3 weeks, with 78% returning to full activities before clinical union. They also found that the average time for return to work in patients in employment was 12.1 weeks with 82.5% returning to work before clinical union.

Table 6.1 shows broad agreement between surgeons who have analysed the use of reamed nails in closed and Gustilo type I and II open fractures. It is obvious that if Gustilo type III fractures are excluded from analysis the infection rate should be below 4% and in most series will be below 2%. Not only is the non-union incidence low but it is easily treated by exchange nailing (Court-Brown *et al.*, 1990a) or by open bone grafting (Klemm and Borner, 1986; Alho *et al.*, 1990). Malunion is avoidable by meticulous attention to technique. It is often caused by failure to lock statically an intramedullary nail. It is always wise to err on the side of too much rather than too little static locking. It is recommended that static locking be used if there is any comminution, if the fracture configuration is spiral or if the fracture is in the proximal or distal quarters of the tibial diaphysis.

The incidence of joint stiffness depends on the type of fracture being treated. Locked reamed nailing allows early weight bearing without a supportive cast and therefore the patient can mobilize the lower limb joints from an early stage. Hooper *et al.* (1991) suggested good joint movement may return by 6 weeks, and although this is possible in low velocity injuries, the return of joint function may take a considerable period, particularly if Tscherne C2 and C3 fractures are being treated. In Court-Brown's series there was a 7.2% incidence of joint stiffness at one year but a number of patients had either had hindfoot damage at the time of injury or had had a compartment syndrome. Comparison of hindfoot motion with that gained following cast or brace management (Digby *et al.*, 1983; Oni *et al.*, 1988) or plate fixation (Van der Linden and Larsson, 1979) shows that nailing allows much better hindfoot motion.

The use of reamed intramedullary nailing in Gustilo grade III open tibial fractures remains somewhat contentious, although its popularity is increasing. Opponents of this technique suggest that the intramedullary vascular damage associated with reaming added to the soft tissue damage caused by the injury means that the prognosis is poor and that there will be a high incidence of infection and non-union.

The work of Bone and Johnson (1986) is often used to support this view. These surgeons treated 112 tibial fractures with reamed nailing and had a 25% infection rate in type II and III open fractures. However, only 26 were open fractures treated primarily with reamed nailing and only one of these was type III in severity. In addition, 84 of the

Table 6.2   Time to union for the different Tscherne grades of closed tibial diaphyseal fracture. The importance of the associated soft tissue damage is highlighted by the increasing time to union

Fracture grade	Definition	No.	Mean time to union (wk)
C0	Simple fracture configuration with little or no soft tissue injury	16	12.5
C1	Superficial abrasion; mild to moderate soft tissue damage; severe fracture configuration	59	16.2
C2	Deep contaminated abrasion with local damage to skin or muscle; moderately severe fracture configuration	30	18.7
C3	Extensive contusion or crushing of skin or destruction of muscle; severe fracture	9	23.7

fractures were treated with a standard unlocked AO nail. In fact, very little literature exists regarding the use of reamed interlocking nails for Gustilo type III fractures. Court-Brown *et al.* (1991) reported on the use of the reamed Grosse–Kempf nail in the treatment of 27 type III fractures. This group consisted of 14 type IIIa fractures and 13 IIIb type fractures. The mean time to union was 27.2 weeks for the IIIa fractures and 50.1 weeks for the IIIb fractures. The IIIa subgroup showed no infection, no cases of malunion and no open bone grafting was required, although 5 patients required exchange nailing to stimulate union. In the IIIb subgroup there were 3 infections and 2 malunions. The need for open bone grafting was dictated by the length of bone loss. Where this exceeded 2 cm and 50% of the bone circumference, it was found that open bone grafting was essential and the authors advocated that this be performed at about 6 weeks once the soft tissue envelope was complete. Lesser bony defects were successfully treated by exchange nailing.

A later analysis of type III open fractures (Court-Brown *et al.*, 1992a) showed similar results but the overall infection rate for the type III fractures had dropped to 8.8%, again with no infection in the IIIa subgroup. A third analysis of the results of reamed intramedullary nailing and the management of Gustilo type III open fractures in the Edinburgh Orthopaedic Trauma Unit was carried out in January 1994. By this time 55 such fractures had been treated by primary nailing using the Grosse–Kempf system. There were 27 type IIIa and 28 IIIb fractures. Analysis of the results with respect to infection showed no infections in the type IIIa fractures and a 10.7% infection rate in the IIIb group. The overall infection rate for type III Gustilo fractures was therefore 5.4%.

Further review of the data showed there had been no infection in Gustilo type III fractures since July 1989, when the unit introduced a rigorous protocol for the management of these fractures. Careful attention to the technique of debridement combined with flap cover has therefore reduced the incidence of infection in these fractures to virtually zero. Comparative analysis of Edinburgh data in the early 1980s is interesting. Court-Brown *et al.* (1990b) documented their results of the use of external skeletal fixation in open tibial fractures and quoted a 37.5% incidence of infection in Gustilo type III fractures. It is interesting to observe that over a 15-year period the infection rate in type IIIb open tibial fractures has fallen from 35.7% to virtually zero. The major operative

change has been the use of reamed intramedullary nailing as opposed to external skeletal fixation, but it is highly unlikely that this has caused the reduction in infection. The use of a rigid protocol with aggressive debridement of both soft tissue and bone combined with early flap closure, usually within 48–72 hours, has ensured that the results have improved. Analysis of mean time to union in the 55 Gustilo type III fractures shows an average union time of 22.3 weeks for the IIIa fracture and 47.7 weeks for the IIIb fracture. Those IIIb fractures with insignificant bone loss united in an average of 37.5 weeks while the fractures with significant bone loss took 56.1 weeks. This represents an improvement over the 1991 analysis, probably being associated with the decreased infection rate.

Complications of reamed nailing

As with all fracture treatment techniques, there are a number of complications associated with the use of reamed tibial nailing. Koval *et al.* (1991) stated that 58% of reamed tibial nailing operations were associated with a complication, but their study was retrospective and a number of the complications were probably produced by the fact that they performed intramedullary nailing on average 10 days after injury. A number of the complications that they detail are almost certainly secondary to nailing, whether done using a reamed or unreamed technique.

Other authors have examined the complications of reamed nailing in some detail (Alho *et al.*, 1990; Court-Brown *et al.*, 1990a; Habernek *et al.*, 1992) and it is now possible to list accurately the complications of this procedure.

Knee pain

The main complication of tibial nailing is knee pain. This occurred in 40.8% of prospective series detailed by Court-Brown *et al.* (1990a). However, a more detailed analysis of the incidence and effect of knee pain following tibial nailing was undertaken by Court-Brown *et al.* (1996a). They undertook an in-depth analysis of 169 patients who had had their tibial fractures primarily treated with the reamed Grosse–Kempf nail. Using a ten-point pain analogue scale and a structured questionnaire, it was seen that 105 (62.1%) of the patients actually complained of some knee pain, although it was felt that in 10 patients knee pain was secondary to intra-articular performance and not related to the nail. However, in 95 (56.2%) of patients it was considered that the knee pain was secondary to the nail. Sixty-four (37.9%) patients had no knee pain at all. Further analysis of the 66.2% of patients with nail-related pain showed that 39.6% of the group had mild pain (analogue < 4), 11.8% had moderate pain (analogue 4–6) and 4.7% had severe pain (analogue > 6). Therefore, of the 169 patients 79.5% had either no pain or minor pain and 16.5% had moderate or severe pain. Despite this, 82.1% of the patients who complained of nail-related pain experienced pain on kneeling, 54.7% experienced pain on squatting, 50.5% had pain on running and 42.1% had walking-related pain. It is therefore obvious despite there being relatively few patients who had moderate or severe pain that the activities of the patients were restricted. Comparison of those patients with no pain and those patients with nail-related pain showed no difference in the type of fracture, the incidence of multiple injury, the location of the skin incision, the presence or absence of a proximal locking screw or whether the incision was medial to or through the patella tendon. The only significant difference between the two groups was that the group who had no knee pain had an average age of 31 years whereas the group with nail-related pain had an average age of 44 years. Nail removal either relieved or abolished the knee-related pain in over 75% of patients and it is recommended that the tibial nail be removed if the patient complains of nail-related pain. It must always be remembered that the patient may well have had damage to the knee as a result of the same injury that caused tibial fracture, and if there is any suggestion of other causes of knee pain appropriate investigations should be undertaken. There is as yet no satisfactory explanation as to why patients get knee pain following tibial nailing. In some incidences the nail is clearly left long (Figure 6.3) and this undoubtedly can be associated with pain on kneeling or knee flexion. In most cases, however, the nail is either buried or left so that only a few millimetres protrudes from the proximal tibial and in these patients we have been unable to correlate the degree of nail protrusion with the amount of knee pain. An alternative explanation is that the gliding tissues below the knee are altered by the dissection involved in introducing the nail. If this were the case one would expect that further surgery to remove the nail would increase the pain and this clearly does not happen. Other authors have also found a relatively high incidence of knee pain, this varying between 15% (Alho *et al.*, 1990) and 55% (Haddad *et al.*, 1996).

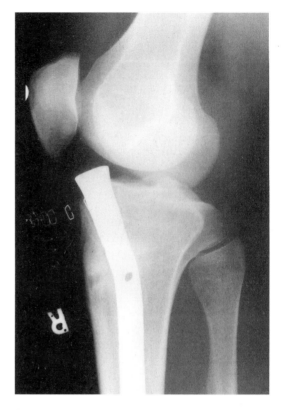

Figure 6.3 Knee pain is the commonest complication of tibial nailing. Prominent nails are associated with pain but frequently it is difficult to correlate the X-ray appearances with the patient's symptoms

Compartment syndrome

Prior to the establishment of reamed tibial nailing as a routine procedure there was some disquiet about the possibility that intramedullary reaming caused raising intracompartmental pressures and thereby compartment syndrome. Some surgeons believe that if reamed nailing is to be used for the management of tibial fractures it should be delayed to allow the soft tissue swelling to settle, thereby minimizing the risk of compartment syndrome.

These fears have, however, proved groundless. Table 6.1 shows that the incidence of compartment syndrome varies between 0.4% and 3.4%. Collective analysis of the 647 fractures detailed in Table 6.1 shows a mean incidence of compartment syndrome following reamed intramedullary nailing of 1.7%.

The relationship of reaming and nailing to compartment pressures was studied in great detail by McQueen *et al.* (1990). They measured the anterior compartment pressures in 67 legs undergoing reamed nailing of the tibia. They showed that reaming and nailing were responsible for a transient rise in intracompartmental pressure, but that the rise in pressure was not sustained and the pressure fell after nailing. They also showed that delayed nailing was not associated with lower intra- or postoperative compartment pressures and they concluded that reamed tibial nailing did not increase the risk of compartment syndrome. These findings were supported by the work of Tischenko and Goodman (1990) and Roger *et al.* (1992). Compartment syndrome is discussed further in Chapter 8.

Neurological damage

Koval *et al.* (1991) stated that 30% of their patients had neurological problems after nailing, although many of these were relatively minor. However, this figure is considerably in excess of that encountered by other workers. The most serious neurological complication associated with tibial nailing is a neuropraxia of the common peroneal nerve (Klemm and Borner, 1986; Koval *et al.*, 1991; Habernek *et al.*, 1992) or posterior tibial nerve (Sarangi and Karachallios, 1993). This complication is reported to have an incidence of between 1.1% (Klemm and Borner, 1986) and 2.7% (Habernek *et al.*, 1992). The prognosis is usually good, with most neuropraxias recovering spontaneously.

There is little evidence in the literature as to why these lesions occur but it is likely that they are associated with excessive preoperative traction, a prolonged delay before surgery which allows excessive tibial shortening or by distraction of the fracture site during nailing. It is of interest that in Edinburgh where early nailing is practised, peroneal nerve palsy has only been seen five times in over 700 tibial nailing procedures. It is often difficult to determine whether a common peroneal nerve palsy has followed the fracture or the nailing procedure. The surgeon should also be aware that there may have been damage to the fibular head and neck or to the proximal tibiofibula joint as a result of the initial injury and that this may have caused the peroneal nerve palsy.

Other neurological problems are usually related to the position of the cross screws or traction pins. Court-Brown *et al.* (1990a) recorded three cases of saphenous or sural nerve damage with distal cross screws. These authors have also seen one case of a lateral plantar neuroma caused by placement of the calcaneal transfixion pin.

Vascular damage

Rarely injudicious drilling or proximal screw placement may cause popliteal artery damage (Browner, 1986). Fortunately this complication is extremely rare, but if it occurs urgent vascular reconstruction is required.

Proximal comminution

As with femoral nailing, the use of an incorrect entry point in the tibia may be associated with proximal comminution. This is rarely a serious problem and is associated with the learning curve inherent in any technique. Court-Brown *et al.* (1990a) noted proximal comminution in 3.2% of the fractures but correct positioning of the proximal cross screws meant that it did not provide a clinical problem. Very occasionally a tongue of bone may be raised from the point of entry of the nail to a distal point in the tibia. This may be produced by failure to flex the knee to at least 90°, thereby imposing stresses on the anterior tibia.

Screw discomfort

The anteroposterior proximal cross screws and any distal screw inserted on the medial border of the tibia are subcutaneous and the patient may complain of significant discomfort within a few weeks of nailing. This occurred in 13.6% of the series of Court-Brown *et al.* (1990a). It is rarely a severe problem as most screws can be removed under local anaesthetic within 2–3 months of fracture.

Unreamed tibial nailing

In the past 2 or 3 years there has been a considerable resurgence of interest in unreamed tibial nailing using interlocking nails (Figure 6.4). The Lottes unreamed nail has continued to be used in the USA but a recent study on its usefulness in closed and open tibial diaphyseal fractures (Howard *et al.*, 1992) showed that while acceptable results were gained in closed and Gustilo type I and II open fractures, the infection rate in Gustilo type III open tibial fractures was 41.2%. This is not too surprising when one considers the degree of bone loss and instability that frequently accompanies Gustilo type III open tibial fractures. This study confirms the view that unlocked nails, whether reamed or unreamed, should not be used to treat Gustilo type III open tibial fractures.

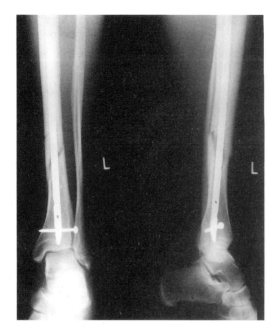

Figure 6.4 An unreamed Synthes nail. It has been statically locked. Note the difference in diameter between the intramedullary canal and the nail. Union was successful and the patient achieved a full range of joint movement

The recent introduction of interlocking unreamed intramedullary nails has allowed all open fractures to be adequately stabilized. The theoretical advantage of such nails is that there is less damage to the intramedullary circulation without the necessity of reaming and therefore lower nonunion and infection rates. In addition, it is also suggested that the absence of reaming will lower the incidence of compartment syndrome. The theoretical effect on the intramedullary blood supply is supported by animal work carried out by Klein *et al.* (1990), who indicated that reaming of the canine tibia diminished the cortical blood supply by 45–85%. This compared with the use of unreamed nails, which altered the cortical blood supply by between 15 and 30%. Further evidence for this was presented by Schemitsch *et al.* (1994). Using a spiral fracture model in sheep tibiae they showed that cortical revascularization occurred within six weeks of the passage of an unreamed nail. When a reamed nail was used revascularization was not complete until 12 weeks.

Reichert *et al.* (1995) took an opposing view. They suggested that reaming is beneficial to fracture healing. Using intact sheep tibiae and labelled microspheres they demonstrated that intramedullary reaming induced a six-fold increase in the periosteal circulation within 30 minutes. They did not demonstrate a rise in the overall blood supply and postulated that an increased periosteal supply compensated for any decrease in the intramedullary circulation. This finding confirmed the earlier work of Danckwardt-Lillestrom (1969) and also suggested that Trueta's hypothesis that the direction of blood flow can reverse from centrifugal to centripetal after loss of the endosteal supply (Trueta, 1972) is correct. The inherent problem with all of the papers discussing laboratory studies related to reaming is that they all tend to concentrate on one particular facet of the complex problem of bone vascularity and union. While the results of a particular paper may be valid it is often impossible to extrapolate the results to the clinical situation. It will fall to clinical trials to show whether unreamed nails are associated with lower complication rates than reamed nails this being particularly important in Gustilo type III open fractures where the nutrient artery, and therefore the intramedullary circulation, is invariably damaged.

As yet there are very few papers in the literature discussing the clinical usefulness of interlocking unreamed nails. Oedekoven *et al.* (1993) treated 100 tibial fractures with either an AO or Russell-Taylor unreamed nail. Fifty-six were closed and 44 were open, these including all Gustilo grades up to IIIb. They followed up 86 patients and showed a delayed union rate of 11.6% and a non-union incidence of 7%. Over 80% of their cases healed without further surgical intervention. There were no deep infections and two (2.3%) superficial infections. However, they had a 9% incidence of compartment syndrome and an 11.6% malunion rate. A further 18.6% of the fractures showed implant problems, this usually being breakage or bending of the screws (Figure 6.5). Renner *et al.* (1993) also had no infection in 17 open and closed tibial fractures. They had a 5.9% malunion rate, an 11.8% incidence of compartment syndrome and a 17.6% screw breakage rate.

Haas *et al.* (1993) examined the use of the AO unreamed nail in Tscherne C2 and C3 closed fractures and Gustilo type II and III open fractures. Again no deep infections were reported but 42% of the patients had a fasciotomy, although it is not reported whether these were prophylactic or therapeutic. In addition, there was a 13.7% incidence of peroneal nerve palsy, a 13.7% incidence of screw breakage and a malunion rate of 23.5%.

Singer and Kellam (1994) reported less satisfactory results using unreamed locked intramedullary nailing over a 3-year period. They evaluated

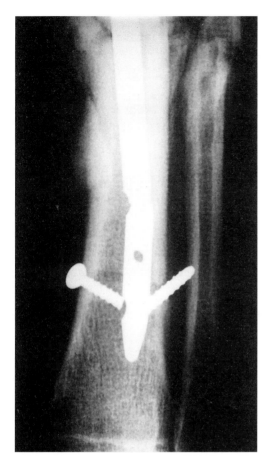

Figure 6.5 The major problem associated with unreamed nails is breakage of both cross screws and nails. Both are shown here

41 high energy open tibial fractures in 39 patients, of which 24 were Gustilo type III in severity. They achieved a 90% union rate in an average of 5.6 months but stressed that 46% of their fractures required an additional procedure to achieve union.

Their complication rates were relatively high, including 49% malunion, 12% deep infection, 41% screw breakage and 20% compartment syndrome. Sanders and Gregory (1995) reported better results from the use of unreamed nails in the management of 47 unstable closed tibial fractures. They found that 87% of the fractures had united by 6 months and that there was no joint stiffness except in patients who had had associated joint injuries. Their complications were few. However Duwelius *et al.* (1995) had a somewhat different experience. They treated 49 displaced tibial fractures of which 31 were closed. They encountered significant problems with delayed and non-union and suggested that dynamization or exchange nailing be considered to hasten union and avoid screw failure.

Whittle *et al.* (1992) examined the use of the unreamed Russell-Taylor nail in Gustilo type III open fractures. They did not use the nail for the treatment of fractures in the distal quarter of the tibia and like the other proponents of unreamed nailing they relied on cast or brace support for a period post-operatively.

They examined 50 fractures, of which 34 were Gustilo grade III in severity. They employed early bone grafting as part of their protocol of management and 96% of their fractures united. Their

Table 6.3 Incidence of aseptic non-union and the requirement for exchange nailing following primary reamed intramedullary nailing of the tibia

Fracture type	No.	Uninfected fracture	Aseptic non-unions (No.)	(%)	Exchange nailings	Bone grafting
Closed						
C0	38	38	0	0	0	0
C1	261	256	8	3.1	8	0
C2	110	109	6	5.5	6	0
C3	29	29	1	3.4	1	0
Total	438	432	15	3.5	15	0
Open						
GI	29	28	2	7.1	2	0
GII	30	27	2	7.1	2	0
GIIIA	23	23	5	21.7	5	0
GIIIB$_1$	15	13	5	38.5	5	1
GIIIB$_2$	12	11	11	100	4	11

The closed fractures are divided into Tscherne grades and the open fractures into Gustilo types and subtypes. GIIIB$_1$ refers to Gustilo IIIB fractures with insignificant bone loss and GIIIB$_2$ to those with significant loss.

infection rate for Gustilo type IIIa fractures was 4.5% with a 25% incidence of infection in the type IIIb fractures. They had a malunion rate of 4%, with a 10% breakage rate of the locking screws and 6% breakage of the nail.

As far as the complications of unreamed nailing are concerned these have not been examined in the same detail as those of reamed nailing and there is as yet little information available as to the incidence of vascular injury, neurological damage or screw discomfort. However, it seems logical that many of the reported complications for reamed nailing will in fact prove to be complications of nailing irrespective of whether the nail is inserted using a reamed or unreamed method. This was confirmed by Court-Brown *et al.* (1996b) who showed no difference in the incidence of knee pain between reamed and unreamed nails. There is no doubt however that the main problem associated with unreamed nailing is equipment failure. These nails are thinner and both nails and cross screws break. Cross screw breakage is usually only a problem when nail removal is undertaken but broken nails can be difficult to remove particularly if the nail is solid. Broken solid nails usually require open removal.

Reamed or unreamed nailing?

As yet there are very few prospective studies comparing the use of reamed and unreamed nails in either closed or open tibial fractures. Court-Brown *et al.* (1996b) carried out a prospective randomized trial comparing the reamed Grosse–Kempf nail with the unreamed AO UTN nail in the management of Tscherne C1 fractures, these being the commonest closed tibial fractures that orthopaedic surgeons have to treat. They analysed the conventional outcome criteria of union time, non-union, malunion, infection and the requirement for secondary surgery. In addition they also looked at joint movement at 26 and 52 weeks as well as the time it took patients to return to a range of common activities. The results showed that the time to union was significantly prolonged in the unreamed nail group ($P > 0.01$) and the reason for this was that five (20%) of the fractures required exchange nailing with a reamed nail to secure union. They found no difference in joint movement or return to basic activities. The only other major difference was in the incidence of screw breakage which was 4% for the unreamed nails and 52% in the unreamed group. The authors concluded that there

was no clinical indication to use unreamed nails in the management of Tscherne C1 tibial fractures.

The only prospective study comparing reamed and unreamed nails in the management of open tibial fractures has been undertaken by Keating *et al.* (1997). They randomized 94 patients with 96 fractures to treatment either with a reamed Grosse–Kempf nail or an unreamed Delta nail. They analysed their results in considerable detail and showed no significant difference in the incidence of compartment syndrome, infection, malunion or patient function. The time to union for the different Gustilo fracture types was similar and the only significant difference was in the incidence of implant failure where they noted a 7% incidence of screw breakage in reamed nails compared with a 27% incidence in the unreamed group.

Most authorities now agree that the incidence of infection in open tibial fractures is governed by the adequacy of soft tissue treatment. Thus the initial debridement and later flap cover are the two most important operations. It seems likely that in Gustilo type III fractures the severity of the soft tissue injury dictates the prognosis of the fracture and any osteogenic benefit derived from reaming is heavily outweighed by the deleterious effect of the injury on the overall bone and soft tissue circulation. In closed fractures, particularly the common Tscherne C1 fracture, this is not the case and there appears to be an osteogenic effect from reaming. It is interesting to note that Kempf *et al.* (1969) compared unlocked reamed and unreamed nails and their decision to favour reamed nailing was based mainly on the lower incidence of non-union with this technique. It would appear that the conclusions from the work of Court-Brown *et al.* (1996) using locked nails are very similar.

Treatment of infection

Orthopaedic surgeons still tend to evaluate the efficacy of fracture fixation techniques by the use of two basic parameters, namely, the incidence of infection and of non-union. However, the incidence of infection following nailing of closed and Gustilo I, II and IIIa open fractures should be very low. Gustilo IIIb fractures have a higher infection rate but it compares favourably with external skeletal fixation (Court-Brown *et al.*, 1991).

One of the striking features common to all the major papers dealing with tibial nailing is that any infection that occurs is usually successfully treated, and indeed if the infection is detected sufficiently early any increased morbidity associated with the infection can be minimized.

There is as yet little literature dealing with the management of infection associated with nailed tibias. Court-Brown *et al.* (1992b) reviewed the results of tibial nailing over a 5-year period. During that time they encountered seven deep infections in closed or Gustilo type I open fractures out of 391 nailed tibias. There were five infections in Gustilo type II and III open fractures out of 68 nailed fractures. In seven closed and type I open fractures there were three groups presenting at different stages or with different clinical findings. Group I patients presented early with local and systemic signs of infection but without a detectable pyogenic collection. In group II the patients also presented early but with a pyogenic collection and in group III the presentation was late with the patients having an established sinus.

Treatment in the group I patients consisted of intravenous antibiotics followed by nail removal with reaming of the intramedullary pyogenic membrane after union. In the group II patients the pyogenic collection was drained and an exchange nailing procedure performed. As in the group I patients the nail was removed and the medullary canal reamed after union. The group III patients required resection of both the unstable soft tissues and infected bone followed by extensive soft tissue and bone reconstruction. The importance of early detection is highlighted by the fact that in the group I patients union occurred at a time appropriate for their Tscherne group whereas in the group II and III patients union was delayed. The treatment of infection associated with severe open fractures is the same as that for the group III patients already described. A protocol for the treatment of infection associated with intramedullary nailing is presented in Figure 6.6.

Although Court-Brown *et al.* (1992b) advocated the maintenance of the intramedullary nail, it is obvious that other methods of bone fixation may be used. Ven and Shih (1992) examined 20 cases of osteomyelitis following tibial nailing using a similar protocol to that used in the group III patients of Court-Brown *et al.* (1992b). This resulted in union in 8 patients. The remaining 12 then had external fixation and bone grafting.

Infection following tibial intramedullary nailing has a reputation for being difficult to eradicate and for causing infection throughout the diaphysis. If basic orthopaedic principles are followed, neither of these beliefs is true. It is in fact relatively straightforward to treat infection, particularly if it is detected early and appropriate therapy administered.

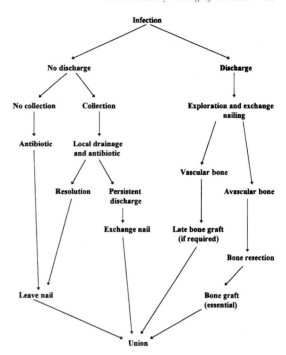

Figure 6.6   A suggested protocol for the management of infection associated with intramedullary nailing

Radiation

Surgeons have been understandably concerned about the amount of radiation that they might be exposed to during tibial nailing. This is a theoretical problem which can be minimized by the development of expertise with the procedure and by the use of modern image intensifiers that incorporate a memory. Such machines deliver negligible radiation during isolated exposures and the surgeon is only at risk during screening. Using such a system Court-Brown *et al.* (1990a) achieved an average fluoroscopy time of less than 6 seconds over 50 consecutive patients with tibial fractures. The greatest exposure to radiation is during distal cross screw insertion and experience with this technique will greatly reduce radiation time. Sanders *et al.* (1993) looked at radiation exposure in orthopaedic surgery. They had an average exposure time of 1.65 minutes but negligible radiation. The addition of a distal lock increased the radiation dose but the authors' estimate that a surgeon could safely perform 20 000 tibial nailings a year without risk. It would therefore appear that radiation exposure is not a significant problem in intramedullary nailing of the tibia.

Treatment of non-union

Intramedullary tibial nailing is associated with a high rate of union (Table 6.1). However, non-unions occur with any treatment method and surgeons will be faced with the problem of treating both atrophic and hypertrophic non-unions in nailed tibias. Obviously standard orthopaedic procedures such as corticocancellous bone grafting or partial fibulectomy can be used to secure union but intramedullary nailing allows for the operation of exchange nailing to be performed. This operation consists of removing the intramedullary nail, reaming the intramedullary canal, usually by an extra 1 mm, and then reinserting a larger nail. Experience in Edinburgh with a group of 33 cases of aseptic tibial non-union in nailed tibias suggests that the technique is very useful (Court-Brown *et al.*, 1995). Analysis of 557 tibial diaphyseal fractures treated by primary reamed intramedullary nailing between August 1986 and June 1992 in the Edinburgh Orthopaedic Trauma Unit allowed the incidences of aseptic non-union for the different Tscherne groups and Gustilo fracture types to be calculated. These are shown in Table 6.3. Table 6.3 also shows the numbers of exchange nailing procedures and bone grafting operations that were required to secure union in these fractures and it is obvious that exchange nailing, without an associated partial fibulectomy, promoted union in all closed fractures and in all open fractures except for Gustilo type IIIb. In these fractures the requirement for open bone graft depended on the size of the bone defects. Where there was significant bone loss measuring more than 50% of the circumference and 2 cm in length, open bone grafting was always required.

The technique of exchange nailing is simpler than that of primary nailing as cross screws are rarely required. In the Edinburgh series 82% of the nails were exchanged without the use of cross screws and there were no malunions. The only complication that appeared to be specific to exchange nailing was superficial infection of the nail entry wounds. Court-Brown *et al.* (1990a) had shown the incidence of this complication to be 1.6% following primary nailing but it rose to 12.1% following exchange nailing. The reason for this is not known.

Sequential external fixation and intramedullary nailing

A number of surgeons have recognized the advantages of intramedullary nailing but prefer to use external fixation for the initial management of their tibial fractures. There has been considerable interest in the potential complication of introducing a nail into a tibia which has previously been stabilized with an external fixation device which may well have been associated with pin track sepsis.

Table 6.4 shows the results of a number of studies examining the success of this sequential technique. There is clearly a dichotomy of opinion, with four of the papers listed in Table 6.4 having a low infection rate and the other three a comparatively high incidence of infection. Interestingly, the only obvious correlation is with the delay between the removal of the external fixator and subsequent nailing of the tibia. Where the delay is relatively short, perhaps less than 2 weeks, the infection rate is low. The longer the delay the greater the incidence of infection, culminating in Tornquist's (1990) study where there was an average delay of 218 days and a 66% infection rate. Court-Brown and Wheelwright (1990b) advocated waiting until the pin tracks granulated before nailing and this policy is used by a number of other surgeons (Figure 6.7).

Siebenrock *et al.* (1993) examined three groups of patients. Group 1 used external fixation through-

Table 6.4 Results from the literature for the sequential technique of primary external fixation and secondary intramedullary nailing

	No.	Duration of ex. fix. (d)	Time before nailing (d)	Pin track sepsis (%)	Infection rate (%)
McGraw and Lim (1988)	16	59.5	21	44	44
Maurer *et al.* (1989)	24	52	65	29	25
Johnson *et al.* (1990)	16	84	13	12.5	0
Blachut *et al.* (1990)	41	17	9	5	5
Tornquist (1990)	6	72	218	100	66
Wheelwright and Court-Brown (1992)	21	57.4	11.7	33.3	4.8
Siebenrock *et al.* (1993)	24	45	?	0	4

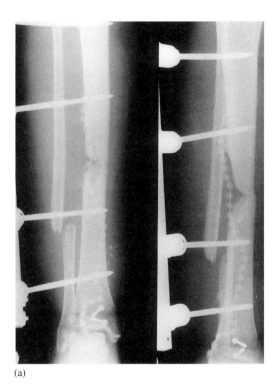

(a)

(b)

Figure 6.7 The sequential technique of external fixation and nailing. (a) A Gustilo IIIB open fracture treated initially with external fixation. Infection occurred during the period of external fixation. (b) After the soft tissues healed a reamed nail was introduced. There was no further infection and the fracture united about 1 year after the injury

out the tibial fracture management, group 2 used primary external fixation and secondary plating and group 3 used sequential external fixation and intramedullary nailing. The distribution of different fracture types between the three groups is not known but they stated that group 3 patients had the lowest incidence of infection, non-union and malunion as well as the shortest time to union.

The comparison of external fixation, intramedullary nailing and sequential external fixation and intramedullary nailing was published by Wheelwright and Court-Brown (1992). All of the different techniques were carried out in one unit. The results are shown in Table 6.5. They indicate the superiority of intramedullary nailing in closed and type I open fractures but there is similarity of

Table 6.5 Results of the use of external fixation, intramedullary nailing and the sequential technique in the Edinburgh Orthopaedic Trauma Unit

| Grade | Time to union (wk) | | |
	External fixation	Combined method	IM nailing
Closed and type I	29.2[1]	27.3	16.7[2]
Type II	26.7[1]	22.5	23.5[4]
Type III	36.7[3]	32.5	38.2[4]

*Comparison of the results is interesting, but it must be remembered that the studies were carried out at different times.
Series: [1]Court-Brown and Hughes (1985); [2]Court-Brown *et al.* (1990a); [3]Court-Brown *et al.* (1990b); [4]Court-Brown *et al.* (1991).

time to union between the three techniques in the more severe fractures.

Comparative studies

Both Hooper *et al.* (1991) and Alho *et al.* (1992) have compared interlocking intramedullary tibial nailing with non-operative management, although as yet only Hooper *et al.* (1991) have carried out a prospective randomized trial of the two techniques.

Alho *et al.* (1992) compared nailing with the use of a functional brace. They found increased infection in the nail group compared with the brace group but there was a markedly decreased incidence of delayed non-union in the nailed group.

Analysis of function in the nail group suggested that this group showed much better results than the braced group.

Hooper *et al.* (1991) examined a number of parameters following both intramedullary nailing and non-operative management. They showed a significant improvement in time to union, time off work, time in hospital, outpatient visits and the number of radiographs between the two groups. They also showed decreased malunion and improved function following nailing. Such was the strength of their views that their initial intention to recruit 100 patients into their trial was not followed up and they concluded that closed intramedullary nailing was a far more effective method of treating tibial shaft fractures than non-operative management.

Flexible intramedullary nailing

There is a considerable tradition of using flexible unreamed small diameter nails to stabilize tibial fractures (see Figure 6.2). These were first popularized by the Rush family in the USA and their philosophy regarding the use of Rush pins in tibial fractures has been adopted by a number of surgeons since. Rush (1955) detailed the technique of using both single and double flexible nails in different types of tibial fracture. The single pin was adopted for most mid-diaphyseal fractures with double pins being used for proximal and distal fractures. They recognized that the inherent problems of this technique are failure to control rotation in spiral fractures and to preserve length in comminuted fractures. They therefore advocated the use of postoperative casts where fracture instability existed after flexible nailing.

Despite the apparent success of Rush pins, most recent publications have involved the use of Ender nails. Ender nails are similar to Rush pins except that they can be stacked and more than two nails may be used (Wiss, 1986).

Flexible nails are usually introduced through small incisions over the medial and lateral tibial condyles. Their introduction and use is usually straightforward and good results may be obtained in a number of fracture configurations. Wiss (1986) suggested that contraindications to the techniques were fractures that involved the proximal or distal tibia within 7.5 cm of the knee or ankle joints as well as fractures with extensive bicortical or circumferential comminution. He also counselled against their use in Gustilo grade III open fractures. Wiss analysed 111 fractures and reported good results, with a 6.3% rate of non-union, 7.2% of malunion and 3.6% of infection. However, his patients used the casts or orthoses until union, and functional outcome was not discussed. More recently Abramowitz *et al.* (1993) have discussed the use of Ender nails in open tibial fractures. Again, however, the problem is control of rotationally unstable fractures and this mitigates against the use of Ender's nails in most Gustilo type IIIb fractures. Whitelaw *et al.* (1990) compared Ender's nails with external fixation and showed that the use of Ender nails was associated with significantly fewer complications in Gustilo type I, II and IIIa open fractures.

The technique of flexible tibial nailing, although superficially attractive has a number of major drawbacks. Many patients require a supportive cast or brace postoperatively and, although joint function following combined flexible nailing and bracing has not been examined, it is highly likely that there will be increased joint stiffness. Many tibial fractures are rotationally unstable and therefore unsuitable for flexible nailing and it is suggested that if this technique is to be used it should be confined to AO type A2 and A3 fractures or to isolated tibial fractures.

References

Abramowitz, A., Wetzler, M.J., Levy, A.S. and Whitelaw, G.P. (1993) Treatment of open fractures with Ender nails. *Clin. Orthop.*, **293**, 246–55

Alho, A., Benterud, J.G., Hoguvold, H.E., Ekeland, A. and Stromsoe, K. (1992) Comparison of functional bracing and locked intramedullary nailing in the treatment of displaced tibial shaft fractures. *Clin. Orthop.*, **277**, 243–50

Alho, A., Ekelund, A., Stromsoe, K., Folleras, G. and Thoresen, B.O. (1990) Locked intramedullary nailing for displaced tibial shaft fractures. *J. Bone Joint Surg.*, **72B**, 805–9

Blachut, P.A., Meek, R.N. and O'Brien, P.J. (1990) External fixation and delayed intramedullary nailing of open fractures of the tibial shaft. A sequential practice. *J. Bone Joint Surg.*, **72A**, 729–35

Bone, L.B. and Johnson K.D. (1986) Treatment of tibial fractures by reaming and intramedullary nailing. *J. Bone Joint Surg.* **68A**, 877–87

Browner, B.D. (1986) Pitfalls, errors and complications in the use of locking Kuntscher nails. *Clin. Orthop.*, **212**, 192–208

Court-Brown, C.M. and Hughes, S.P.F. (1985) Hughes external fixator in treatment of tibial fractures. *J. R. Soc. Med.*, **78**, 830–7

Court-Brown, C.M., Christie, J. and McQueen, M.M. (1990a) Closed intramedullary tibial nailing. Its use in closed and type I open fractures. *J. Bone Joint Surg.*, **72B**, 605–11

Court-Brown, C.M., Wheelwright, E.F., Christie, J. and McQueen, M.M. (1990b) External fixation for type III open tibial fractures. *J. Bone Joint Surg.*, **72B**, 801–4

Court-Brown, C.M., McQueen, M.M., Quaba, A.A. and Christie, J. (1991) Locked intramedullary nailing of open tibial fractures. *J. Bone Joint Surg.*, **73B**, 959–64

Court-Brown, C.M., McQueen, M.M., Quaba, A.A. and Christie, J. (1992a) *Reamed Intramedullary Nailing of Grade III Open Tibial Fractures*, AAOS, Washington, DC

Court-Brown, C.M., Keating, J.F. and McQueen, M.M. (1992b) Infection after intramedullary nailing of the tibia. Incidence and protocol for management. *J. Bone Joint Surg.*, **74B**, 770–4

Court-Brown, C.M., Keating, J.F., Christie, J. and McQueen, M.M. (1995) Exchange intramedullary nailing. Its use in aseptic tibial non-union. *J. Bone Joint Surg.*, **77B**, 407–11

Court-Brown, C.M., Gustilo, T. and Shaw, A. (1996a) Knee pain following intramedullary nailing of the tibia. *J. Orthop. Trauma*, **II**, 103–5

Court-Brown, C.M., Will, E., Christie, J. and McQueen M.M. (1996b) Reamed or unreamed nailing for closed tibial fractures. A prospective study in Tscherne C1 fractures. *J. Bone Joint Surg.*, **78B**, 580–3

Danckwardt-Lillestrom, G. (1969) Reaming of the medullary cavity and its effect on diaphyseal bone. *Acta Orthop. Scand* Suppl **128**, 1–53

Digby, J.M., Holloway, G.M.N. and Webb, J.K. (1983) A study of function after tibial cast bracing. *Injury*, **14**, 432–9

Donald, G. and Seligson, D. (1983) Treatment of tibial shaft fractures by percutaneous Kuntscher nailing. *Clin. Orthop.*, **178**, 64–73

Duwelius, P.J., Schmidt, A.H., Rubinstein, R.A. and Green, J.M. (1995) Non-reamed interlocking intramedullary tibial nailing: one community's experience. *Clin. Orthop.* **315**, 104–13

Gregory, P. and Sanders, R. (1995) The treatment of closed, unstable tibial shaft fractures with unreamed interlocking nails. *Clin. Orthop.*, **315**, 48–55

Haas, N., Krettek, C., Schandelmaier, P., Frigg, R. and Tscherne, M. (1993) A new solid unreamed tibial nail for shaft fractures with severe soft tissue injury. *Injury*, **24**, 49–54

Habernek, H., Kwasny, O., Schmid, L. and Ortner, F. (1992) Complication of interlocking nailing for lower leg fractures: a 3-year follow-up of 102 cases. *J. Trauma*, **33**, 863–9

Henley, M.B. (1989) Intramedullary devices for tibial fracture stabilisation. *Clin. Orthop.*, **240**, 87–96

Hooper, G.J., Keddell, R.G. and Penny, I.D. (1991) Conservative management of closed nailing for tibial shaft fractures. *J. Bone Joint Surg.*, **73B**, 83–5

Howard, M.W., Zinar, D.M. and Stryker, W.S. (1992) The use of the Lottes nail in the treatment of closed and open tibial shaft fractures. *Clin. Orthop.*, **279**, 246–53

Johnson, E.E., Simpson, L.A. and Helfet, D.L. (1990) Delayed intramedullary nailing after failed external fixation of the tibia. *Clin. Orthop.*, **253**, 251–7

Keating, J.F., O'Brien, P.J., Blachut, P.A., Meek, R.N. and Broekhuyse, H.M. (1997) Interlocking intramedullary nailing of open fractures of the tibia. A prospective randomised comparison of reamed and unreamed nails. *J. Bone Joint Surg.*, **79A**, 334–41

Kempf, I., Gonzalo-Vivar, F., Copin, G. and Jaeck, D. (1969) L'enclovage centro-medullaire avec ou sans alesage: traitement de choux des fractures recents diaphysaires ouverts et fermes de jambe. *Ann. Chir.*, **24**, 303–9

Kempf, I., Grosse, A. and Laffourge, D. (1978) L'apport du verouilage dans l'enclouge centromedullaire des os longs. *Rev. Chir. Orthop.*, **64**, 635

Klein, M.P.M., Rahn, B.A., Frigg, R., Kessler, S. and Perren, S.M. (1990) Reaming versus non-reaming in medullary nailing: interference with control circulation of the canine tibia. *Arch. Orthop. Trauma. Surg.*, **109**, 314–16

Klemm, K. and Schellmann, W.D. (1972) Dynamische and statische Verriegelung des Marknagels. *Monatsschr. Unfallheilk.*, **75**, 568

Klemm, K.W. and Borner, M. (1986) Interlocking nailing of complex fractures of the femur and tibia. *Clin. Orthop.*, **212**, 89–100

Koval, K.J., Clapper, M.F., Brumback, R.J. *et al.* (1991) Complications of reamed nailing of the tibia. *J. Orthop. Trauma*, **5**, 184–9

Lottes, J.O. (1952) Intramedullary fixation for fractures of the shaft of the tibia. *South. Med. J.*, **407**, 14

Lottes, J.O. (1974) Medullary nailing of the tibia with the triflange nail. *Clin. Orthop.*, **105**, 253–266

Maurer, D.J., Merkow, R.C. and Gustilo, R.B. (1989) Infection after intramedullary nailing of severe open tibial fractures initially treated with external fixation. *J. Bone Joint Surg.*, **71A**, 835–8

McGraw, J.M. and Lim, E.V.A. (1988) Treatment of open tibial shaft fractures. External fixation and secondary intramedullary nailing. *J. Bone Joint Surg.*, **70A**, 900–11

McQueen, M.M., Christie, J. and Court-Brown, C.M. (1990) Compartment pressures after intramedullary nailing of tibia. *J. Bone Joint Surg.*, **72B**, 395–7

Merle d'Aubigne, R., Maurer, P., Zucman, P. and Masse, Y. (1974) Blind intramedullary nailing for tibial fractures. *Clin. Orthop.*, **105**, 267–75

Müller, M.E., Allgöwer, M. and Willenegger, H. (1965) *Technique of Internal Fixation of Fractures*, Springer-Verlag, Berlin

Oedehoven, G., Claudi, B. and Frigg, R. (1993) Treatment of open and closed tibial fractures with unreamed interlocking tibial nails. *Orthop. Traumatol.*, **2**, 115–28

Oni, O.O.A., Hui, A. and Gregg, P.J. (1988) The healing of closed tibial shaft fractures: the natural history of union with closed treatment. *J. Bone Joint Surg.*, **70B**, 787–90

Puno, R.M., Taynor, J.T., Nagano, J. and Gustilo, R.B. (1986) Critical analysis of results of treatment of 201 tibial shaft fractures. *Clin. Orthop.*, **212**, 113–21

Reichert, I.L.H., McCarthy, I.D. and Hughes, S.P.F. (1995) The acute vascular response to intramedullary nailing: microsphere estimation of blood flow in the intact ovine tibia. *J. Bone Joint Surg.*; **77B**, 490–493

Renner, N., Regazzoni, P., Babst, R. and Rosso, R. (1993)

Initial experiences with the unreamed tibial nail. *Helv. Chir. Acta*, **59**, 665–8

Roger, D.J., Tromanhauser, S., Kropp, W.E., Durman, J. and Guchs, M.D. (1992) Compartment pressures of the leg following intramedullary fixation of the tibia. *Orthop. Rev.*, **21**, 1221–5

Rush, L.V. (1955) *Atlas of Rush Pin Techniques*, Berivon Company, Meridian, Mississippi

Sanders, R., Koval, K.J., DiPasquale, T. *et al.* (1993) Exposure of the orthopaedic surgeon to radiation. *J. Bone Joint Surg.*, **75A**, 326–30

Sarangi, P.P. and Karachallios, T. (1993) Posterior tibial nerve palsy after intramedullary nailing. *Int. Orthop.*, **17**, 125–6

Schemitsch, E.H., Kowalski, M.J., Swiontkowski, M.F. and Senft, D. (1994) Cortical bone blood flow in reamed and unreamed locked intramedullary nailing: a fractured tibia model in sheep. *J. Orthop. Trauma*, **8**, 373–82

Siebenrock, K.A., Schillig, B. and Jakob, R.P. (1993) Treatment of complex tibial shaft fractures: arguments for early secondary intramedullary nailing. *Clin. Orthop.*, **290**, 269–74

Singer, R.W. and Kellam, J.F. (1994) Open tibial diaphyseal fractures. Results of unreamed locked intramedullary nailing. *Clin. Orthop.*, **315**, 114–18

Tischenko, G.J. and Goodman, S.B. (1990) Compartment syndrome after intramedullary nailing of the tibia. *J. Bone Joint Surg.*, **72A**, 41–4

Tornquist, H. (1990) Tibia non-unions treated by interlocking nailing: increased risk of infection after previous external fixation. *J. Orthop. Trauma*, **4**, 109–14

Trueta, J. (1974) Blood supply and the rate of healing of tibial fractures. *Clin. Orthop.*, **105**, 11–26

Van der Linden, W. and Larsson, K. (1979) Plate fixation versus conservative treatment of tibial shaft fractures: a randomised trial. *J. Bone Joint Surg.*, **61A**, 873–8

Ven, W.N. and Shih, C.H. (1992) Management of infected tibial intramedullary nailing using an organised treatment practical. *J. Formosan Med. Assoc.*, **91**, 879–85

Weller, S., Kuner, E. and Schweikert, C.H. (1979) Medullary nailing according to Swiss study group principles. *Clin. Orthop.*, **138**, 45–55

Wheelwright, E.F. and Court-Brown, C.M. (1992) Primary external fixation and secondary intramedullary nailing in the treatment of tibial fractures. *Injury*, **23**, 373–6

Whitelaw, G.P., Wetzler, M., Nelson, A. *et al.* (1990) Ender rods versus external fixation in the treatment of open tibial fractures. *Clin. Orthop.*, **253**, 258–69

Whittle, A.P., Russell, T.A., Taylor, J.C. and Lavelle, D.G. (1992) Treatment of open fractures of the tibial shaft with the use of interlocking nailing without reaming. *J. Bone Joint Surg.*, **74A**, 1162–71

Wiss, D.A. (1986) Flexible medullary nailing of acute tibial shaft fractures. *Clin. Orthop.*, **212**, 122–32

Zucman, J. and Maurer, P. (1970) Primary medullary nailing of the tibia for fractures of the shaft in adults. *Injury*, **2**, 84–92

7

External fixation of the tibia

D. Pennig

Introduction

The use of external skeletal fixation in the management of tibial diaphyseal fractures is an attractive concept as the soft tissue dissection that is required for pin insertion is minimal and the load-bearing device can be constructed outside the soft tissue envelope (Lambotte, 1908; Pennig, 1991). Currently three basic designs of external fixators exist, these being unilateral devices, circular devices and two or three-dimensional frames (Behrens and Searls, 1986). In recent publications there has clearly been a move away from complex three-dimensional frames to simpler unilateral frames (Burny, 1983; De Bastiani *et al.*, 1984; Gotzen *et al.*, 1984; Behrens and Searls, 1986; Evans *et al.*, 1988; Finlay *et al.*, 1987; Méléndez and Colón, 1989; Aro and Chao, 1990a, b; Keating *et al.*, 1991; Aro and Chao, 1993). Unilateral frames permit dynamization and therefore allow micromovement at the fracture site. This has been shown to have experimental (Tayton and Bradley, 1982; Goodship and Kenwright, 1985; Huiskes and Chao, 1986; Pennig *et al.*, 1989; Kenwright *et al.*, 1991; Klein and Pennig, 1992) and clinical advantages (Lambotte, 1908; De Bastiani *et al.*, 1984; Marsh and Nepola, 1990; Marsh *et al.*, 1991).

Development of external fixation

The first comprehensive system of unilateral fixators was designed and studied by Albin Lambotte from Belgium early this century. In his original 1902 paper Lambotte described unilateral external fixation in his system of fixation devices which also included screws, plates and cerclage wires (Figure 7.1). External fixation was used predominantly in fractures of the tibia, femur and humerus and was regarded by Lambotte as the method of choice for all long-bone fractures. Depending on the degree of fracture instability, Lambotte would use 4 or 6 pins, placing the pins near the fracture site in the proximal and distal tibial fragments (Figure 7.2). Lambotte's main objective in surgically stabilizing long-bone fractures was the rapid restoration of limb function, ideally within 4 weeks. After more than 400 operations of this kind Lambotte stated that 'the intervention is no more dangerous than the surgical treatment of hernias' (Lambotte, 1908).

A circular fixator was first described in 1923 by Hempel and Block (Klapp and Block, 1930). It had

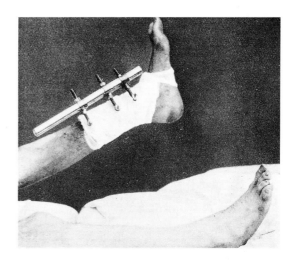

Figure 7.1 The Lambotte unilateral external fixator applied in a distal tibial fracture

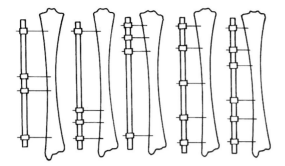

Figure 7.2 Different applications of the Lambotte fixator in tibial fractures; the more unstable the fracture the more pins are employed. Also note the neutralization of the longer fragment by an additional pin at a distance from the fracture

a rectangular design and utilized tension wires to transfix the tibia. The fixator was subsequently improved by adopting a ring construct for better mechanical stability. Wittmoser, a pupil of Böhler in Vienna, used tension wires in a circular frame devised in 1944. This frame also incorporated hinges to allow for asymmetrical compression and distraction if required (Wittmoser, 1953). In recent years Ilizarov has received considerable attention for the successful use of this type of ring fixator in severe malunion, non-union and bone loss (Ilizarov, 1989a,b).

In 1933 an external fixator patent was granted to Renevey from Switzerland. Tensioned transfixion wires were used in a frame incorporating ball joints on all four corners in addition to distraction-compression rods (Renevey, 1934). In 1938 Hoffmann, also from Switzerland, introduced his frame fixator using larger diameter transfixion pins and universal clamps (Hoffmann, 1954). This device has been used extensively over the years and many configurations with different biomechanical properties have been described (Vidal, 1980; Burny, 1983; Schroder *et al.*, 1986; Finlay *et al.*, 1987; Rommens *et al.*, 1989).

However the disadvantages of using transfixion pins soon became established and safe corridors for pin insertion were described for the tibia (Behrens and Searls, 1986) (Figure 7.3). With complex fractures the assessment and management of associated soft tissue damage is difficult and if flap cover is required this may be considerably hindered by the presence of transfixion pins. This problem together with others such as the need for an extensive array of hardware, prolonged application time and difficult postoperative mobilization led to a careful examination of the fixator rigidity

provided by three-dimensional configurations (Court-Brown *et al.*, 1990a). An improved understanding of the relationship between soft tissue healing and bone union has also permitted the

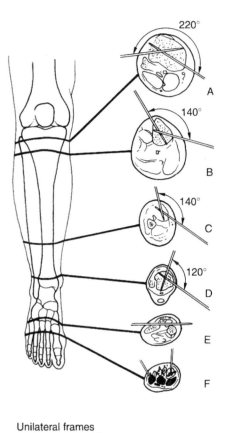

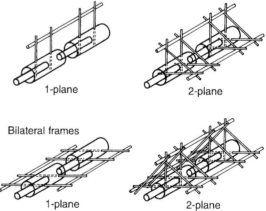

Figure 7.3 (a) 'Safe corridor' for pin insertion in the lower leg. Note that unilateral fixators have a safety margin ranging from 120° to 220° which makes application of these devices less risky than biplanar or three-dimensional fixators. (b) Basic frame configurations. (After Behrens and Searls, 1986)

design of simpler external fixators which allow improved access to the soft tissues (Broekhuizen, 1988; Broekhuizen *et al.*, 1988; Chao and Hein, 1988; Bonar and Marsh, 1993). The biology of fracture repair and callus formation has been extensively researched and there are indications that a degree of elasticity promotes callus formation (Goodship and Kenwright, 1985; Kenwright *et al.*, 1991; Pennig, 1990).

Immediately after a fracture occurs there is a complete loss of the structural integrity of the bone which must be replaced by the external construct. This requires a certain degree of rigidity which may be reduced as soon as periosteal callus provides for a degree of fixation at the fracture site (Nicoll, 1964). The controlled reduction of rigidity allows more weight to be taken by the bone and increased load transmission across the fracture (Burny, 1983; De Bastiani, *et al.*, 1984; Watkins *et al.*, 1988; De Bastiani *et al.*, 1989; Aro and Chao, 1993). Micromovements occurring at the fracture also promote healing (Goodship and Kenwright, 1985; Kenwright *et al.*, 1991). The process involving an increased load transmission across the fracture is described as dynamization (Chao and Hein, 1988; Pennig *et al.*, 1989; Kershaw *et al.*, 1993; Klein and Pennig, 1992). The principle of dynamization involves the reduction of the rigidity of the external fixator construct. This seems to contribute to the high union rates achieved with this method (De Bastiani *et al.*, 1989).

Biomechanical requirements of fixator design

A large number of different external fixators exist and to make a rational choice the surgeon needs to have knowledge of the biomechanical characteristics of the different frames. In trauma work, speed of application (Pannike *et al.*, 1981; Johnson *et al.*, 1985), ease of handling and unobstructed access to the soft tissues are of paramount importance (Broekhuizen *et al.*, 1988; Brug *et al.*, 1989; Pennig, 1991 and unpublished data; Pennig *et al.*, 1988a,b). Therefore unilateral devices would appear to be more advantageous than the more complex circular frames which might be more appropriately used in post-traumatic bone reconstruction (Putti, 1921; Ilizarov, 1989a,b; Saleh, personal communication). Comparative biomechanical studies show that a unilateral fixator utilizing 5 mm pins fulfils the appropriate biomechanical requirements of fracture healing (Figure

7.4) (Broekhuizen, 1988; Broekhuizen *et al.*, 1988). Some fixators, however, when subjected to higher loads, show increased instability by slippage of the pins in the clamps (Seligson and Kristiansen, 1978; Dabezies *et al.*, 1984; Broekhuizen, 1988; Broekhuizen *et al.*, 1988). It is important that an external fixator prevents the occurrence of angular deformities during healing and weight bearing and a stable unilateral device performs significantly better in this respect than a bilateral frame. Whereas the unilateral fixator allows axial loading after dynamization bending is reduced to a minimum. Only a three-dimensional frame offers a similar rigidity but at the expense of bulkiness and the obvious problems of soft tissue care (Broekhuizen, 1988; Broekhuizen *et al.*, 1988).

Anatomical alignment following fracture reduction creates a more favourable environment for

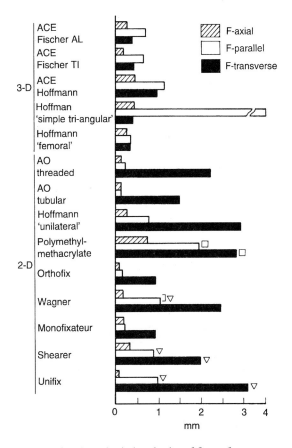

Figure 7.4 Biomechanical evaluation of fixator frames. Note the high stability provided by unilateral frames (e.g. Orthofix) which can only be matched by three-dimensional constructs (After Broekhuizen *et al.*, 1988)

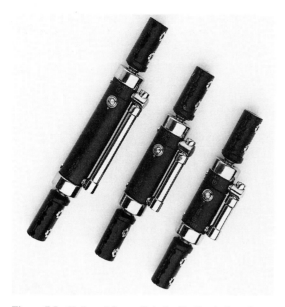

Figure 7.5 Unilateral fixator Orthofix (De Bastiani *et al.*, 1984, 1989) with two ball joints, a telescope and compression/distraction unit. The pin clusters are in line with the long axis of the fixator

fracture healing. Ball joints greatly facilitate the manoeuvres required for fracture reduction (Pennig, 1991) and they also seem to reduce the stress put on the pins by forceful frame handling (Figure 7.5) (De Bastiani *et al.*, 1984, 1989). When employing a unilateral fixator with ball joints the clamps holding the fixator pins should be in line with the long axis of the fixator body. This makes fracture reduction much easier than in devices which employ pin clusters outside the long axis of the bone (Pennig, 1991). Such a device also utilizes less space and if applied on the anteromedial surface of the tibia it allows unobstructive anteroposterior and lateral radiographs to be taken (Pennig, 1991). Pin clusters placed outside the axis of the fixator create shear forces across the fracture after dynamization and these shear forces may well play an important role in the development of non-union (Pauwels, 1965).

The number of fixator components necessary for external fixator application should be limited to help surgeons, theatre nurses and sterilizing staff (Figure 7.6). This makes a unilateral modular

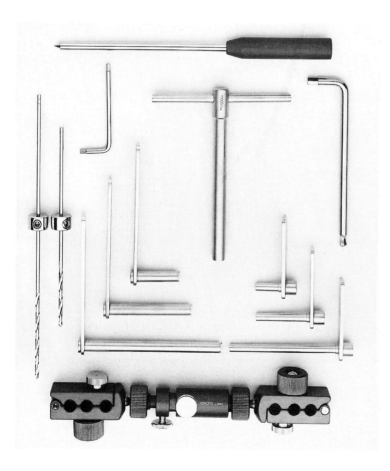

Figure 7.6 Basic instrumentation for pin placement in unilateral fixators. A template (*bottom*) allows parallel unstrained placement of fixator pins which are pre-drilled and guided by appropriate sleeves

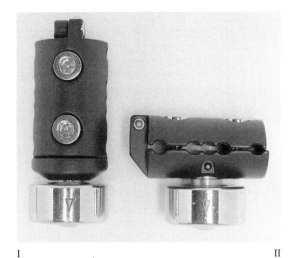

I

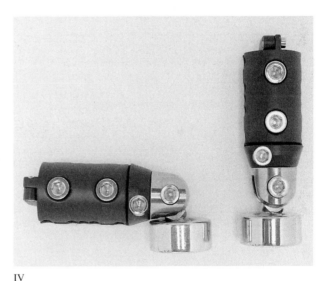

Figure 7.7 Four different clamp types, to be used in the shaft (I), in perarticular application (II), in the metaphysis (III), and for oblique insertion in the femoral neck (IV)

II

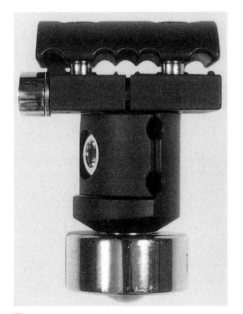

IV

III

system attractive. The fixator should cater for the treatment of a variety of fracture types and permit pin placement close or parallel to the joint lines (Figure 7.7). Also coupling of fixators should be possible in those fractures that may require bridging of a joint (Figure 7.8). The fixator axis itself should be parallel to the long axis of the bone to allow fracture dynamization (Figure 7.9) (Chao and Hein, 1988; Aro and Chao, 1990a,b, Pennig, 1991).

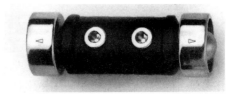

Figure 7.8 A coupling clamp allows easy construction of a fixator link combining two main fixator components

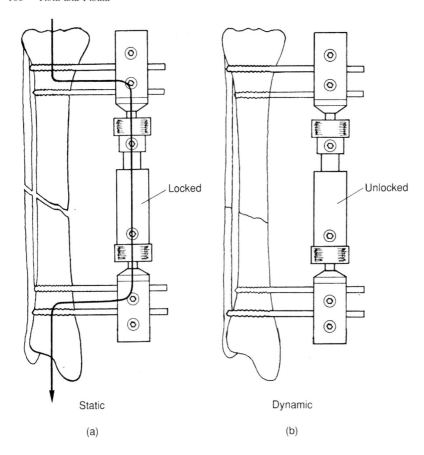

Figure 7.9 (a) Loading of a tibial fracture stabilized by a unilateral fixator in the static mode (telescope locked). Note the load being diverted from the tibial axis and borne by the fixator. (b) After dynamization (unlocking of the telescope) the load is transferred through the tibia and the fracture with the fixator acting as a bypass

Locked

Unlocked

Static

Dynamic

(a)

(b)

Design of fixator pins

The success of external fixation in tibial fractures largely depends on the pin–bone interface. Selection of pins and their appropriate placement are key elements in avoiding pin loosening and other complications (Figure 7.10) (Mathews *et al.*, 1984). Many standard tibial fixation pins have a diameter of 4 mm (Burny, 1983) and several different thread designs have been used. A pin may only be threaded distally to engage the far cortex or a longer thread may engage both cortices. Fixator pins with a conical thread geometry have the advantage of creating a new thread depth with every turn improving the engagement of the smaller tip in the distal cortex (De Bastiani *et al.*, 1989). The disadvantage of a conical shape lies in the fact that the pin cannot be backed out without loosening it (Pennig, 1991). Pin introduction may be at right-angles to the long axis of the bone or oblique to it. In oblique drilling the tip of the drill

bit hits the inner table of the far cortex and has a tendency to slide along this table and therefore bend. If this happens the hole in the near cortex is enlarged which may lead to early pin loosening and infection (Prinz *et al.*, 1989). Different internal fixation screws exist for both cortical and cancellous bone and the use of similar designs for external fixation pins seemed logical (De Bastiani *et al.*, 1984, 1989).

In selecting the correct pin size the surgeon should be aware that the threaded portion should safely engage both cortices. The skin however should be penetrated by the smooth portion of the pin and not by the threaded portion. This facilitates later pin care. The pins should be stiff in order to reduce their number and thereby the number of pin-tracks which require supervision. A 6 mm shank with a threaded portion of 5–6 mm seems advantageous (De Bastiani *et al.*, 1984, 1989).

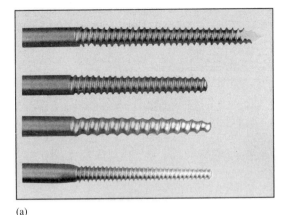

(a)

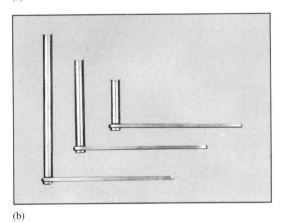

(b)

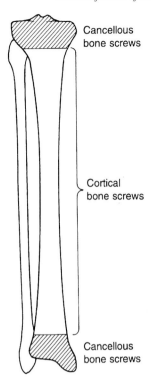

Cancellous
bone screws

Cortical
bone screws

Cancellous
bone screws

Figure 7.11 Guide to screw selection in the tibia. In the epiphysis and proximal metaphysis cancellous screws are used, whereas in the diaphysis and the adjacent portion of the metaphysis cortical bone screws are recommended

Figure 7.10 (a) Different bone screws for unilateral fixators. *Top*, self-cutting, self-tapping bone screw for pelvic applications, *second*, cortical bone screw; *third*, cancellous bone screw; *fourth*, reduced diameter cortical bone screw for the smaller shaft. (b) Screw guides of different length allowing safe insertion of fixator pins in smaller or larger soft tissue envelopes

Tibial pin placement

The subcutaneous anteromedial aspect of the tibia seems to be the most suitable position for the application of a unilateral fixator (see Figure 7.3). The pins can be inserted at 45 ° to the frontal plane which makes injuries to nerves and vessels unlikely. The use of different sizes of drill bits for cortical and cancellous bones is advised (see Figure 7.6), and surgeons must guard against the forceful insertion of self-cutting pins through the thick cortex of the tibial diaphysis as considerable heat may be generated (Mathews *et al.*, 1984). Pin introduction should be undertaken using a template to facilitate parallel pin placement. The fixator itself can often be used as a template, the advan-

tage being that once the pins have been inserted the clamp can be tightened avoiding stress at the pin bone interface. In the tibia the pins should be introduced through a skin incision twice as wide as the pin diameter with the pin sitting centrally in the incision. The areas suitable for cortical and cancellous pins are illustrated in Figure 7.11.

Operative technique

In closed tibial fractures the use of a tourniquet is unnecessary. With open fractures the surgeon may choose to use a tourniquet to control bleeding. When preparing the leg for surgery the skin should be cleaned from just below the knee to the metatarsals. The surgeon (S1) is positioned opposite the injured leg and the contralateral uninjured leg is lowered 5–10 cm to allow the lateral X-ray to be taken (Figure 7.12). The image intensifier (I) is located on the side of the injury. With the assistance of the image intensifier the area of the fracture and the adjacent bone is marked on the skin.

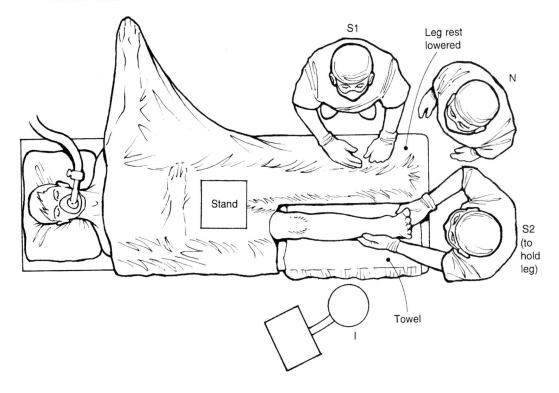

Figure 7.12 Positioning for the management of tibial fractures by unilateral external fixation. The surgeon (S1) with the nurse (N) are positioned opposite the injured leg. The assistant surgeon (S2) controls the rotation and the image intensifier (I) operates from the injured side. The opposite leg should be lowered by 5–10 cm in order to obtain an unobstructed lateral view

The pin closest to the fracture should be placed at a distance of about 3 cm. In an open injury where a free flap, random patterned flap or local muscle flap may be necessary the closest fixator pin may have to be further from the fracture (Caudle and Stern, 1987). The fixator is mounted on the antero-medial aspect of the tibia about 45° to the frontal plane but the exact location is dictated by the extent and location of any coexisting soft tissue injury.

The assistant surgeon (S2) should stand at the end of the leg to control rotation. A rolled-up towel is placed under the Achilles tendon to minimize the risk of any recurvatum of the distal fragments. An appropriate fixator template is then used to determine the pin positions above and below the fracture. Generally speaking the initial screws to be inserted are in the shorter fragment with the screw nearest the adjacent joint being inserted first (Figure 7.13). Placing the external fixator pins adjacent to a joint should be avoided if possible as there is increased skin and soft tissue movement in this location. Once the position of the transfixion screw has been selected the skin should be marked and an incision twice as wide as the pin shaft diameter be

made (Figure 7.14). The soft tissues are separated down to the level of the bone detaching the perios-teum from the bone (Figure 7.15). An appropriately sharp drill bit should be used as blunt drills gener-ate heat causing osteonecrosis and are therefore a potential cause for early pin loosening. It is impor-tant to place the transfixion pin centrally through the medullary canal as an eccentric location through the periphery of the bone will ensure that the sur-geon only drills through hard cortical bone. This will cause inappropriate heat generation at the drill tip. To locate the centre of the bone a screw guide and trocar are recommended (Figure 7.16). The screw guide should be equipped with sharp teeth for optimal cortical purchase (Figure 7.17). Using a drill guide (Figure 7.18) both cortices are penetrated (Figure 7.19) and the correct length of cortical screw length is selected (Figure 7.20). The thread length should be sufficient just to get purchase in both cortices but the thread ideally should not pro-trude through the skin since cleaning of the thread is more difficult than that of the polished shaft (Figure 7.20). The pin itself should not be too long as this can interfere with later patient ambulation.

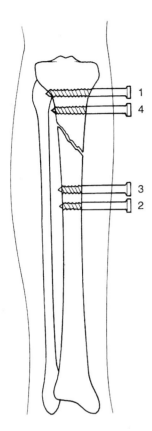

Figure 7.13 Sequence of pin insertion in a proximal tibial fracture. The pin closest to the joint in the shorter fragment is introduced first

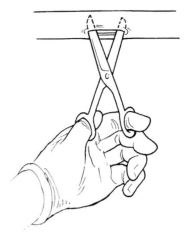

Figure 7.15 Scissors are used to separate the soft tissues down to the bone

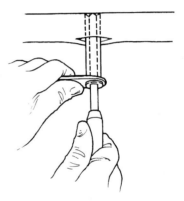

Figure 7.16 With a screw guide and a trocar, the centre of the bone is identified

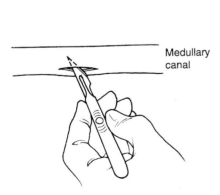

Medullary canal

Figure 7.14 Stab incision using a number 11 knife. The incision is made twice as wide as the shaft diameter of the bone screw

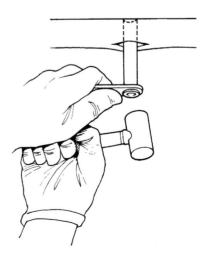

Figure 7.17 A trocar is anchored by lightly tapping on it

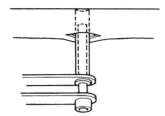

Figure 7.18   A drill guide helps to centralize the drill bit

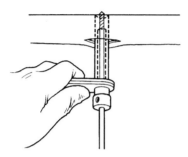

Figure 7.19   Drilling of both cortices with an appropriate drill bit. Note that there are different drill sizes for cortical and cancellous bone

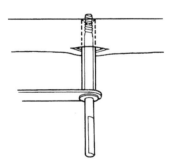

Figure 7.20   Insertion of a bone screw. Note that the threaded portion does not protrude from the skin

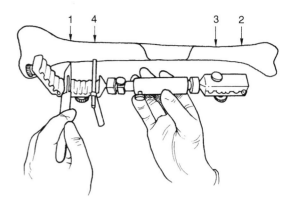

Figure 7.21   After the first bone screw has been inserted, a template is used for placement of the following bone screws

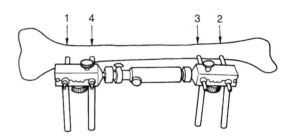

Figure 7.22   With the template, provisional stabilization of the fracture and radiographic control can be carried out

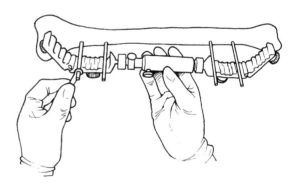

Figure 7.23   Removal of the template and the screw guide

The screw guide is left in position on the initial screw and one end of the template is then applied to it (Figure 7.21). The second screw to be inserted should be in the other main fracture fragment furthest away from the fracture itself (Figure 7.21). After this second screw is inserted the template can be used for temporary reduction, this being checked with the image intensifier in both planes (Figure 7.22). Following this the two inner screws closest to the fracture are inserted and usually two screws per clamp are sufficient. There are a number of situations where the use of three pins per clamp is advisable. This can be considered if there

is considerable bone loss, the fracture is such that a prolonged time in the fixator can be expected or the bone is very osteoporotic. After removal of the template and the screw guides (Figure 7.23) the correct penetration of the opposite cortex by the fixator pins can be checked radiologically and the definitive fixator applied (Figure 7.24).

After the fixator has been applied the pin sites should be checked to see if there is any skin tension

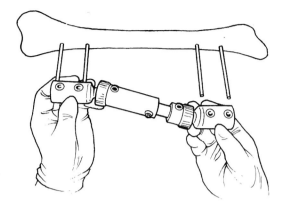

Figure 7.24 The template is replaced by the definitive fixator. The distance from the skin should be approximately 20 mm

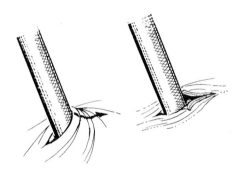

Figure 7.25 Mobilization of the adjacent joints after definitive reduction and stabilization of the fracture. Any tethering of the skin requires release to avoid pin track problems

around the screws. To assess if this is a problem the knee and ankle joints should be moved through their range and a soft tissue release is recommended if tethering is observed (Figure 7.25).

It is always recommended that when reducing a fracture with an external fixator the aim should be to achieve anatomical alignment. Any residual displacement, particularly if there is a varus or valgus deformity, may lead to a delay in union. Only correct axial alignment with optimal contact of the fragments will allow for early weight bearing, early dynamization and thereby early callus formation with rapid union.

Proximal tibial fractures

Proximal fractures of the tibial diaphysis can be challenging as locked nailing is not an easy option (Alho *et al.*, 1990; Court-Brown *et al.*, 1990b; Court-Brown, 1991) and the contour and cross-section of the area does not lend itself easily to plate fixation (Allgöwer and Perren, 1982). Conservative management is difficult because of the proximity to the joint (Nicoll, 1964; Sarmiento and Latta, 1981; Sarmiento *et al.*, 1989).

Traditionally external fixators have been used with pin clusters placed along the axis of the bone or at right-angles to it (De Bastiani *et al.*, 1984, 1989). However this may be disadvantageous mechanically as fixator pins in one plane only are less stable than if they are placed in two planes. A metaphyseal clamp which allows pin placement both in the horizontal as well as the vertical plane has both biomechanical and clinical advantages (Pennig, unpublished data). In addition, the proximal and distal metaphyses of the tibia are not located centrally on the shaft, there being an offset of several millimetres. A metaphyseal clamp (see Figure 7.27) with an asymmetrical design takes care of this anatomical problem (Figure 7.26). If the metaphyseal clamp is being used the first screws to be inserted are the ones closest to the joint (Figure 7.27a). Pins are placed at 45° to the frontal plane and care has to be taken when drilling through the opposite cortex in order to avoid injuries to the adjacent neurovascular structures. The most distal screw is then inserted below the fracture line followed by the screw closest to the fracture line in the distal pin group (Figure 7.27b,c).

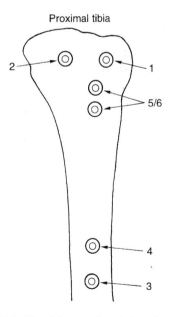

Figure 7.26 Use of the metaphyseal clamp in the proximal tibia. Note the sequence of screw insertion, starting with the periarticular screws first

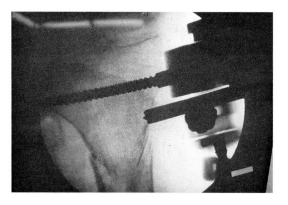

Figure 7.27(a)   Intraoperative radiograph of pin insertion in a proximal tibial fracture. The two proximal screws are inserted. The vertical screw site has been occupied by a screw guide to create a triangular bone screw assembly

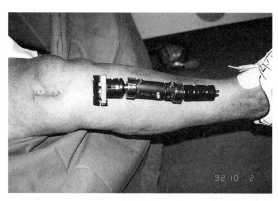

Figure 7.27(c)   Clinical photograph showing the metaphyseal clamp proximally and a straight clamp distally

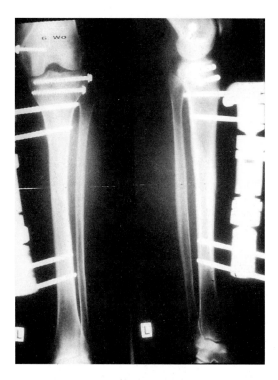

Figure 7.27(b)   Postoperative radiograph showing neutralization of a proximal tibial fracture with intra-articular involvement in the lateral tibial plateau stabilized by two lag screws

A template should be used for preliminary reduction of the fracture. After the reduction has been checked in both planes with the image intensifier one or both pin sites in the vertical part of the metaphyseal clamp can be filled. Definitive reduction is performed after the fixator itself has been attached to the pins and after checking the pin penetration of the opposite cortex. If the proximal fragment is too small for a metaphyseal clamp the vertical clamp seats may be left empty or a standard T-clamp be used (Figure 7.28).

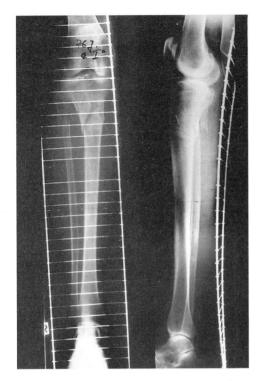

Figure 7.28(a) Proximal extra-articular fracture in a 67-year-old female patient; Gustilo type I fracture

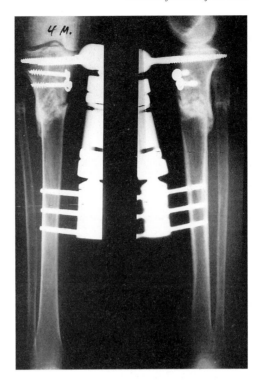

Figure 7.28(c) Consolidation after 4 months with adequate callus formation. Removal of the fixator

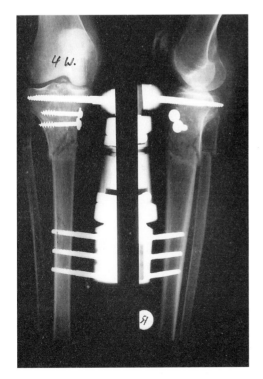

Figure 7.28(b) Closed reduction and additional stabilization with two lag screws and washers. Correct alignment of the axis

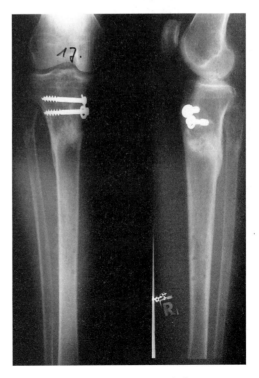

Figure 7.28(d) Postoperative control after one year, showing remodelling of the callus

Distal tibial fractures

The distal tibial metaphysis has the added disadvantage of having a smaller cross-section than the proximal metaphysis (Breitfuss *et al.*, 1988; Saleh *et al.*, 1993). Therefore precise pin placement is necessary and again the screws parallel to the joint should be inserted first when a metaphyseal clamp is used (Figure 7.29). The two screws proximal to the fracture line are then inserted and the template is used again for preliminary reduction. One or two of the vertical pin sites in the metaphyseal clamp

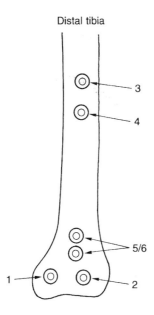

Distal tibia

Figure 7.29 Use of the metaphyseal clamp in the distal tibia. Note the perarticular screws being inserted first

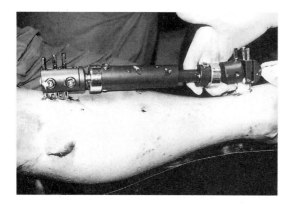

Figure 7.30 Clinical example of the use of a metaphyseal clamp in the distal tibia in a fracture with a CL III soft tissue injury

are then filled. In the distal tibia one has to avoid the tibiofibular syndesmosis since ossification may result if this is damaged. If the pins are inserted from the anteromedial side tethering of the tendons is unlikely (Figure 7.30). After reduction has been achieved the knee and ankle joints should be moved and any skin tension around the pins is released.

Meta-diaphyseal fractures with articular involvement

Fractures of the metaphysis and the diaphysis should always be examined for any associated intra-articular involvement. Thus it is essential in any tibial diaphyseal fracture to have X-rays displaying both the knee and ankle joints. In general intra-articular involvement with a tibial diaphyseal or metaphyseal fracture is uncommon, and when present is often undisplaced.

Joint reconstruction always takes priority in the management of these fractures (Keating *et al.*, 1991). If the intra-articular fracture is displaced open reduction may be necessary and internal fixation using lag screws can be performed. In undisplaced fractures percutaneous placement of a reduction clamp is followed by percutaneous insertion of cannulated or non-cannulated cancellous screws (Figure 7.31). If the nature of the intra-articular fracture is such that plate fixation is required the combination with external fixation may only be considered if there is a minimum of 5 cm between the pins and the plate and there is no subcutaneous communication between the pin site and the plate location.

Following the intra-articular reconstruction the main diaphyseal fracture can be stabilized. The fixator should be placed on the anteromedial aspect of the tibia if this is possible. However the nature of the injury may require different positioning of the fixator and it is worth remembering that this combination of fractures represents a relative indication for the use of an internal fixator.

External fixation bridging the knee or ankle joint

Where possible transarticular fixation across a joint should be avoided as permanent joint stiffness may result. If there is a dislocation of the knee or ankle joint together with an open tibial diaphyseal fracture associated with severe soft tissue injury transarticular fixation may be necessary. Using a unilateral frame this can be achieved by

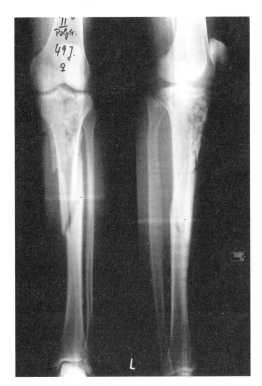

Figure 7.31 (a)   Midshaft and proximal tibial fracture involving the lateral tibial plateau, severe comminution of the anterior metaphyseal region; Gustilo type II compound fracture

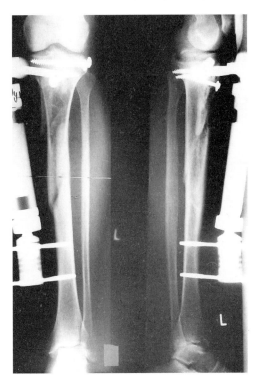

Figure 7.31 (c)   Radiograph after 8 weeks showing early signs of callus formation in the diaphysis

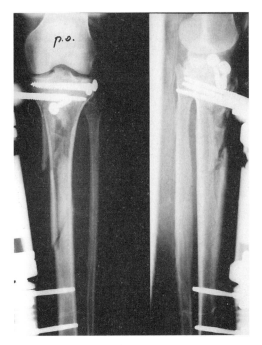

Figure 7.31 (b)   Stabilization with the unilateral external fixator and supplementary lag screws for fixation of the plateau fracture and reattachment of the tibial tuberosity

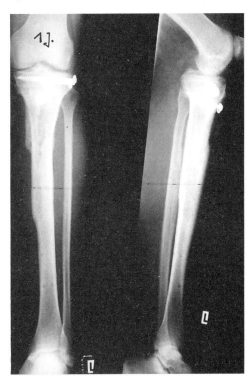

Figure 7.31 (d)   One-year control showing full consolidation of the metaphyseal and diaphyseal fracture

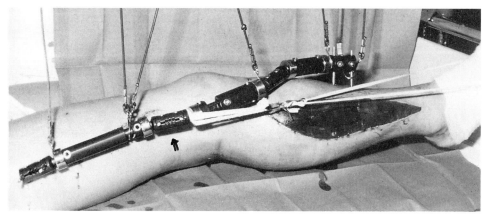

Figure 7.32 Use of a coupling clamp (*arrow*) to combine two fixator components. Use for the stabilization of a proximal tibial epiphysiolysis with a femoral fixator employed for stabilization of a femoral shaft fracture

either using a coupling clamp which connects two fixator components or by using fixator pins with longer shafts to allow placement of a second clamp on top of the first. Crossing the knee joint involves careful planning of the pin positions in the distal femur and an anterolateral location is associated with fewest disadvantages.

In similar fractures in the distal tibia the fixator can be extended down to the calcaneus (Schweiberer *et al.*, 1987; Baranowski *et al.*, 1990; Saleh *et al.*, 1993). Pin placement in the calcaneus is best carried out open with pins being inserted from the medial side carefully avoiding the neurovascular structures. Again a coupling clamp may be used to connect two fixator components (Figure 7.32) or the second fixator may be built up on the longer pins of the main fixator unit. As soon as the state of the soft tissue and bone allows the transarticular fixators should be removed and joint mobilization thereby facilitated.

Circular frames

Circular frames are usually used in reconstructive surgery and there are few indications in acute tibial diaphyseal fractures for their use (Pennig, 1991; Watson, 1994). The disadvantages of circular frames are that the assembly time is prolonged compared with simple unilateral frames. In addition, it is more awkward to treat the soft tissues, and in particular, the use of skin flaps.

Postoperative management

Postoperatively, the leg should be elevated about 5 cm above the mattress using hooks which can be

attached to both the fixator and the bed-mounted frame. This serves to reduce the pressure on the posterior tibial compartments. The ankle should be stabilized in a neutral position and a foot plate can be attached to the fixator to prevent an equinus deformity (Figure 7.33).

The success of external skeletal fixation depends on the integrity of the pin bone interface and meticulous pin care is crucial. Daily pin care is best performed with a supervised protocol and detailed instructions for the patient. Coloured antiseptics should be avoided since they stain the skin and make early detection of inflammation difficult. With tibial external fixators dressings are rarely necessary after 10–14 days but the pin sites still have to be cleaned at least every other day and incisions may have to be extended should there be skin tension around the pins. Using this approach a number of workers have shown that pin site

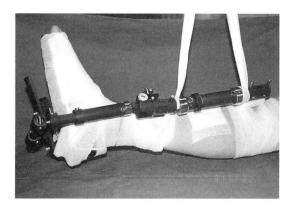

Figure 7.33 A tibial fixator with a connected foot plate to prevent equinus deformity

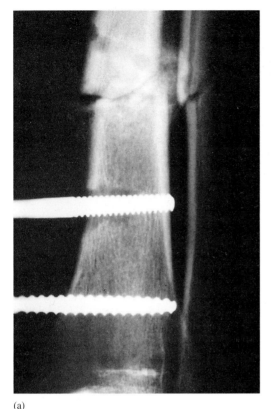

(a)

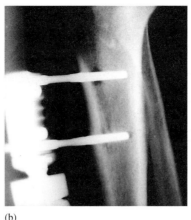

(b)

Figure 7.34 (a) Pin loosening in the near cortex with adequate purchase in the the far cortex. This usually responds to improved pin care but requires close observation. If osteolysis in the far cortex occurs re-siting of the pin may be required. (b) Osteolysis due to improper pin placement in the proximal pin. The distal pin is not engaged in the far cortex, increasing the load on the near cortex

problems can be virtually eliminated. An incidence of 2.9% pin track complications (De Bastiani *et al.*, 1984, 1989) has been reported compared with 36% if bilateral or three-dimensional frames are used (Schroder *et al.*, 1986). Should severe inflammation occur around the pin site an X-ray is advisable (Figure 7.34). If marked osteolysis is seen it may be advisable to re-site the pin.

Mobilization of the patient and dynamization

If unilateral external fixation is used mobilization of the patient should be carried out as soon as the soft tissues have healed (Figure 7.35). Thus on the day after surgery or after the soft tissues have healed weight bearing with 15 kg in both stable and unstable tibial fractures is permitted. Loading of the fracture may be permitted by dynamization and in some fixators this can be controlled although in others it is unrestricted (Table 7.1). Full weight bearing should be achieved within 4 weeks after dynamization provided shortening is avoided by the use of dynamization control mechanisms (Figure

7.36). In very unstable fractures full weight bearing may have to be delayed to avoid excessive straining of the pin-bone interface. Should excessive shortening occur distraction will be required. Some unilateral fixators have a distraction unit which can be placed between the pin clamps. Other fixators have an inbuilt distraction facility.

Follow-up includes radiological assessment of fracture position at weekly intervals for the first 4 weeks. Should there be any loss of alignment this can be corrected during the first 2–3 weeks without much effort. Thereafter the callus becomes too stiff and closed reduction is usually impossible. After the first 4 weeks it is recommended that X-ray assessment be performed every 3–4 weeks.

Table 7.1 Postoperative protocol for the Orthofix unilateral fixator

Procedure	Stable fracture	Unstable fracture
15 kg weight bearing	Day 1 Soft tissues healed	Day 1 Soft tissures healed
Dynamization	Day 14	Day 14/DYN-A-ring
Full weight bearing	Within 4 weeks after dynamization	Within 4–6 weeks after dynamization

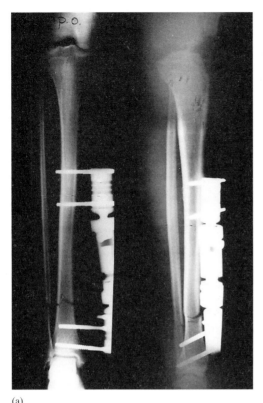

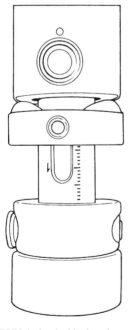

(a)

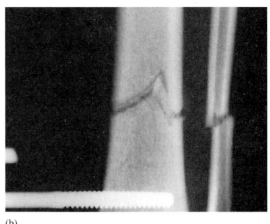

(b)

Figure 7.35   (a) Distal tibial fracture postoperatively with persistent distraction of the fracture site. (b) Dynamization and weight bearing leads to closure of the gap

Figure 7.36   DYN-A-ring inside the telescope of a fixator. The arrows indicate the silicon cushions which allow 1–2 mm compression during weight bearing. This creates micromovements and prevents collapse especially in the uncooperative patient

Indications for external fixation in tibial fractures

Originally external fixation was conceived as the last resort in difficult tibial diaphyseal fractures (Gustilo and Anderson, 1976; Caudle and Stern, 1987; Court-Brown *et al.*, 1990a) and not infrequently a change to internal fixation was often required because of the delayed union which is associated with complex and very rigid frames (Blick *et al.*, 1989; Blachut *et al.*, 1990). With improved external fixator and pin design unilateral external fixation has become a definitive treatment (De Bastiano *et al.*, 1984, 1989; Pennig *et al.*, 1988; Pennig, 1991) (Table 7.2).

Table 7.2   Key factors in tibial fractures managed with external fixation

competent debridement of soft tissues and bone
anatomical alignment
early soft tissue cover
meticulous pin care
early partial weight bearing
early bone grafting if necessary
dynamization
early full weight bearing

Open fractures

The anteromedial border of the tibia is subcutaneous and the result of this is that there is a higher incidence of open tibial fractures than in any other long-bone. In Gustilo type II and III fractures (Gustilo and Anderson, 1976) the rationale for the use of unilateral external fixation is that it is associated with minimal additional operative trauma, there is no implant at the fracture site, it is easy to apply and provides excellent access to the soft tissues. In these cases fracture stabilization is carried out immediately after a thorough wound debridement with inspection of the vascular supply of the bone fragments (Russell *et al.*, 1990). Even large bone fragments with insufficient soft tissue attachments should be removed. If a bony defect is left after debridement it may be necessary to shorten the tibia to achieve a stable contact between the bone fragments (Figure 7.37). Shortening of up to 5 cm is possible and this has the added benefit of reducing the soft tissue tension and making soft tissue cover easier (Saleh, personal communication). After the soft tissues have healed and bony consolidation has been achieved a lengthening procedure may be undertaken (Figure 7.38). The importance of the initial debridement cannot be over-emphasized. Decisions regarding the viability of soft tissues and bone require the expertise of an experienced senior surgeon as decisions made at primary operation frequently determine the final outcome. After debridement the fixator pins should

be placed in healthy skin on the anteromedial border of the tibia (Figure 7.39). It is important to attempt to get an anatomical fracture alignment and once this has been achieved the soft tissue viability should be reassessed. As a general rule wound closure should not be done primarily. In a retrospective series comparing primary closure to delayed closure the infection rate in primary closure was 20% compared with 3% in delayed closure (Russell *et al.*, 1990). Wound closure is frequently undertaken using a local muscle flap or a fasciocutaneous flap. This should ideally be performed within 4–5 days of the injury. With larger soft tissue defects a free flap may well be required and again it is important that the use of such a flap should not be delayed to avoid secondary necrosis of bone and tendons.

The decision regarding the necessity for bone grafting is ideally made during the initial debridement (Figure 7.40). Bone grafting should be undertaken about 6 weeks after the injury (Blick *et al.*, 1989). Corticocancellous chips are usually used and since the grafted material has to be vascularized the posterolateral approach should be used if this is possible (Simpson *et al.*, 1990). Anteromedial grafts seem to be less successful. After bone grafting the fixator should not be dynamized for 3–4 weeks to avoid irritation of the soft tissues and to provide better conditions for graft incorporation (Lin *et al.*, 1990). There is no place for primary bone grafting in open tibial fractures because of the risk of infection.

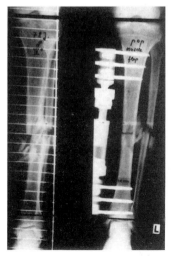 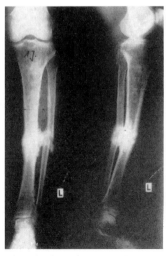

Figure 7.37 A 78-year-old male patient with the type IIIB compound fracture of the left and type IIIA fracture of the right tibia as well as other injuries. Marked comminution of the initial radiograph (*left*); squaring of the bone ends was carried out in order to transform an unstable into a relatively stable fracture (*right*). (a) Weight bearing was subsequently possible, union was reached after 5.5 months without grafting; (b) Late radiograph after one year

(a)   (b)

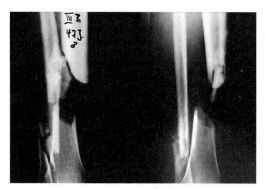

(a)

Figure 7.38 (a) Segmental bone loss in a type IIIB fracture in a 47-year-old male patient. This situation can be considered as an indication for primary shortening to release the soft tissue tension and facilitates soft tissue coverage. (b) After correct alignment of the axis, a limb reconstruction system is applied and shortening of the tibia is carried out. The fibula has to be shortened as well. (c) Compression results in contact of the bone ends distally. After soft tissue repair a corticotomy between the proximal and the intermediate pin group is carried out. (d) Callus distraction leads to a restoration of tibial length while the distal fracture consolidates

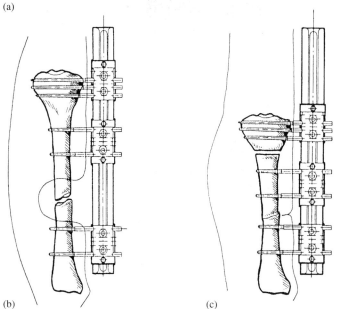

(b)

(c)

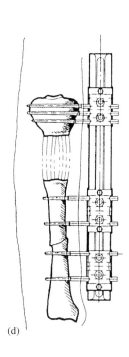

(d)

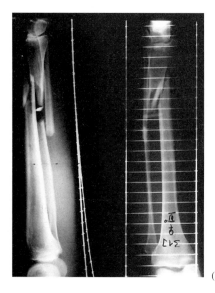

(a)

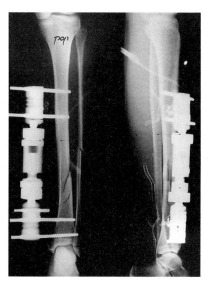

(b)

Figure 7.39 (a) Gustilo type II compound fracture in a 30-year-old woman with one major and several smaller bone fragments. (b) Stabilization with unilateral fixator and discarding of the smaller fragment. Note the larger fragment between tibia and fibula. (c) Union was achieved after 5 months. The radiograph after 15 months shows sound consolidation and incorporation of the larger remaining fragment between tibia and fibula

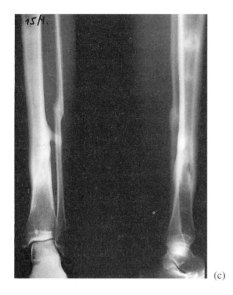

(c)

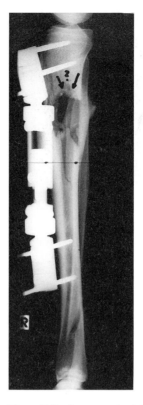

Figure 7.40 Large proximal defect in a compound tibial fracture. This type of defect requires grafting after 6 weeks provided the soft tissue situation is adequate

Open fractures are often associated with delayed union or non-union (Bier, 1923; Gustilo and Anderson, 1976; Brug *et al.*, 1989; Court-Brown *et al.*, 1990a). The cause of this may be periosteal stripping, soft tissue damage and/or bone loss. In periosteal stripping revascularization largely takes place endosteally and if there is combination with bone loss a delay in union is predictable. Bone grafting plays an important role in promoting union in these fractures and after soft tissue healing has been achieved the procedure should not be delayed for more than 6 weeks.

Even if bony contact does not exist partial weight bearing should be allowed as soon as the condition of the soft tissue permits. For dynamization the bone has to be able to take some of the load during weight bearing. This fact means that early grafting in the presence of comminution or bone loss is a necessary step on the way to union. The technique of bone grafting is illustrated in Chapter 11.

Closed fractures

In closed fractures there are several treatment options ranging from non-operative management (Nicoll, 1964; Sarmiento and Latta, 1981; Sarmiento *et al.*, 1989) to open reduction and internal fixation (Allgöwer and Perren, 1982). Internal fixation is more comfortable for the patient but does frequently require a second hospitalization and anaesthetic for implant removal. External fixation has some advantages in those closed fractures that are associated with significant soft tissue damage (Tscherne type C2 or C3 fractures) (Gotzen *et al.*, 1984). In these cases external fixation has the added benefit of combining stable fixation with minimal surgical trauma and it is not necessary to wait for an improvement in the condition of the soft tissues before implementing treatment (Tischenko and Goodmann, 1990; Pennig, 1991) (Figure 7.41).

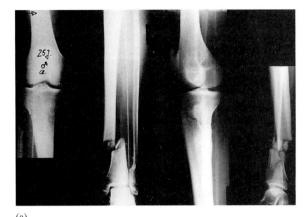

(a)

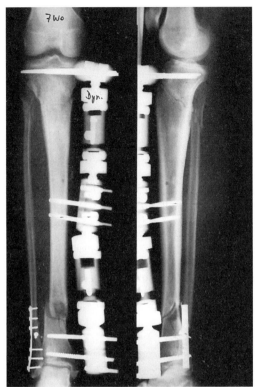

(b)

Figure 7.41   (a) Segmental fracture involving the proximal metaphysis and a displaced distal tibial fracture type C2. (b) Reduction and stabilization of both fractures with a proximal T-clamp, a coupling clamp in the middle segment and a straight distal clamp; the fibula is plated

Supplementary internal fixation in the diaphysis

Supplementary internal fixation is not recommended in the tibial diaphysis since this means that a combination of rigid and elastic fixation will be used (Brug *et al.*, 1989; Pennig, 1991). In addition exposure of the bone ends, extra soft tissue dissection and drilling may cause further vascular damage and thereby increase the risk of infection. With the exception of intra-articular fractures screws and short plates should be avoided when one is using external skeletal fixation as this method of management relies on micromovement after dynamization. Clinical (Krettek *et al.*, 1991) and experimental (Ostrum *et al.*, 1994) evidence indicates that the complication rate with regards to infection and refracture is increased if supplementary internal fixation is used in the diaphysis together with external skeletal fixation.

Delayed union in external fixation

External fixation devices have been accused of contributing to delay in union (Court-Brown, 1985). However many of the fractures treated with these

devices are severe and union may well be delayed. It is often difficult to assess whether the device itself has contributed to delayed union (McKibbin, 1978). Healing of unstable fractures requires an initial high stability and, as callus forms, the rigidity of the fixator should be decreased to stimulate further callus formation and maturation (Aro and Chao, 1990a,b; De Bastiani, personal communication). Shear forces are detrimental to fracture healing and these can be observed after loading in the sagittal plane with simple bilateral frames as well as with complex Vidal type configurations (Pauwels, 1965; Brockhuizen *et al.*, 1988). Stable unilateral fixators perform significantly better in this respect.

In 1955 Yamagishi and Yoshimura described in their experimental study of the biomechanics of fracture healing that moderate compression as well as distraction promotes callus formation. For optimal healing they found that moderate intermittent compression of the organizing tissue at the fracture surface was necessary. This is the basic principle which is known as dynamization today. Load is applied during weight bearing and is taken off when the patient lifts his or her leg. If these principles are followed high union rates can be expected (De Bastiani *et al.*, 1984).

If delayed union is encountered six factors merit consideration. These are periosteal stripping, fracture location, comminution, alignment, the state of the fibula and the presence of peripheral vascular disease. If the periosteum is stripped the primary cell source for bone healing is absent and slower endosteal healing has to replace it (Pennig, 1990). Distal fractures of the tibia have a poorer blood supply because of the distribution of the nutrient artery. In combination with a damaged periosteal blood supply union delay is predictable. If there is severe comminution early bone grafting has to be considered to achieve fracture healing. Poor axial alignment may cause shear forces across the fracture and thereby contribute to a delay in union. The fibula, if intact or united at an early stage, can prevent effective dynamization taking place (Sárváry and Berentey, 1984; Karabi and Reis, 1986; Morrison *et al.*, 1991). A resection of 2 cm of fibula at the level of the tibial fracture should be considered in cases where the tibial callus response is absent or inadequate after 6 weeks. This should be followed by full weight bearing after dynamization. In cases of peripheral vascular disease there is generally impaired perfusion of the limb. In this situation the

blood flow is reduced and this may well contribute to delayed union (see Chapter 11).

Unilateral external fixators incorporating a compression-distraction device may be used clinically to apply the experimental results of Yamagishi and Yoshimura (1955). The fracture is gradually distracted by 1 mm per day for 7–10 days (tension) after fibular resection and subsequently closed at the same rate (compression) (Figure 7.42). This enhances callus formation, particularly in hypertrophic and oligotrophic non-unions and should be followed by dynamization and weight bearing. Bone grafting is an established method of encouraging union with external fixation and if required should be performed at an early stage, preferably within 6 weeks after injury (see Figure 7.40) (Blick *et al.*, 1989).

Relative contraindications to unilateral external fixation

Certain clinical conditions make the use of external fixators in the tibia less advisable (Moran *et al.*, 1990; Pennig, 1992). These are:

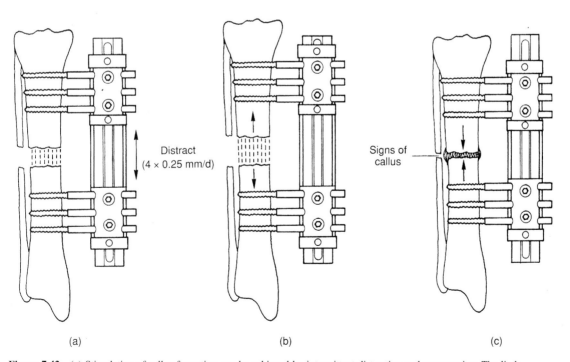

(a)	(b)	(c)

Figure 7.42 (a) Stimulation of callus formation can be achieved by intermittent distraction and compression. The limb reconstruction system (LRS) fixator may be used in cases with no malalignment. (b) The fracture site is distracted for 7–10 days at 1 mm per day. (c) Recompression results in formation of callus

1 Severe osteoporosis (Singh *et al.*, 1970)
2 Poorly controlled diabetes
3 Predictable poor patient compliance
4 Hemiplegic, paraplegic and tetraplegic patients
5 HIV positive and hepatitis patients
6 A known allergy to medical grade stainless steel. An alternative is to use titanium pins
7 Severe peripheral vascular disease

These conditions do not exclude the use of external fixation but other treatment alternatives should be considered (Brug and Pennig, 1990).

Nailing after unilateral external fixation

Nowadays external fixation using a modern unilateral device is recognized as being a definitive treatment in both open and closed tibial fractures (De Bastiani *et al.*, 1984; Broekhuizen *et al.*, 1988; De Bastiani *et al.*, 1989; Marsh *et al.*, 1991; Pennig, 1991). There is no requirement to change the treatment method to internal fixation or cast bracing. A number of authors have used sequential external fixation followed by internal fixation and have had poor results (Olerud and Karlstrom, 1972; McGraw and Lim, 1988; Riemer and Butterfield, 1993). McGraw and Lim quoted an infection rate of 44% with 50% non-union in external fixation followed by nailing. A more recent report (Blachut *et al.*, 1990) emphasizes a period of external fixation averaging 17 days to allow soft tissue healing followed by reamed locked nailing. The infection rate was 12.8% including two deep infections (5%). However the vast majority of these fractures were relatively straightforward with 87.2% of the fractures being either Gustilo I, II or IIIa in severity. The available results make the routine use of the sequential protocol after external fixation open to question (Baker *et al.*, 1992). This sequential method of management is discussed further in the chapter on intramedullary nailing. There are a number of indications for nailing after external fixation. The most important are severe osteoporosis and the non-compliant patient. The prerequisites for the procedure are:

1 To carry out the intramedullary nailing procedure as early as possible. Ideally this should be within 4 weeks after the application of the external fixator.
2 The soft tissue should be healed.
3 There should be no evidence of pin track sepsis.
4 The nails should not be inserted until the pin

tracks have healed. This may require a period in a cast or traction.
5 There should be no suspicion of a sequestrum in the pin track on conventional X-rays or scans.
6 Antibiotics should be given pre- and postoperatively.
7 Reaming should not be excessive.
8 Statically locked nailing should be used.

If the surgeon plans sequential external fixation and intramedullary nailing this treatment protocol should be discussed with the patient.

Temporary use of external fixation for intraoperative fracture reduction

External fixators with a mechanical distraction facility may be used to assist with open reduction and internal fixation of fractures of the tibial plateau and tibial pilon (Saleh *et al.*, 1993). External fixation may also be used for the alignment of tibial shaft fractures if a traction table is not available or cannot be used.

Depending on the morphology of the fracture site in the tibial plateau the fixator is applied either from the medial or the lateral side (Figure 7.43).

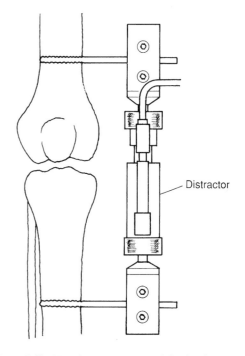

Distractor

Figure 7.43 Use of temporary external fixation for intraoperative reduction in tibial plateau fractures followed by internal fixation

Only one pin per clamp is required since the external fixator is only applied temporarily during the operation. The fixator pins are inserted at right angles to the long axis of the bone and care is taken not to interfere with the necessary incision used for the articular reconstruction. The principle of ligamentotaxis is applied and axial alignment is achieved with the external fixator. Temporary over-distraction of a joint may be necessary, especially if surgery is delayed, to allow elevation of articular fragments and grafting.

In tibial pilon fractures similar principles can be followed but with these fractures there is an option to use the external fixator to provide supplementary fixation when limited internal fixation has been used (see Chapter 13).

An external fixator may be used as a distracter for tibial nailing. The fixator pins are inserted from the posteromedial side in order to avoid obstruction of the lateral X-ray and to neutralize the forces during nail insertion. Proximally the pins are placed in the centre of the metaphysis, the distal pin being about 5 mm from the articular surface (Figure 7.44). After fracture reduction has been achieved a guidewire is inserted, the intramedullary canal is reamed and the nail inserted. At the end of the procedure the fixator is removed.

The distraction capacity of an external fixation device seems to be helpful in the reconstruction of complex injuries of the skeleton. External fixators that incorporate ball joints are particularly useful in allowing a three-dimensional manipulation of a fracture. It is, however, important to plan the use of the distraction device preoperatively and to place the device and the pins in such a position that it does not obstruct the use of the chosen implant.

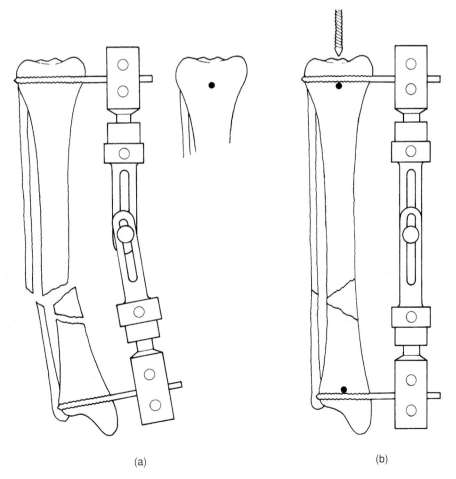

(a)   (b)

Figure 7.44　(a) Use of external fixation to obtain alignment prior to guidewire insertion and nailing (b)

Results

It is often difficult to compare clinical series because of the variables that are involved with different external fixation devices. In 27 severe tibial fractures treated with the Hoffmann external fixator Kimmel (1982) obtained an 87% union rate with a 39% incidence of malunion. Bone grafting was required in 45% of the patients and 50% showed evidence of pin site drainage.

Rommens *et al.* (1989), in their 8-year study of the Hoffmann–Vidal–Adrey frame, documented an average of 6 months in the fixator in 119 closed and open tibial shaft fractures. To increase fracture stability internal fixation was used in the diaphysis. In one-third of the patients frame removal was followed by cast application for an average of 5 months. The non-union rate was 13%, deep infection occurred in 4% and pin loosening in 7%. In 15% of the patients the external fixation device was changed to plate or intramedullary fixation and the incidence of bone grafting was recorded at 21%. Behrens and Searls (1986) reported on 75 fractures treated with the AO external fixator. Bone grafting was used in 75 and pin track infection observed in 12% of the patients. There was one refracture.

De Bastiani *et al.* (1984) demonstrated a union rate of 91% in 91 closed tibial fractures. The incidence of pin track sepsis was less than 1% and the time to union was 3.6 months. Thirty-five out of the 40 open tibial fractures united with an average time of 5.2 months to clinical union.

Meléndes and Colón (1989) studied 44 patients with 45 open tibial fractures. Eighty-nine percent of the fractures were Gustilo type III. All fractures united except one and the average time to union was 22.6 weeks. They used an Orthofix fixator and dynamization was carried out after 8.1 weeks. They recorded that 58% of the patients required bone grafting and their overall union rate was 98%. The authors emphasized the importance of adequate initial reduction, correct pin placement, additional stabilization of large segments with supplementary pins and they also highlighted the importance of satisfactory pin care. In addition they addressed the importance of early dynamization to shorten the union time.

Marsh *et al.* (1991), in a series of 101 cases of open tibial fractures treated with the unilateral Orthofix fixator, had a union rate of 95%. The average time to union was 24.4 weeks with a range of 12–50 weeks. Despite the fact that there were 63 Gustilo type III fractures (24 IIIa, 33 IIIb and

6 IIIc) there were only six fracture site infections during the course of treatment.

Conclusion

External fixation, whether this be a unilateral frame or a more complex construct required for treatment of complex fractures, has provided a useful addition to the arnamentarium for the treatment of tibial fractures. De Bastiani emphasized the importance of respecting the physiology and not compromising the vascularity of the fracture. He stressed the importance of preserving the haematoma, allowing early weight bearing and inducing micromovements by controlled dynamization. A prerequisite for uneventful healing is anatomical alignment of the fractures. DeSouza (1987) demonstrated in 124 tibial fractures that early unrestricted weight bearing led to union after an average of 10 weeks. This series included both closed and open injuries but unfortunately had a high incidence of malunion. However early weight bearing seems to be an important factor for early

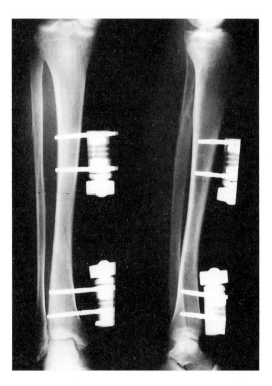

Figure 7.45 Tibial fracture healing without visible callus formation. Routinely after union first the telescope is removed. The patient is seen one week later and removal of the remaining hardware is carried out if no changes are reported

union. Nature will tend to heal fractures and surgical interference should be as limited as possible. The role of the surgeon is to take care of the anatomical alignment whereas the biology of bone healing will look after fracture union.

The mechanical demand of the fracture changes during the healing process and the fixation employed should permit a similar flexible response. There is no doubt that other techniques such as nailing and plating can give good results in centres experienced in these techniques. Unilateral external fixation can save time and equipment (Shaw, 1991) and the patient may be saved a second hospitalization for implant removal (Figure 7.45). The indication is not strictly limited to the tibial diaphysis but the same fixator may be used for metaphyseal and transarticular applications (Pennig, 1993).

References

Alho, A., Ekeland, A., Stromsoe, K. *et al.* (1990) Locked intramedullary nailing for displaced tibial shaft fractures. *J. Bone Joint Surg.*, **72B**, 805

Allgöwer, M. and Perren, S. (1982) Voraussetzungen und Indikatinen der operativen Behandlung von Tibiafrakturen. *Akt. Chir.*, **17**, 1

Aro, H.T. and Chao, E.Y.S. (1990a) Biomechanics of external fixation Part I. *Surg. Rounds Orthop.*, **6**, 17

Aro, H.T. and Chao, E.Y.S. (1990b) Biomechanics of external fixation Part II. *Surg. Rounds Orthop.*, **7**, 43

Aro, H.T. and Chao, E.Y.S. (1993) Bone-healing patterns affected by loading, fracture fragment stability, fracture type and fracture site compression. *Clin. Orthop. Rel. Res.*, **293**, 8

Baker, J.T., McKinney, L.A., Costa, A.S. *et al.* (1992) Comparison of infected rates in contaminated tibial fractures stabilized with internal vs external skeletal fixation in rabbits. *J. Orthop. Trauma*, **6**, 509

Baranowski, D. and Pennig, D. (1988) Grenzindikationen der Verriegelungsnagelung. In *Osteosynthese International*. (eds H.C. Nonnemann, V. Vécsei, R. Lindholm), Schnetztor-Verlag, Konstanz, p. 419

Baranowski, D., Pennig, D. and Borchardt, W. (1990) Komplementär-Osteosynthese und dynamisch-axiale Fixation an der distalen Tibia. *Unfallchirurg.*, **93**, 270

Behrens, F. and Searls, K. (1986) External fixation of the tibia. *J. Bone Joint Surg.*, **68B**, 246

Bier, A. (1923) Über Knochenregeneration, über Pseudarthrosen und über Knochentransplantation. *Arch. Klin. Chir.*, **127**, 1

Blachut, P.A., Meek, R.N. and O'Brien, P.J. (1990) External fixation and delayed intramedullary nailing of open fractures of the tibial shaft. *J. Bone Joint Surg.*, **72A**, 729

Blick, S.S., Brumback, R.J., Lakatos, R. *et al.* (1989) Early prophylactic bone grafting of high energy tibial fractures. *Clin. Orthop.*, **240**, 21

Bonar, S.K. and Marsh, J.L. (1993) Unilateral external fixation for severe pilon fractures. *Foot Ankle*, **14**(2), 57

Breitfuss, H., Muhr, G., Neumann, K. *et al.* (1988) Prognose und Therapie geschlossener, distaler, intraartikularer Unterschenkelbrüche. *Unfallchirurg.*, **91**, 557

Broekhuizen, A.H. (1988) Femoral fractures – indication and biomechanics of external fixation. Thesis, Rotterdam Erasmus University

Broekhuizen, A.H., Boxma, H., van der Meulen, P.A. *et al.* (1988) Performance of external fixation devices in femoral fractures: the ultimate challenge? *Injury*, **21**, 145

Brug, E., and Pennig, D. (1990) Indikation zur Verriegelungsnagelung. *Unfallchirurg.*, **93**, 492

Brug, E., Klein, W. and Pennig, D. (1989) The management of compound tibial fractures with regard to dynamic axial fixation. In *La fissazione esterna*, (ed Pipino) OIC Medical Press, Florence, p. 95

Burny, F. (1983) Principles of external fixation of the tibial fractures. A study of 1421 cases. In *External Fixation* (eds A.F. Brooker and C.C. Edwards), Williams and Wilkins, Baltimore, p. 55

Chao, E.Y.S. and Hein, T.J. (1988) Mechanical performance of the standard Orthofix external fixator. *Orthopaedics*, **11**, 1057

Caudle, R.J. and Stern, P.J. (1987) Severe open fractures of the tibia. *J. Bone Joint Surg.*, **69A**, 801

Court-Brown, C.M. (1985) An analysis of the Hughes fixator in the treatment of tibial fractures. *J. Bone Joint Surg.*, **67B**, 845

Court-Brown, C.M., (1991) *An Atlas of Closed Nailing of the Tibia and Femur*, Martin Dunitz, London

Court-Brown, C.M., Wheelwright, E.F., Christie, J. *et al.* (1990a) External fixation for type III open tibial fractures. *J. Bone Joint Surg.*, **72B**, 801

Court-Brown, C.M., Christie, J. and McQueen, M.M. (1990b) Closed intramedullary tibial nailing. *J. Bone Joint Surg.*, **72B**, 605

Dabezies, E.J., d'Ambrosia, R., Shoki, H. *et al.* (1984) Fractures of the femur treated with the Wagner device. *J. Bone Joint Surg.*, **66A**, 360

De Bastiani, G., Aldegheri, R. and Renzi-Brivio, L. (1984) Treatment of fractures with a dynamic axial fixator. *J. Bone Joint Surg.*, **66B**, 538

De Bastiani, G., Aldegheri, R., Renzi-Brivio, L. *et al.* (1989) Dynamic axial external fixation. *Automedica*, **10**, 235

De Souza, L.J. (1987) Healing time of tibial fractures in Ugandan Africans. *J. Bone Joint Surg.*, **69B**, 56

Evans, G., McLaren, M. and Shearer, J.R. (1988) External fixation of fractures of the tibia: clinical experiences of a new device. *Injury*, **19**, 73

Finlay, J.B., Moroz, T.K., Rorabeck, C.H. *et al.* (1987) Stability of ten configurations of the Hoffmann external fixation frame. *J. Bone Joint Surg.*, **69A**, 734

Goodship, A.E. and Kenwright, J. (1985) The influence of induced micromovements upon the healing of experimental tibial fractures. *J. Bone Joint Surg.*, **67B**, 650

Gotzen, L., Haas, N. and Schlenzka, R. (1984) Der Einsatz des Monofixateurs bei geschlossenen Unterschenkelfrakturen. *Orthopade*, **13**, 287

Gustilo, R.B. and Anderson, J.T. (1976) Prevention of infection in the treatment of 1025 open fractures of long bones. *J. Bone Joint Surg.*, **58A**, 453

Hoffmann, R. (1954) Osteotaxis. Osteosynthèse externe par fiches et rotules. *Acta Chir. Scand.*, **107**, 72

Huiskes, R. and Chao, E.Y.S. (1986) Guidelines for external fixation frame rigidity and stresses. *J. Orthop. Res.*, **4**, 68

Ilizarov, G. (1989a) Angular deformities with shortening. In *External Fixation and Functional Bracing* (eds R. Coombs, S. Green and A. Sarmiento), Orthotext, London, p. 359

Ilizarov, G. (1989b) Fractures and non unions. In *External Fixation and Functional Bracing* (eds R. Coombs, S. Green, R. Sarmiento), Orthotext, London, p. 347

Johnson, K.D., Cadambi, A. and Seibert, G.B. (1985) Incidence of adult respiratory distress syndrome in patients with multiple musculoskeletal injuries: effect of early operative stabilization of fractures. *J. Trauma*, **25**, 375

Karkabi, S. and Reis, N.D. (1986) Fibular bowing due to tibial shortening in isolated fracture of the tibia. *Arch. Orthop. Trauma Surg.*, **106**, 61

Keating, J.F., Gardner, E., Leach, W.J. *et al.* (1991) Management of tibial fractures with the Orthofix dynamic external fixator. *J. R. Coll. Surg. Edinb.*, **36**(4), 272

Kenwright, J., Richardson, J.B., Cunningham, J.L. *et al.* (1991) Axial movement and tibial fractures. A controlled randomised trial of treatment. *J. Bone Joint Surg.*, **73B**(4), 654

Kershaw, C.J., Cunningham, J.L. and Kenwright, J. (1993) Tibial external fixation, weight bearing and fracture movement. *Clin. Orthop. Rel. Res.*, **293**, 28

Kimmel, R.B. (1982) Results of treatment using the Hoffmann external fixator for fractures of the tibial diaphysis. *J. Trauma*, **22**, 960

Klapp, R. and Block, W. (1930) *Die Knochenbruchbehandlung mit Drahtzugen*, Ferdinand-Encke-Verlag, Stuttgart

Klein, W. and Pennig, D. (1992) Untersuchungen zur Dynamisierung des Fixateurs. In *Osteosynthese International* (eds V. Vécsei and H.C. Nonnemann), Schnetztor-Verlag, Konstanz, p. 305

Krettek, C., Haas, N. and Tscherne, H. (1991) The role of supplemental lag-screw fixation for open fractures of the tibial shaft treated with external fixation. *J. Bone Joint Surg.*, **73A**(6), 893

Lambotte, A. (1908) Sur l'osteosynthèse. *La Belgique Medicale*, **20**, 231

Lin, K.Y., Bartlett, S.R., Yaremchuck, M.J. *et al.* (1990) The effect of rigid fixation on the survival of onlay bone grafts: an experimental study. *Plast. Reconstr. Surg.*, **86**, 449

Marsh, J.L. and Nepola, J.V. (1990) External fixation for open tibia fractures. A management strategy. *Orthop. Rev.*, **19**(3), 273

Marsh, J.L., Nepola, J.V., Wuest, T.K. *et al.* (1991) Unilateral external fixation until healing with the dynamic axial fixator for severe open tibial fractures. *J. Orthop. Trauma*, **5**(3), 341

Matthews, L.S., Green, C.A. and Goldstein, S.A. (1984) The thermal effects of skeletal fixation-pin insertion in bone. *J. Bone Joint Surg.*, 66A, 1077

McKibbin, B. (1978) The biology of fracture healing in long bones. *J. Bone Joint Surg.*, **60B**, 150

McGraw, J.M. and Lim, E.V.A. (1988) Treatment of open tibial shaft fractures. External fixation and secondary intramedullary nailing. *J. Bone Joint Surg.*, **70A**, 900

Meléndez, E.M. and Colón, C. (1989) Treatment of open tibial fractures with the Orthofix fixator. *Clin. Orthop. Rel. Res.*, **241**, 224

Moran, C.G., Gibson, M.J. and Cross, A.T. (1990) Intramedullary locking nails for femoral shaft fractures in elderly patients. *J. Bone Joint Surg.*, **72B**, 19

Morrison, K.M., Ebraheim, N.A., Southworth, S.R. *et al.* (1991) Plating of the fibula. Its potential value as an adjunct to external fixation of the tibia. *Clin. Orthop. Rel. Res.*, **266**, 209

Nicoll, E.A. (1964) Fractures of the tibial shaft. A survey of 705 cases. *J. Bone Joint Surg.*, **46B**(3), 373

Oestern, H.J. and Tscherne, H. (1984) Pathophysiology and classification of soft tissue injuries associated with fractures. In *Fractures with Soft Tissue Injuries* (eds H. Tscherne and L. Gotzen), Springer-Verlag, Berlin

Olerud, S. and Karlstrom, G. (1972) Secondary intramedullary nailing of tibial fractures. *J. Bone Joint Surg.*, **54A**, 1419

Ostrum, R.F., Litsky, A.S. and Anson, L.W. (1994) Limited internal fixation of the tibia with external fixation: an *in vivo* canine study. *J. Orthop. Trauma*, **8**(1), 50

Pannike, A., Siebert, H., Kron, H. *et al.* (1981) Behandlungsgrundsätze und Prioritäten des Polytraumas in der Unfallchirurgie. *Unfallchirurg.*, **7**, 76

Pauwels, F. (1965) *Gesammelte Abhandlungen zur funktionellen Anatomie des Bewegungsapparates*, Springer-Verlag, Berlin

Pennig, D. (1990) Zur Biologie des Knochens und der Knochenbruchheilung. *Unfallchirurg.*, **93**, 488

Pennig, D. (1991) The place of unilateral external fixation in the treatment of tibial fractures. *Int. J. Orthop. Trauma*, **1**(3), 161

Pennig, D. (1992) Principles of fracture management in elderly patients. In *Orthogeriatrics* (ed. R.J. Newman), Butterworth-Heinemann, Oxford, p. 175

Pennig, D. (1993) The place of anterior external fixation in the stabilization of pelvic ring disruptions. *Suppl. Int. J. Orthop. Trauma*, **3**(3), 44

Pennig, D., Podbielska, H., Klein, W. *et al.* (1989) Laserholographische Analyse der mechanischen Reaktion bei axialer Belastung und monolateraler Fixateurstabilisierung der Tibia. *Hefte Unfallheilk.*, **207**, 319

Pennig, D., Klein, W., Baranowski, D. *et al.* (1988a) Dynamisch-axiale Fixation als primär definitive Osteosynthese bei der Unterschenkelfraktur. *Hefte Unfallheilk.*, **200**, 294

Pennig, D., Stedtfeld, H.W., Baranowski, E. *et al.* (1988b) Die primär-definitive Versorgung der Tibiafraktur durch externe Fixation. In *Osteosynthese International* (eds H.C. Nonnemann, V. Vécsei, and R. Lindholm), Schnetztor-Verlag, Konstanz, p. 486

Prinz, H., Blomer, A. and Echterhoff, M. (1989) Pin-track infection. In *External Fixation and Functional Bracing* (eds R. Coombs, S. Green and A. Sarmiento), Orthotext, London, p. 49

Putti, V. (1921) The operative lengthening of the femur. *JAMA*, **12**, 934

Renevey, E. (1934) *Apparatus for the Treatment of Bone Fractures*. Patent Specification, United Kingdom, 421 788

Riemer, B.L. and Butterfield, S.L. (1993) Comparison of reamed and unreamed solid core nailing of the tibial diaphysis after external fixation: a preliminary report. *J. Orthop. Trauma*, **7**(3), 279

Rommens, P., Gielen, J., Broos, P. *et al.* (1989) Intrinsic problems with the external fixation device of Hoffmann–Vidal–Adrey. *J. Trauma*, **29**, 630

Russell, G.G., Henderson, R. and Arnett, G. (1990) Primary or delayed closure for open tibial fractures. *J. Bone Joint Surg.*, **72B**, 125

Saleh, M., Shanahan, M.D. and Fern, E.D. (1993) Intra-articular fractures of the distal tibia: surgical management by limited internal fixation and articulated distraction. *Injury*, **24**(1), 37

Sarmiento, A., Gerstein, L.M., Sobol, P.A. *et al.* (1989) Tibial shaft fractures treated with functional braces. *J. Bone Joint Surg.*, **71B**, 602

Sarmiento, A. and Latta, L. (1981) *Closed Functional Treatment of Fractures*, Springer-Verlag, Berlin

Sárváry, A. and Berentey, G. (1984) Die Rolle der Fibula in der Statik des Unterschenkels. *Unfallchirurg.*, 10 (3), 145

Schroder, H.A., Christoffersen, H., Sorensen, T.S. *et al.* (1986) Fractures of the shaft of the tibia treated with Hoffmann external fixation. *Arch. Orthop. Trauma. Surg.*, **105**, 28

Schweiberer, L., Betz, A., Nast-Kolb, D. *et al.* (1987) Spezielle Behandlungstechnik am distalen Unterschenkel und bei Pilonfraktur. *Unfallchirurg.*, **90**, 253

Seligson, D. and Kristiansen, T.K. (1978) Use of the Wagner apparatus in complicated fractures of the femur. *J. Trauma*, **18**, 795

Shaw, D. (1991) The use and cost effectiveness of a dynamic axial fixator. Paper presented at the Royal College of Surgeons Course on External Fixation in Trauma and Orthopaedics, London

Simpson, J.M., Ebraheim, N.A., An, H.S. *et al.* (1990) Posterolateral bone graft of the tibia. *Clin. Orthop. Rel. Res.*, **251**, 200

Singh, M., Nagrath, A.R. and Maini, P.S. (1970) Changes in trabecular pattern of the upper end of the femur as an index of osteoporosis. *J. Bone Joint Surg.*, **52A**, 457

Tayton, K. and Bradley, J. (1982) How stiff should semi-rigid fixation of the human tibia be? *J. Bone Joint Surg.*, **64B**, 105

Tischenko, G.L. and Goodmann, S.B. (1990) Compartment syndrome after intramedullary nailing of the tibia. *J. Bone Joint Surg.*, **72A**, 41

Van Linge, B. (1985) Fracturen statistiek van het Gemeenschappelijk Administratiekantoor. *Ned. Tijdschr. Geneeskd.*, **130**, 2019

Vidal, J. (1980) Historique et perspectives d'avenir de la fixation externe. In *Proceedings of the 7th International Conferences on the Hoffmann External Fixation* (ed. J. Vidal), Diffinco SA, Geneva, p. 5

Watkins, P.E., Kelly, D.J., Rigby, H.S. *et al.* (1988) External fixation for fracture stabilization: what is the optimal mechanical environment? *J. Bone Joint Surg.*, **70B**, 154

Watson, J.T. (1994) Current concepts review: Treatment of unstable fractures of the shaft of the tibia. *J. Bone Joint Surg.*, **76A**, 1575

Wittmoser, R. (1953) Zur Druckosteosynthese. *Arch. Klin. Chir.*, 229

Yamagishi, M. and Yoshimura, Y. (1955) The biomechanics of fracture healing. *J. Bone Joint Surg.*, **37A**, 1035

8

Acute compartment syndrome in tibial fractures

M. McQueen

An acute compartment syndrome is a condition in which the circulation and function of tissues within a closed space are compromised by increased pressure within that space. If untreated this condition leads to ischaemia of muscle and nerve and eventually to disabling contractures, sensory changes and muscle weakness. It is now well over a century since the first description of ischaemic muscle contractures was published. This was attributed to Hamilton in 1850 by Hildebrand (1906) but Hamilton's original description has never been found. The credit for the first full description belongs to Richard von Volkmann (1881) and in deference to this the end stage of acute compartment syndrome is termed Volkmann's ischaemic contracture.

Volkmann believed that contractures were caused by too tight bandaging of the forearm and hand, were ischaemic in nature and were caused by prolonged blocking of arterial blood. In 1888 this aetiology was doubted by Peterson, who reported a case of ischaemic contracture occurring in the absence of bandaging. The first suggestion of raised pressure was made by Hildebrand (1906) who suggested that after injury or tight bandaging an 'oedematous saturation' of muscles occurred which caused raised pressure in the area eventually resulting in compression of the major vessels and muscle ischaemia.

Bardenheuer (1911) published a remarkably similar account of the sequence of events to that which is known today. He described the presence of fascial compartments and differentiated between acute ischaemia caused by major vessel rupture, acute ischaemia caused by 'subfascial tension', the late stage of ischaemic contracture and the sepa-

rate concept of nerve involvement. He was the first to describe the incision of fascia or fasciotomy to relieve pressure and pointed out that this should not be delayed until the pulse disappears or cyanosis develops. A few years later, Murphy (1914) stressed the importance of prophylaxis of ischaemic contracture by fasciotomy performed within 24–36 hours. Jepson (1926) developed this idea further and demonstrated prevention of the development of contractures in animal models by fasciotomy.

During the Second World War several authors considered that ischaemic contractures were caused by arterial spasm (Griffiths, 1940; Foisie, 1942; Sirbu et al., 1944). Griffiths recommended excision of the affected artery and his successful results are undoubtedly due to the fact that fasciotomy was carried out simultaneously. An unfortunate legacy of this belief persists today in still surprisingly widely held but dangerously mistaken view that an acute compartment syndrome cannot exist in the presence of normal peripheral pulses.

The first major report on lower limb ischaemic contractures in 16 cases (Seddon, 1966) included 4 cases of tibial fractures. Seddon noted early and gross swelling in all cases and palpable peripheral pulses in 50%. He recommended early fasciotomy for all cases. McQuillan and Nolan (1968) clearly differentiated between ischaemia caused by major vessel disruption and 'local ischaemia'. Of 15 cases of local ischaemia or acute compartment syndrome 9 were due to tibial fracture.

Matsen (1975) drew all these concepts together defining compartmental syndrome as a condition in which the circulation and function of tissues within a closed space is compromised by increased pressure within that space and pointing out that the underlying features of all compartment syndromes are the same irrespective of the aetiology or location. This concept is now accepted as the basic mechanism giving rise to the acute compartment syndrome (Matsen and Clawson, 1975; Rorabeck and McNab, 1975; Whitesides *et al.*, 1975; Mubarak *et al.*, 1976; Heppenstall *et al.*, 1988; Bourne and Rorabeck, 1989).

Pathogenesis

Acute compartment syndrome reduces blood flow to all the tissues in the compartment including muscle, nerve and bone. Although it is accepted that muscle blood flow is reduced there remains considerable debate as to the mechanism of vessel shut-down. This includes proponents of a critical closing pressure with a combination of active arteriolar closure and passive capillary compression (Ashton, 1975), reduction of local arterio-venous pressure (Matsen, 1980) and capillary occlusion (Hargens *et al.*, 1978).

Regardless of the mechanism of vessel shutdown the effect is to cause acute tissue ischaemia. Muscle blood flow has been studied extensively (Rorabeck *et al.*, 1972; Sheridan and Matsen, 1975; Clayton *et al.*, 1977; Rorabeck and Clarke, 1978; Matsen *et al.*, 1979; Reneman *et al.*, 1980; Matsen *et al.*, 1981) and there is universal agreement that increasing compartmental pressure results in decreasing muscle blood flow with an abrupt drop occurring when intracompartmental pressure reaches 60 mmHg, even for a short time. Clayton and his colleagues (1977) have studied muscle blood flow clinically and found that muscle blood flow reduced as the difference between compartment pressure and diastolic pressure reduced.

The length of time for which pressure has been applied also has a significant influence on muscle ischaemia. A pressure which is tolerated over a period of a few hours may lead to significant muscle ischaemia over a longer period (Rorabeck and Clarke, 1978). Other factors that reduce the tolerance of muscle to raised compartment pressure are hypotension, hypoxia, arterial occlusion and halothane anaesthesia (Matsen *et al.*, 1981).

All authors agree that loss of neuromuscular function occurs in the acute compartment syndrome, although there remains debate about the level and duration of applied pressure that causes irreversible damage (Sheridan *et al.*, 1977; Matsen *et al.*, 1977; Gelberman *et al.*, 1983). Matsen and

his co-authors examined the effects of raised pressure on peripheral nerve function in human subjects and noted considerable variation of pressure tolerance. Recommended pressure levels for decompression vary from 30 mmHg (Hargens *et al.*, 1979) to 55 mmHg (Gelberman *et al.*, 1983) in normotensive patients to prevent permanent neuromuscular deficit.

Bone union after fracture is also affected by raised compartmental pressures. Karlstrom and his co-authors (1975) and DeLee and Stiehl (1981) noted a high incidence of delayed or non-union in tibial fractures complicated by acute compartment syndrome. In a retrospective study (Court-Brown and McQueen, 1987), a series of tibial fractures in adults complicated by acute compartment syndrome took an average of 34 weeks to unite compared to 15 weeks in a matched uncomplicated group. A recent prospective study of 25 tibial fractures complicated by acute compartment syndrome has confirmed this finding (McQueen, 1995) with cases of acute compartment syndrome with sequelae taking twice as long to unite their tibial fractures as those without sequelae. Increasing the delay to fasciotomy significantly increased the union time of tibial diaphyseal fractures. This is attributed to an effect on bone blood flow.

Epidemiology of acute compartment syndrome

There are many underlying causes of the acute compartment syndrome. The commonest reported cause is fracture, with incidences ranging from 30% (Sheridan and Matsen, 1976) to 70% (Mubarak and Carroll, 1979). In a recent prospective study of 68 acute compartment syndromes presenting to the Edinburgh Orthopaedic Trauma Unit 75% of the cases were due to fractures, half of these being tibial fractures (McQueen, 1995). The proportion of cases caused by fracture varies, however, with varying patient populations.

In Edinburgh in the period from January 1988 to July 1992 there were 25 acute compartment syndromes in tibial fractures giving an incidence of 4% in all tibial fractures and 1% in open tibial fractures. Of the 25 patients there were 23 males and 2 females with an average age of 28 years. The age/sex distribution does not show the usual bimodal distribution of trauma cases but is unimodal (Figure 8.1). The two females were older but were underperfused due to multiple injuries.

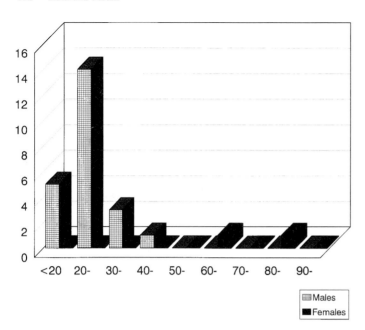

Figure 8.1 Age/sex distribution of acute compartment syndrome in tibial diaphyseal fractures

In the under 35-year-old age group the incidence is 6.5% compared with 1.7% in the over 35-year-old age group. This difference is statistically significant. The younger patient is therefore at greater risk of acute compartment syndrome after tibial fracture. In the whole group the majority of the fractures (64%) had been caused by sporting injuries; 28% were caused by road accidents. The incidence of acute compartment syndrome did not differ between low and high energy injury, which implies equal risk of acute compartment syndrome after tibial fracture regardless of the severity of the injury.

It is possible that there is a genetic predisposition to the development of acute compartment syndrome in tibial fractures after injury in patients with relatively small compartment size compared to the bulk of their muscles. This would explain the lower incidence in older patients, who are more likely to have atrophic muscle.

Clinical diagnosis

The clinical symptoms and signs of acute compartment syndrome are those of muscle and nerve ischaemia. The commonest and most reliable symptom is pain that is out of proportion to the clinical situation (Eaton and Green, 1975; DeLee and Stiehl, 1981; Bourne and Rorabeck, 1989). Rollins and his co-authors (1981) found pain to be present in 83% of their patients requiring fasciotomy, while in the Edinburgh series 95% of conscious patients had significant pain (McQueen, 1995). However, pain can be an unreliable symptom as it can be very variable in degree (Whitesides *et al.*, 1975; Eaton and Green, 1975; Matsen and Krugmire, 1978). Acute compartment syndrome may be painless either in association with nerve injury (Holden, 1979; Wright *et al.*, 1989) or in its early stages (McQueen *et al.*, 1990). In the deep posterior compartment syndrome pain may be minimal (Matsen and Clawson, 1975; Matsen and Krugmire, 1978) while pain is not a useful symptom in the unconscious patient. Pain is normally increased by passive stretching of the affected muscle group but this may often be confused by muscle injury which will cause similar findings.

Sensory symptoms and signs are usually the first indication of nerve ischaemia, with paraesthesia or anaesthesia in the territory of the nerves running through the affected compartments (Matsen and Krugmire, 1978; Bourne and Rorabeck, 1989). Sensory deficit is reported in 42–100% of cases (Rollins *et al.*, 1981; DeLee and Stiehl, 1981; Rorabeck, 1984). In the Edinburgh series, 30% had sensory deficits prior to fasciotomy (McQueen, 1995).

Progression of nerve ischaemia causes paralysis of muscles, which is reported in varying frequency in different series. It is generally believed that motor deficit is a late finding and is associated with irreversible damage to muscle and nerve (Willis and Rorabeck, 1990). Fifteen per cent of patients had developed motor weakness at the time of fasciotomy in the Edinburgh series. There was a statistically significant increase in permanent sequelae in these patients (McQueen, 1995).

A potentially disastrous error in the clinical diagnosis of the acute compartment syndrome is to underestimate the severity of the condition because peripheral pulses are present. Compartment pressure is only rarely high enough to occlude a major vessel and the acute compartment syndrome often occurs with pressure lower than the diastolic pressure (Whitesides *et al.*, 1975; Mubarak, 1983; Bourne and Rorabeck, 1989; Symes, 1991; McQueen, 1995). The only exception to this is in associated arterial injury, where the absent pulse is due to arterial damage rather than high compartment pressure. Distal ischaemia and absent pulses are an indication for arteriography.

Swelling or tenseness is a common sign of acute compartment syndrome provided it is possible to palpate the compartment. However in cases where the leg is encased in plasters or dressings or where there is marked peripheral oedema, this sign may be difficult to elicit.

The early diagnosis of the acute compartment syndrome is of paramount importance. Delay in diagnosis is often due either to inexperience and insufficient awareness of the condition, or to an indefinite and confusing clinical presentation with unreliable clinical signs. Delay in treatment can lead to catastrophic consequences, including contracture, infection and occasionally amputation, and is cited as the single most important cause of failure (McQuillan and Nolan, 1968; Matsen and Clawson, 1975; DeLee and Stiehl, 1981; Rorabeck, 1984; McQueen, 1995).

Anatomy of the leg compartments

A knowledge of the anatomy of the leg compartments is essential for any surgeon managing tibial fractures. The clinical findings can be correlated with the anatomy to allow an accurate assessment of the compartments involved. Adequate decompression of all compartments relies on a clear understanding of their anatomy. There are four compartments in the leg – anterior, superficial posterior, deep posterior and lateral (Figure 8.2).

The anterior compartment is bound anteriorly by skin and fascia, laterally by the anterior inter-

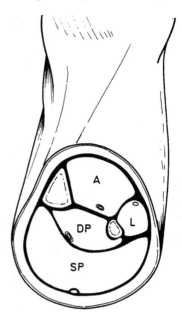

Figure 8.2   The four compartments of the leg. A, anterior; SP, superficial posterior; L, lateral; DP, deep posterior

muscular septum, posteriorly by the fibula and interosseous membrane and medially by the tibia. It contains the dorsiflexors of the foot (tibialis anterior, extensor digitorum longus, extensor hallucis longus, peroneus tertius), the anterior tibial nerve (deep peroneal nerve) and the anterior tibial artery. Thus an acute anterior compartment syndrome will cause pain on stretching the extensors by passive flexion of the toes or ankle and numbness in the first web space where sensation is supplied by the anterior tibial nerve. Progression of the compartment syndrome causes paralysis of the foot and toe dorsiflexors.

The lateral compartment is bounded laterally by skin and fascia, posteriorly by the posterior intermuscular septum, medially by the fibula and anteriorly by the anterior intermuscular septum. It contains the peroneus longus and brevis and the superficial peroneal nerve. An acute compartment syndrome affecting the lateral compartment causes pain on passive stretching of the peronei by passive inversion of the foot and sensory change on the dorsum of the foot which is supplied by the superficial peroneal nerve. Weakness of the peronei is generally a later sign. Theoretically numbness may occur in the first web space as the deep peroneal nerve passes through the lateral compartment before entering the anterior compartment.

The superficial posterior compartment is bounded

anteriorly by the intermuscular septum between the superficial and deep compartments and posteriorly by skin and fascia. It contains the soleus, gastrocnemius and plantaris muscles and the sural nerve. Thus the signs of acute compartment syndrome affecting the superficial posterior compartment are pain on passive dorsiflexion of the ankle, numbness on the dorsolateral aspect of the foot and weakness of ankle plantar flexion.

The deep posterior compartment is limited anteriorly by the tibia and interosseous membrane, laterally by the fibula, posteriorly by the intermuscular septum separating it from the superficial posterior compartment and medially distally in the leg by skin and fascia. It contains tibialis posterior, flexor hallucis longus and flexor digitorum longus along with the posterior tibial nerve. Acute compartment syndrome in this compartment causes pain on passive extension of the toes and ankle or eversion of the foot which stretches tibialis posterior. Numbness may be found on the sole of the foot and in later stages weakness of toe flexion, plantar flexion and inversion of the foot may be found.

Monitoring of intracompartmental pressure

Because of the unreliability of the clinical diagnosis of the acute compartment syndrome methods of measuring pressure within the muscle compartment have been developed. The first method reported was the needle manometer method (Whitesides *et al.*, 1975) but this technique has been criticized by several authors because of the potential for falsely high readings caused by injection of saline (Mubarak *et al.*, 1976), the impossibility of continuous pressure readings (Reneman, 1968) and the awkwardness of observing an air fluid meniscus and a manometer simultaneously with possible inter-observer error (Matsen *et al.*, 1976).

Matsen *et al.* (1976) described a continuous infusion method of monitoring pressure which relies on measurement of the pressure required to infuse fluid slowly into the muscle compartment. Matsen and his colleagues concluded that the method is simple to use and accurate to within 2 mmHg. The main disadvantages are a slow response time and the risk of aggravating swelling by continuous infusion (Rorabeck *et al.*, 1981).

The wick catheter technique (Mubarak *et al.*, 1976) depends on braided Dexon wicks which pro-

trude from the end of an epidural catheter and provide an extensive contact area preventing obstruction of the catheter tip. Mubarak and his co-authors found the method to be accurate and reproducible and to allow continuous long-term measurement. A possible disadvantage of this technique is the risk of leaving part of the catheter in situ.

The slit catheter technique (Rorabeck *et al.*, 1981) depends on slits being cut at the tip of a catheter resulting in a large surface area preventing occlusion by muscle. A continuous infusion is therefore not required but a disadvantage of this technique is its susceptibility to the presence of an air bubble at the tip of the catheter reducing catheter response to changes in intracompartmental pressure (Mubarak, 1983).

It is possible to set up a compartment monitoring system with equipment which is readily available in the operating theatre. The assistance of an interested anaesthetist is invaluable as the equipment is used on a daily basis by anaesthetic departments. A slit catheter is simple to manufacture by using a 20 gauge 6-inch central venous pressure catheter and cutting two slits in its tip (Figure 8.3). This is then inserted into the appropriate compartment and the trocar withdrawn. A small amount of sterile saline is used to fill the catheter which is then connected to an external dome transducer via a length of saline-filled manometer tubing. The transducer is connected to a pressure monitor and zeroed to atmospheric pressure, ensuring that the transducer is placed at the same level as the catheter tip. Care must be taken to exclude air bubbles from the system otherwise falsely low pressure levels will be recorded. The patency of the system should be confirmed by squeezing the calf which should elicit an immediate rise in compartment pressure. If this does not occur the system should be disconnected and refilled with saline. Saline should not be injected through the catheter as this will result in a rise in compartment pressure. It is important that there should be a continuous record of the compartment pressures and this is achieved in Edinburgh by a

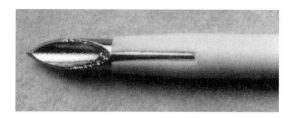

Figure 8.3   A slit catheter

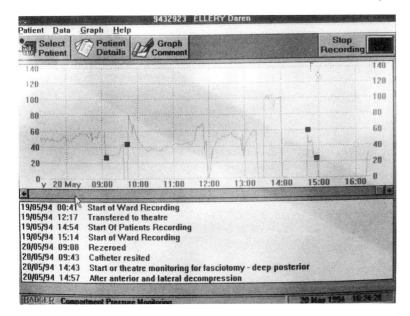

19/05/94 00:41	Start of Ward Recording
19/05/94 12:17	Transfered to theatre
19/05/94 14:54	Start Of Patients Recording
19/05/94 15:14	Start of Ward Recording
20/05/94 09:08	Rezeroed
20/05/94 09:43	Catheter resited
20/05/94 14:43	Start or theatre monitoring for fasciotomy - deep posterior
20/05/94 14:57	After anterior and lateral decompression

Figure 8.4 A computer screen showing a continuous graph of pressure measurements

computerized recording system (Figure 8.4). It is possible to place the catheter in any of the four leg compartments without difficulty. In practice the anterior compartment is most often monitored. The catheter is introduced from an entry point approximately 7.5 cm distal to the tibial tuberosity and 2.5 cm lateral to the subcutaneous border of the tibia (Figure 8.5). As in all compartments a characteristic 'give' is felt as the trocar penetrates the tough fascial layer after which it should be advanced so that the catheter lies at approximately the level of the fracture. This ensures that the highest possible compartment pressure will be measured (Heckmann *et al.*, 1994). The lateral compartment and superficial posterior compartments are both superficial and easily entered either lateral to the fibula for the lateral compartment or in the mid-line posteriorly for the superficial posterior compartment.

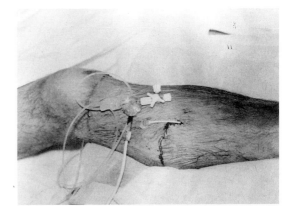

Figure 8.5 A slit catheter in the anterior compartment

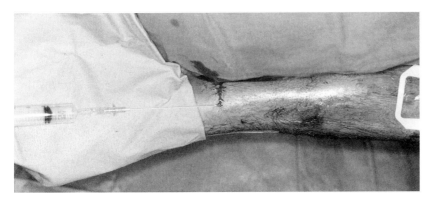

Figure 8.6 Insertion of a catheter into the deep posterior compartment from the distal end of the leg

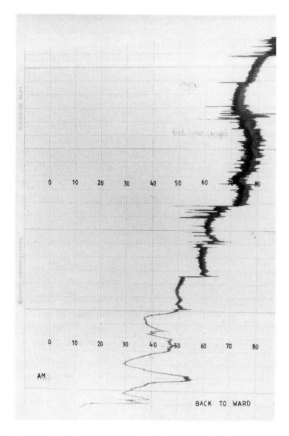

Figure 8.7 A pressure recording showing a developing acute compartment syndrome

The deep posterior compartment is entered distally in the leg where it becomes superficial on the medial border of the distal tibia. The surgeon stands at the patient's feet and the trocar is inserted alongside the subcutaneous border of the distal tibia (Figure 8.6). The trocar is then 'walked' along the posteromedial edge of the tibia until it no longer makes contact with bone at which point the tip should be lying well within the muscle compartment.

Tissue pressure thresholds for decompression

There is considerable debate about the pressure level over which muscle compartments should be decompressed. Whitesides and his co-authors (1975) stress the importance of relating the tissue pressure to the systemic blood pressure and stated that ischaemia begins when the tissue pressure rises

to within 10–30 mmHg of the diastolic pressure. This statement was supported by Heckmann and his co-authors (1993) who studied the effect of varying differences between the compartment pressure and the diastolic pressure (Δp) on canine muscle and concluded that a Δp of 10–20 mmHg was an indication for fasciotomy. Other authors have quoted critical tissue pressures of 30 mmHg (Mubarak *et al.*, 1978, Hargens *et al.*, 1989), 40 mmHg (Matsen *et al.*, 1976; Koman *et al.*, 1981; McDermott *et al.*, 1984; Schwartz *et al.*, 1989) to 45 mmHg (Matsen *et al.*, 1980). Some of this variation may be explained by differing techniques and some by failure to take the patient's blood pressure into account. It is recognized that there is considerable variation in the individual's tolerance of increased tissue pressure (Mubarak *et al.*, 1978; Matsen *et al.*, 1980) and that the use of a single absolute pressure as an indication for fasciotomy may result in unnecessary decompressions (Blick *et al.*, 1986).

A series of 116 patients with tibial diaphyseal fractures underwent continuous compartment monitoring in the Edinburgh Orthopaedic Trauma Unit (McQueen, 1995). Continuous pressure monitoring of the anterior compartment was carried out for at least 24 hours using the slit catheter method. Review was carried out at an average of 15 months after injury to document the incidence of late contracture. There were three acute compartment syndromes with Δp levels of 15 mmHg, 10 mmHg and 15 mmHg respectively. The third patient illustrates the use of continuous compartment pressure monitoring. He was a 19-year-old male with a Tscherne Grade C1 (Oestern and Tscherne, 1984) tibial diaphyseal fracture sustained whilst playing football. six hours after injury the fracture was reduced and stabilized with an intramedullary nail and compartment monitoring was commenced. His compartment pressure immediately postoperatively was 45 mmHg (Δp 45 mmHg) (Figure 8.7). The patient was symptom-free after recovery from anaesthetic. Over the following twelve hours the pressure rose to 75 mmHg (Δp 15 mmHg) (Figure 8.7) and the patient developed some stretch pain. Fasciotomy was performed and the surgical findings confirmed the diagnosis (Figure 8.8). Recovery was uneventful and no sequelae of the acute compartment syndrome were found 13 months after injury. This case illustrates that compartment monitoring allows the early diagnosis of compartment syndrome.

In the group of 116 patients a Δp of less than 30 mmHg was taken as an indication for decompression. Fifty-three patients had compartment

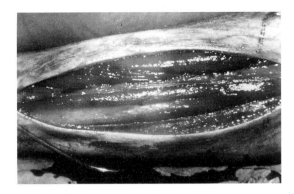

Figure 8.8 The anterior compartment of the patient in Figure 8.7 after decompression

pressures of greater than 30 mmHg and 30 of these had pressures higher than 40 mmHg in the first 12 hours after injury but only one had a Δp of less than 30 mmHg and he had a fasciotomy.

During the second 12 hours after injury 28 patients had pressures over 30 mmHg and 7 had pressures over 40 mmHg. Two patients had Δp levels of less than 30 mmHg and underwent fasciotomy. None of the patients with a Δp of more than 30 mmHg had any sequelae of the acute compartment syndrome at final review. Had a compartment pressure of 30 mmHg been the threshold for decompression 50 patients would have had an unnecessary fasciotomy. Even if a higher threshold of 40 mmHg were used, 27 patients would have had an unnecessary decompression.

Decompression of involved compartments should be performed if the Δp level drops to less than 30 mmHg. It is safe to observe relatively high compartment pressures provided there is the protection of a Δp level of greater than 30 mmHg. Continuous monitoring is essential until the Δp is steadily rising and the compartment pressure is dropping as there may be a lag period between injury and the onset of muscle ischaemia.

Indications for pressure monitoring

Currently accepted indications for pressure monitoring are the unconscious patient (Whitesides *et al.*, 1975; Mubarak *et al.*, 1978; Matsen *et al.*, 1980; Hargens *et al.*, 1989), in patients difficult to assess such as young children (Whitesides *et al.*, 1975; Willis and Rorabeck, 1990), in patients with equivocal symptoms and signs especially in the presence of concomitant nerve injury (Gelberman

et al., 1981; Wright *et al.*, 1989) and in patients with multiple injury (Bourne and Rorabeck, 1989). Compartment monitoring has also been recommended to assess the adequacy of decompressive fasciotomy (Mubarak *et al.*, 1978) and in patients 'at risk' of compartment syndrome. Some authors (Viegas *et al.*, 1988) consider that pressure monitoring should not replace clinical assessment despite stating that clinical findings are well-known to be unreliable while others (Rollins *et al.*, 1981) feel that the usefulness of pressure monitoring is limited because most surgeons would find pressure monitoring cumbersome and the need for fasciotomy is readily apparent clinically. Despite this statement this series had 5 patients with complications of acute compartment syndrome caused by delay in decompression.

Of 25 tibial fractures complicated by acute compartment syndrome presenting to the Edinburgh Orthopaedic Trauma Unit over a period of four and a half years (McQueen, 1995) 13 patients underwent early continuous compartment monitoring and 12 either had no monitoring performed or had a single pressure measurement carried out immediately before fasciotomy to confirm the clinical diagnosis. The choice was dictated by surgeon preference. The severity of injury was not statistically different on comparing the two groups. At review almost one year after injury the monitored group demonstrated no complications of acute compartment syndrome. In contrast in the non-monitored group there were 10 patients with complications of acute compartment syndrome. There was an associated dramatic reduction in delay to fasciotomy in the monitored group.

This clearly demonstrates the effectiveness of compartment pressure monitoring in tibial fractures. Compartment monitoring heightens awareness amongst medical and nursing staff of the possibility of the syndrome developing and acts as an 'early warning system' for cases of impending compartment syndrome. These factors combine to reduce delay and to reduce the long-term sequelae.

Ideally all tibial fractures should undergo compartment pressure monitoring and this is currently part of the routine management of tibial fractures in Edinburgh. It is recognized however that compartment monitoring may be a limited resource in some centres and in these circumstances patients most at risk should be monitored. In the context of tibial fractures the younger patient is at risk of acute compartment syndrome and should undergo continuous pressure measurements to reduce the incidence of disabling consequences.

Management

The only reliable method of treating an established acute compartment syndrome is surgical decompression by incision of overlying fascia or fasciotomy. No other method has been documented which is either sufficiently reliable or rapid in reducing compartment pressures. Impending acute compartment syndromes may on occasions be aborted by release of external limiting envelopes such as dressings or plaster casts. Volkmann (1881) was the first to note that tight bandaging could cause paralysis and contractures in the hands. Garfin and his colleagues (1981) demonstrated a 65% reduction in intracompartmental pressure by splitting and spreading a cast in experimentally elevated compartment pressures and a further 10% reduction by splitting the underlying dressings. The split and spread cast has also been shown to be the only method of casting which can expand to accommodate increasing swelling in a limb (Younger *et al.*, 1990). Figure 8.9 illustrates the effect of splitting a cast on compartment pressures in the clinical situation. In most cases however

splitting of a cast or dressings will not prevent progression from impending to established acute compartment syndrome and fasciotomy is required. Several techniques are available but whichever is employed all authors agree that exposure of all four compartments is necessary (Kelly and Whitesides, 1967; Ernst and Kaufer, 1971; Gaspard and Kohl, 1975; Mubarak and Owen, 1977; Rollins *et al.*, 1981; Rorabeck, 1984).

The double incision four compartment fasciotomy (Mubarak and Owen, 1977) is one of the most commonly used techniques in clinical practice. The anterior and lateral compartments are approached through a longitudinal incision placed just anteriorly to the fibular shaft. The anterior intermuscular septum is identified as a thin white line underlying the skin incision and the skin is retracted anteriorly to allow a longitudinal incision in the fascia which should be placed halfway between the septum and the lateral border of the tibia and should extend the whole length of the compartment (Figure 8.10). The skin is then retracted posteriorly and a longitudinal fasciotomy made in line with the fibular shaft, taking care not

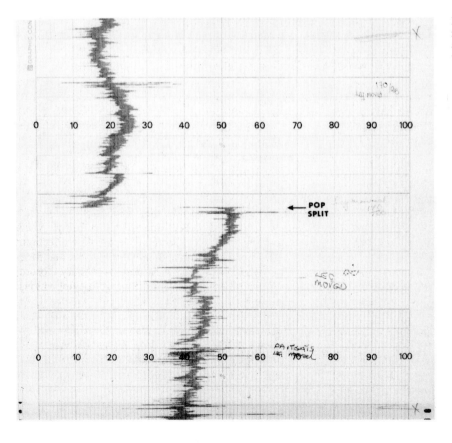

Figure 8.9 A pressure recording showing an abrupt drop in pressure when a cast is split

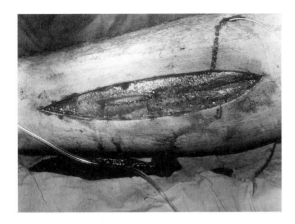

Figure 8.10 The skin incision for decompression of the anterior compartment

to injure the superficial peroneal nerve which pierces the fascia and lies superficial to it in the distal third of the leg.

A second incision is then made longitudinally and approximately 2.5 cm medial to the medial border of the tibia. The superficial posterior compartment is easily accessible in the proximal two-thirds of the leg and the overlying fascia is incised. The deep posterior compartment is superficial in the distal third immediately posterior to the tibia and is readily accessible. Care must be taken however to protect the saphenous vein and nerve which run just behind the tibia. Generous skin incisions are important as skin has been reported to act as a limiting boundary for acute compartment syndromes (Gaspard and Kohl, 1975; Cohen *et al.*, 1991) and for this reason closed fasciotomy is absolutely contraindicated in the acute compartment syndrome.

Fasciotomy of all four compartments through a single incision has been described (Kelly and Whitesides, 1967; Ernst and Kaufer, 1971; Ngheim and Boland, 1980; Cooper, 1992) and has the advantage of improving the appearance of the leg in the long term. Excision of the fibula was advocated initially to expose all four compartments (Kelly and Whitesides, 1967; Ernst and Kaufer, 1971) but this is unnecessarily destructive, risks damage to the common peroneal nerve and removes any potentially stabilizing influence of the fibula on a tibial fracture.

Single incision fasciotomy of all four compartments without fibulectomy is performed through a lateral incision which allows easy access to the anterior and lateral compartments. Anterior retraction of the peroneal muscles then allows exposure

of the posterior intermuscular septum overlying the superficial posterior compartment. The deep posterior compartment is entered by an incision immediately posterior to the posterolateral border of the fibula.

Double incision fasciotomy is faster and since the fascial incisions are all superficial is probably safer than single incision methods although both appear to be equally effective at reducing compartment pressures (Mubarak and Owen, 1977; Vitale *et al.*, 1988).

Whichever technique is employed it is essential to obtain a clear and complete view of all four muscle compartments. There is no indication for decompression of fewer than four compartments in acute compartment syndrome complicating tibial fracture. Muscle viability must be assessed and necrotic tissue excised. The skin and fascia must then be left open as closure would restore a potential limiting envelope. The leg should be inspected 24–48 hours later for any further muscle necrosis. At this stage secondary closure or skin grafting may be performed.

The method of closure of fasciotomy wounds is a cause for debate. Clearly these wound must never be closed primarily. At the second inspection if the wounds are healthy then they may be covered by split-skin graft. Occasionally delayed closure is possible at this stage but should never be attempted if there is any tension on the skin edges.

Criticisms of the use of split-skin grafting include the need to immobilize the patient, and the inevitably poor cosmetic result with poor sensation in a large area of the leg. Methods of delayed primary closure have been reported most of which employ gradual re-approximation of the skin edges using a shoe lace technique (Harris, 1993; Berman *et al.*, 1994) and achieve cover within five to eleven days. This is a longer period with an open wound than would be expected with split-skin graft coverage and raises concern about the possible introduction of hospital acquired infection. Johnson and his co-authors (1992) found that 51% of patients who had secondary or primary closure of fasciotomy wounds had wound complications compared to only 5% who had split-skin graft cover although they were employing a one-stage secondary closure rather than a shoelace type technique. It is recognized in open fractures that delay in wound coverage leads to poorer results (Gustilo and Anderson, 1976; Chapman and Mahoney, 1979) although the soft tissue injury of an open fracture is not necessarily analogous to that in acute compartment syndrome. Further studies need to be performed to assess the safety of gradual closure of fasciotomy wounds.

Provided fasciotomy is performed expeditiously and wound healing is achieved without complications, there seems to be little support for the possible development of chronic venous insufficiency at a later stage (Ris *et al.*, 1993; Aita *et al.*, 1993).

It is now accepted practice that in the presence of an acute compartment syndrome a tibial fracture should be stabilized by internal or external fixation (Rorabeck, 1984; Gershuni *et al.*, 1987). This facilitates wound care and allows early mobilization of surrounding joints thereby reducing the development of fibrosis and joint stiffness. Internal fixation using an intramedullary nail where possible is preferable as this causes the least further disturbance to the soft tissue and avoids the need for pins transfixing the tissues which may lead to added difficulty with wound closure.

Complications

Complications of the acute compartment syndrome occur when decompression is either late or inadequate and include muscle contractures and paralysis leading to deformity, sensory changes including pain, infection and delayed union of the tibial fracture (Court-Brown and McQueen, 1987; McQueen, 1995).

Muscle necrosis occurs initially and this is then replaced by scar tissue which causes the muscle contracture. The resultant deformity depends on the site of contracture. In the deep posterior compartment involvement of the long toe flexors alone can cause toe clawing but contracture of all the contained muscles can cause a fixed equinovarus deformity (Karlstrom *et al.*, 1975; Matsen and Clawson, 1975; Kikuchi *et al.*, 1978). In the anterior compartment the initial sign of necrosis is a foot drop which may then progress to contracture of tibialis anterior and subsequent loss of plantar flexion of the ankle. Occasionally isolated flexor hallucis longus involvement can result in an extension contracture of the great toe. Deformity from lateral compartment involvement does not seem to occur (Seddon, 1966) while deformity from superficial posterior contractures is rare and causes an equinovarus deformity of the foot.

Assessment of the extent of muscle contractures can be performed by CT scanning (Landi *et al.*, 1989) or MR scanning. Treatment is required in cases of persistent deformity with disability and consists of a combination of procedures including excision of scarred muscle (Manoli *et al.*, 1993), or tendon lengthening (Kikuchi *et al.*, 1978; Manoli *et al.*, 1993) or tendon transfer (Kikuchi *et al.*, 1978). Foot deformities cause serious disability and may require arthrodesis to achieve a plantigrade foot. Amputation may be indicated where muscle necrosis is so extensive that useful function is precluded (Figure 8.11), in the presence of an anaesthetic foot or for severe intractable pain.

Treatment of the complications of acute compartment syndrome is unrewarding and it is clear that the prevention of complications by early diagnosis and urgent decompression is of prime importance.

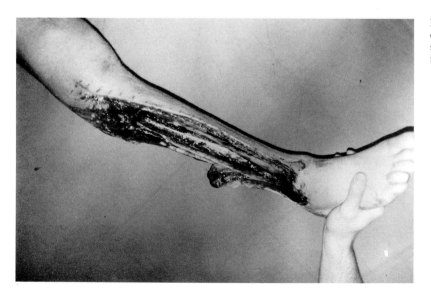

Figure 8.11 A neglected case of acute compartment syndrome with extensive muscle loss

References

Aita, D.J., Kvamme, P., Rice, J.C. and Kerstein, M.D. (1993) Venous insufficiency: a late sequelae of four-compartment fasciotomy in the lower extremity? *Am. Surg.*, **59**, 574–7

Ashton, H. (1975) The effect of increased tissue pressure on blood flow. *Clin. Orthop.*, **113**, 15–26

Bardenheuer, L. (1911) Die Aneang und Behandlung der ischaemische Muskellahnungen und Kontrakturen. *Samml. Klin. Vortrage*, **122**, 437

Berman, S.S., Schilling, J.D., McIntyre, K.E. *et al.* (1994) Shoelace technique for delayed primary closure of fasciotomies. *Am. J. Surg.*, **167**, 435–6

Blick, S.S., Brumback, R.J., Poka, A. *et al.* (1986) Compartment syndrome in open tibial fractures. *J. Bone Joint Surg.*, **68A**, 1348–53

Bourne, R.B. and Rorabeck, C.H. (1989) Compartment syndromes of the lower leg. *Clin. Orthop.*, **240**, 97–104

Chapman, M.W. and Mahoney, M. (1979) The role of early internal fixation in the management of open fractures. *Clin. Orthop.*, **138**, 120–30

Clayton, J.M., Hayes, A.C. and Barnes, R.W. (1977) Tissue pressure and perfusion in the compartment syndrome. *J. Surg. Res.*, **22**, 333–9

Cohen, M.S., Garfin, S.R., Hargens, A.R. and Mubarak, S.J. (1991) Acute compartment syndrome. Effect of dermotomy on fascial decompression in the leg. *J. Bone Joint Surg.*, **73B**, 287–90

Cooper, G.G. (1992) A method of single incision four-compartment fasciotomy of the leg. *Eur. J. Vasc. Surg.*, **6**, 659–61

Court-Brown, C.M. and McQueen, M.M. (1987) Compartment syndrome delays tibial union. *Acta Orthop. Scand.*, **58**, 249–52

DeLee, J.C. and Stiehl, J.B. (1981) Open tibia fracture with compartment syndrome. *Clin. Orthop.*, **160**, 175–84

Eaton, R.G. and Green, W.T. (1975) A volar compartment syndrome of the forearm. *Clin. Orthop.*, **113**, 58–64

Ernst, C.B. and Kaufer, H. (1971) Fibulectomy – fasciotomy. An important adjunct in the management of lower extremity arterial trauma. *J. Trauma*, **11**, 365–80

Foisie, P.S. (1942) Volkmann's ischemic contracture. *N. Engl. J. Med.*, **226**, 671–9

Garfin, S.R., Mubarak, S.J., Evans, K.L., Hargens, A.R. and Akeson, W.H. (1981) Quantification of intracompartmental pressure and volume under plaster casts. *J. Bone Joint Surg.*, **63A**, 449–53

Gaspard, D.J. and Kohl, R.D. (1975) Compartmental syndromes in which the skin is the limiting boundary. *Clin. Orthop.*, **113**, 65–8

Gelberman, R.H., Garfin, S.R., Hergenroeder, P.T., Mubarak, S.J. and Menon, J. (1981) Compartment syndromes of the forearm: diagnosis and treatment. *Clin. Orthop.*, **161**, 252–61

Gelberman, R.H., Szabo, R.M., Williamson, R.V. *et al.* (1983) Tissue pressure threshold for peripheral nerve viability. *Clin. Orthop.*, **178**, 285–91

Gershuni, D.H., Mubarak, S.J., Yani, N.C. and Lee, Y.F. (1987) Fracture of the tibia complicated by acute compartment syndrome. *Clin. Orthop.*, **217**, 221–7

Griffiths, D.L. (1940) Volkmann's ischaemic contracture. *Br. J. Surg.*, **28**, 239–60

Gustilo, R.B. and Anderson, J.T. (1976) Prevention of infection in the treatment of one thousand and twenty-five open fractures of long bones: retrospective and prospective analyses. *J. Bone Joint Surg.*, **58A**, 453–8

Hargens, A.R., Akeson, W.H., Mubarak, S.J. *et al.* (1978) Fluid balance within the canine anterolateral compartment and its relationship to compartment syndromes. *J. Bone Joint Surg.*, **60A**, 499–505

Hargens, A.R., Akeson, W.H., Mubarak, S.J. *et al.* (1989) Kappa Delta Award Paper. Tissue fluid pressures: from basic research tools to clinical applications. *J. Orthop. Res.*, **7**, 902–09

Hargens, A.R., Romine, J.S., Sipe, J.C. *et al.* (1979) Peripheral nerve conduction block by high muscle compartment pressure. *J. Bone Joint Surg.*, **61A**, 192–200

Harris, I. (1993) Gradual closure of fasciotomy wounds using a vessel loop shoelace. *Injury*, **24**, 565–6

Heckmann, M.M., Whitesides, T.E., Grewe, S.R. *et al.* (1993) Histologic determination of the ischaemic threshold of muscle in the canine compartment syndrome model. *J. Orth. Trauma*, **7**, 199–210

Heckmann, M.M., Whitesides, T.E., Grewe, S.R. and Rooks, M.D. (1994) Compartment pressure in association with closed tibial fractures. *J. Bone Joint Surg.*, **76A**, 1285–92

Heppenstall, R.B., Sapega, A.A., Scott, R. *et al.* (1988) The compartment syndrome. An experimental and clinical study of muscular energy metabolism using phosphorus nuclear magnetic resonance spectroscopy. *Clin. Orthop.*, **226**, 138–55

Hildebrand, O. (1906) Die Lehre von den ischamischen Muskellahmungen und Kontrakturen. *Zeitschr. Chirurg.*, **108**, 44–201

Holden, C.E.A. (1979) The pathology and prevention of Volkmann's ischaemic contracture. *J. Bone Joint Surg.*, **61B**, 296–300

Jepson, P.N. (1926) Ischaemic contracture: experimental study. *Ann. Surg.*, **84**, 785–95

Johnson, S.B., Weaver, F.A., Yellin, A.E., Kelly, R. and Bauer, M. (1992) Clinical results of decompressive dermotomy-fasciotomy. *Am. J. Surg.*, **164**, 286–90

Karlstrom, G., Lonnerholm, T. and Olerud, S. (1975) Cavus deformity of the foot after fracture of the tibial shaft. *J. Bone Joint Surg.*, **57A**, 893–900

Kelly, R.P. and Whitesides, T.E. (1967) Transfibular route for fasciotomy of the leg. *J. Bone Joint Surg.*, **49A**, 1022–3

Kikuchi, S., Hasue, M. and Watanabe, M. (1978) Ischaemic contracture in the lower limb. *Clin. Orthop.*, **134**, 185–92

Koman, L.A., Hardaker, W.T. Jr and Goldner, J.L. (1981) Wick catheter in evaluating and treating compartment syndrome. *South. Med. J.*, **73**, 303–9

Landi, A., De Santis, G., Sacchetti, G.L. *et al.* (1989) The use of CT scan in evaluating Volkmann's syndrome in the limbs. *Ital. J. Orth. Traumatol.*, **15**, 521–33

McDermott, A.G.P., Marble, A.E. and Yabsley, R.H. (1984) Monitoring acute compartment pressures with the S.T.I.C. catheter. *Clin. Orthop.*, **190**, 192–8

McQueen, M.M. (1995) MD Thesis, University of Edinburgh

McQueen, M.M., Christie, J. and Court-Brown, C.M. (1990) Compartment pressures after intramedullary nailing of the tibia. *J. Bone Joint Surg.*, **72B**, 395–7

McQuillan, W.M. and Nolan, B. (1968) Ischaemia complicating injury. *J. Bone Joint Surg.*, **50B**, 482–92

Manoli, A., Smith, D.G. and Hansen, S.T. (1993) Scarred muscle excision for the treatment of established ischaemic contracture of the lower extremity. *Clin. Orthop.*, **292**, 309–14

Matsen, F.A. (1975) Compartmental syndrome. An unified concept. *Clin. Orthop.*, **113**, 8–14

Matsen, F.A. (1980) In *Compartmental Syndromes*, Grune & Stratton, New York

Matsen, F.A. and Clawson, D.K. (1975) The deep posterior compartmental syndrome of the leg. *J. Bone Joint Surg.*, **57A**, 34–9

Matsen, F.A. and Krugmire, R.B. (1978) Compartmental syndromes. *Surg. Gynecol. Obstet.*, **147**, 943–9

Matsen, F.A., King, R.V., Krugmire, R.B., Mowery, C.A. and Roche, T. (1979) Physiological effects of increased tissue pressure. *Int. Orthop.*, **3**, 237–44

Matsen, F.A., Mayo, K.Y., Sheridan, G.W. and Krugmire, R.B. (1976) Monitoring of intramuscular pressure. *Surgery*, **79**, 702–9

Matsen, F.A., Mayo, K.A., Krugmire, R.B., Sheridan, G.W. and Kraft, G.H. (1977) A model compartment syndrome in man with particular reference to the quantification of nerve function. *J. Bone Joint Surg.*, **59A**, 648–53

Matsen, F.A., Winquist, R.A. and Krugmire, R.B. (1980) Diagnosis and management of compartmental syndromes. *J. Bone Joint Surg.*, **62A**, 286–91

Matsen, F.A., Wyss, C.R., King, R.V., Barnes, D. and Simmons, C.W. (1981) Factors affecting the tolerance of muscle circulation and function for increased tissue pressure. *Clin. Orthop.*, **155**, 224–30

Mubarak, S.J. (1983) A practical approach to compartmental syndrome. Part II: Diagnosis. *AAOS Instr. Course Lect.*, **32**, 92–102

Mubarak, S.J. and Carroll, N.C. (1979) Volkmann's contracture in children: aetiology and prevention. *J. Bone Joint Surg.*, **61B**, 285–93

Mubarak, S.J. and Owen, C.A. (1977) Double-incision fasciotomy of the leg for decompression in compartment syndromes. *J. Bone Joint Surg.*, **59A**, 184–7

Mubarak, S.J., Hargens, A.R., Owen, C.A., Garetto, L.P. and Akeson, W.H. (1976) The wick catheter technique for measurement of intramuscular pressure. A new research and clinical tool. *J. Bone Joint Surg.*, **58A**, 1016–20

Mubarak, S.J., Owen, C.A., Hargens, A.R., Garetto, L.P. and Akeson, W.H. (1978) Acute compartment syndromes. Diagnosis and treatment with the aid of the wick catheter. *J. Bone Joint Surg.*, **60A**, 1091–5

Murphy, J.B. (1914) Myositis. *JAMA*, **63** (15), 1249–55

Nghiem, D.D. and Boland, J.P. (1980) Four-compartment fasciotomy of the lower extremity without fibulectomy: a new approach. *Am. Surg.*, **46**, 414–17

Oestern, H-J. and Tscherne, H. (1984) Pathophysiology and classification of soft tissue injuries associated with fractures. In *Fractures with Soft Tissue Injuries* (eds H. Tscherne and L. Gotzen), Springer-Verlag, Berlin, pp. 1–9

Peterson, F. (1888) Ueber ischamische Muskellahmung. *Arch. Klin. Chir.*, **37** 675–7

Reneman, R.S. (1968) *The Anterior and the Lateral Compartment Syndrome of the Leg*, Mouton & Co, Paris

Reneman, R.S., Slaaf, D.W., Lindbom, L., Tangelder, G.J. and Arfors., K.E. (1980) Muscle blood flow disturbances produced by simultaneously elevated venous and total muscle tissue pressure. *Microvasc. Res.*, **20**, 307–18

Ris, H-B., Furrer, M., Stronsky, S., Walpoth, B. and Nachbur, B. (1993) Four compartment fasciotomy and venous calf-pump function. Long term results. *Surgery*, **113**, 55–8

Rollins, D.L., Bernhard, V.M. and Towne, J.B. (1981) Fasciotomy: an appraisal of controversial issues. *Arch. Surg.*, **116**, 1474–81

Rorabeck, C.H. (1984) The treatment of compartment syndromes of the leg. *J. Bone Joint Surg.*, **66B**, 93–7

Rorabeck, C.H. and Clarke, K.M. (1978) The pathophysiology of the anterior tibial compartment syndrome. An experimental investigation. *J. Trauma*, **18**(5), 299–304

Rorabeck, C.H. and Macnab, I. (1975) The pathophysiology of the anterior tibial compartmental syndrome. *Clin. Orthop.*, **113**, 52–7

Rorabeck, C.H. and Macnab, I. (1976) Anterior tibial compartment syndrome complicating fractures of the shaft of the tibia. *J. Bone Joint Surg.*, **58A**, 549–50

Rorabeck, C.H., Castle, G.S.P., Hardie, R. and Logan, J. (1981) Compartmental pressure measurements: an experimental investigation using the slit catheter. *J. Trauma*, **21**, 446–9

Rorabeck, C.H., Macnab, I. and Waddell, J.P. (1972) Anterior tibial compartment syndrome: a clinical and experimental review. *Can. J. Surg.*, **15**, 249–56

Schwartz, J.T., Brumback, R.J., Lakatos, R. *et al.* (1989) Acute compartment syndrome of the thigh. *J. Bone Joint Surg.*, **71A**, 392–400

Seddon, H.J. (1966) Volkmann's ischaemia in the lower limb. *J. Bone Joint Surg.*, **48B**, 627–36

Sheridan, G.W. and Matsen, F.A. (1975) An animal model of the compartmental syndrome. *Clin. Orthop.*, **113**, 36–42

Sheridan, G.W. and Matsen, F.A. (1976) Fasciotomy in the treatment of the acute compartment syndrome. *J. Bone Joint Surg.*, **58A**, 112–15

Sheridan, G.W., Matsen, F.A. and Krugmire, R.B. (1977) Further investigations on the pathophysiology of the compartmental syndrome. *Clin. Orthop.*, **123**, 266–70

Sirbu, A.B., Murphy, M.J. and White, A.S. (1944) Soft tissue complications of fracture of the leg. *Calif. West Med.*, **60**, 53–5

Symes, J. (1991) Compartment syndrome. *Can. J. Surg.*, **34**, 307–8

Viegas, S.F., Rimoldi, R., Scarborough, M. and Ballantyne, G.M. (1988) Acute compartment syndrome in the thigh: a case report and a review of the literature. *Clin. Orthop.*, **234**, 232–4

Vitale, G.C., Richardson, J.D., George, S.M. and Miller, F.B. (1988) Fasciotomy for severe, blunt and penetrating trauma of the extremity. *Surg. Gynecol. Obstet.*, **166**, 397–401

Volkmann, R. (1881) Die ischaemischen Muskellahmungen und Kontrakturen. *Centrabl. Chir.*, 51–801

Whitesides, T.E., Haney, T.C., Morimoto, K. and Harada, H. (1975) Tissue pressure measurements as a determinant for the need of fasciotomy. *Clin. Orthop.*, **113**, 43–51

Willis, R.B. and Rorabeck, C.H. (1990) Treatment of compartment syndrome in children. *Orthop. Clin. North Am.*, **21**, 401–12

Wright, J.G., Bogoch, E.R. and Hastings, D.E. (1989) The 'occult' compartment syndrome. *J. Trauma*, **29**, 133–4

Younger, A.S.E., Curran, P. and McQueen, M.M. (1990) Backslabs and plaster casts: which will best accommodate increasing intracompartmental pressures? *Injury*, **21**, 178–81

9

The management of bone loss

M. Saleh

In recent years orthopaedic surgeons have been increasingly faced with the problem of bone loss following open tibial fractures. Advances in fracture fixation techniques and in the handling of soft tissues have meant that many more limbs are now saved. In previous years severe open tibial fractures associated with bone loss were frequently treated by primary or secondary amputation. Recently, however, the incidence of infection following open tibial fracture has dropped dramatically and the problem of how to manage large bone defects is now the most challenging problem that orthopaedic traumatologists encounter.

Occasionally patients will present with a missing bone segment but more commonly it becomes clear at the time of the initial debridement that there is extensive bone damage and periosteal stripping. Consequently the surgeon has to resect bone, thereby creating a bone defect. If this defect is left, a malunion or a non-union will inevitably ensue. Occasionally the orthopaedic surgeon will be faced with a bone defect that has followed bone resection carried out for infected non-union, osteomyelitis or malignancy. The treatment of these secondary defects is the same as for a primary defect that has occurred following a severe open tibial fracture.

In this chapter the various options of treating tibial bone loss are discussed with particular reference to limited bone grafting and the use of callus distraction. Bifocal techniques are described for simultaneous osteosynthesis and bone lengthening. In addition, the technique of primary bone shortening to facilitate union followed by secondary bone lengthening using callus distraction will be described.

Classification

Any classification of bone loss should make the distinction between partial and complete bone loss and any comprehensive description of the problem should include the volume of bone loss or the length of the bone defect. The classification of the Orthopaedic Trauma Association is in widespread use (Figure 9.1). In this classification the type I lesion involves less than 50% of the diameter; type II bone loss is present when there is more than 50% of the diameter missing; in type III bone loss there is complete bone loss involving a circumferential segment (Gustilo, 1991).

The AO classification (Müller et al., 1990) of tibial diaphyseal fractures is described in Chapter 1. The C3 group consists of irregular complex fractures and the C3.3 subgroup is composed of diaphyseal fractures which are associated with significant comminution. Thus many of the tibial fractures that present with bone loss will be C3.3 in severity. Although the degree of bone loss is not selectively defined by the AO classification, an extensive description of the soft tissue and bony damage may be compiled using the various descriptors that are allied to the main AO classification. The Gustilo classification of open fractures (Gustilo and Anderson, 1976; Gustilo et al., 1984) does not address the problem of bone loss but obviously only IIIB and IIIC fractures will be associated with bone loss. There is no current classification for bone shortening but shortening should be described in terms of its location within the bone and its extent, the latter being expressed as a percentage of the current segment length.

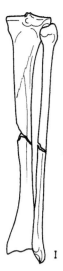
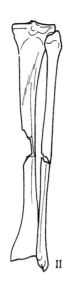
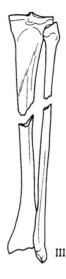

Figure 9.1 The OTA classification of bone loss (Gustilo, 1991). See text for explanation

Management principles for fractures with bone loss

Analysis of data from the Edinburgh Orthopaedic trauma Unit concerning open tibial diaphyseal fractures (Court-Brown and Rose, 1995) has shown that 27% of patients who present with a Gustilo IIIB open tibial fracture are multiply injured and that 70% of these patients have other orthopaedic injuries. It is therefore obvious that many patients who present with tibial bone loss will be seriously injured. It is therefore vital that a surgeon carefully evaluates the overall condition of the patient as well as carries out an adequate assessment of the injured limb. Assessment of the multiply injured patient lies outwith the remit of this book.

Primary examination of the injured limb should involve a careful evaluation of the state of the soft tissues and the bone. If possible, the surgeon should ask about the preoperative physical state of the patient and ascertain whether he or she may have had peripheral vascular disease, diabetes or any other condition that might have affected the viability of the limb. These and other factors such as the amount of muscle damage and the presence of posterior tibial nerve damage may suggest to the surgeon that primary amputation is the treatment of choice. Post-traumatic amputation is discussed further in Chapter 12.

Initial treatment should aim to restore the circulation to the limb by volume replacement, fracture reduction and vascular repair if this is required. It is mandatory that a thorough debride-ment be undertaken and that the surgeon should internally or externally fix the diaphyseal fracture and any related adjacent articular fractures. Keating *et al.* (1994) have shown that 5% of tibial diaphyseal fractures are associated with intra-articular fractures of either the knee or ankle. Failure to treat these adequately will lead to severe disability. Early mobilization of the knee, ankle and subtalar joints is essential and fracture fixation must aim to allow this as soon as possible after surgery. The goal of fracture treatment is not merely to achieve union but to achieve the best possible mobility for the limb and the patient. The surgeon must be particularly aware of the problems of leaving untreated foot fractures. These are frequently ignored and lead to crippling disabilities. Compartment syndrome is addressed in detail in Chapter 8. It is advised that compartment pressure monitoring should be carried out where possible, but if this is not available for the surgeon he or she must have a low threshold for fasciotomy. The effects of compartment syndrome occur rapidly and last for the patient's lifetime.

Initial fracture surgery

The most important part of the initial operation is debridement. It is vital that all devitalized soft tissue and bone be removed at the time of the initial wound exploration. Care must be taken to assess the state of the skin around the open wound and the extent of any associated degloving. The viability of the local musculature must be assessed and all devitalized muscle removed. Failure to do this will greatly increase the risk of infection. It is recommended that gentle lavage be used with appropriate use of intravenous antibiotic prophylaxis. The open wounds should not be closed under any circumstances and can be treated by either secondary closure, split-skin grafting or flap cover at a later time.

All Gustilo type III fractures should be treated by a secondary debridement 24–36 hours after the initial wound inspection. If the wound remains dirty at this time a third debridement must be performed. If by the third debridement the wound still contains devitalized tissues the surgeon must consider whether there has been significant muscle crushing and that it may not be possible to save the limb.

Bone grafting should only be undertaken after good soft tissue healing has been achieved. If bone grafting is undertaken at the time of skin closure or flap cover there is a risk of infection and the bone graft will be lost. The Papineau technique (Papineau *et al.*, 1979) involves packing areas of bone loss with graft and allowing the skin to granulate. With the introduction of improved plastic surgery techniques this technique has now been superseded by either flap cover and corticocancellous grafting or by bone transport. Following initial debridement the treatment principles are bone realignment and stabilization followed by fracture stimulation to secure union (Ribbans *et al.*, 1992; Saleh and Scott, 1992).

Fracture realignment and stabilization

At the time of the initial debridement it may not seem important to realign the bone adequately. However, there is no better time to achieve correct bony alignment. The bone will almost invariably be easily visible in the wound and the surgeon must undertake adequate fracture stabilization with correct alignment.

In the management of severe open tibial fractures associated with bone loss there is no place for the use of casts or braces. Such methods of managing severe open tibial fractures are outdated and should not be used. Three major fixation methods are available to the surgeon. These are bone plating, intramedullary nailing, using either a reamed or unreamed nail, and external skeletal fixation.

The AO group were responsible for revolutionary new ideas in the management of open tibial fractures. They advocated the use of rigid bone plates but it became clear that there were a number of problems associated with this technique. Bone plating is the most difficult of the three techniques to do well as the soft tissues must be stripped away from the bone to allow the plate to be inserted. If this is not done carefully there can be significant bone avascularity and infection and non-union will ensue. Even if done carefully, the use of bone plates in the presence of bone loss means that a very large plate must be applied and considerable soft tissue dissection undertaken.

Other disadvantages of plating were that surgeons often left devitalized bone segments in position to provide structural 'stability'. Bone healing using rigid plate fixation was slow with callus formation being significantly lessened by the rigid nature of the implant. Thus there was a high incidence of non-union and infection with Clifford *et al.* (1988) quoting an infection rate of 7.8% in Gustilo type II fractures and 44.4% in type III open fractures.

Plate fixation of open tibial fractures has now largely been superseded by either intramedullary nailing or external skeletal fixation. There is still debate about the relative merits of intramedullary nailing and external fixation and about whether surgeons should use reamed or unreamed nails if intramedullary nailing is selected. Court-Brown and his co-workers have reported on the use of reamed intramedullary nails in Gustilo type III open fractures over the past four years (Court-Brown *et al.*, 1991; Court-Brown and Rose, 1995). In the initial paper they reported the incidence of infection in Gustilo type III fractures to be 11.1% with the infection rate in the IIIB subgroup being 23%. A later analysis undertaken by Court-Brown and Rose (1995) of intramedullary nailing of open tibial fractures over a 7-year period showed that the overall infection rate in Gustilo type III open tibial fractures had dropped to 5.5% with a 10.7% incidence in the IIIB subgroup. Despite these excellent results the use of nailing in more severe cases is still viewed with caution by many surgeons as they feel that retained devitalized tissue may lead to intramedullary infection which is perceived to be difficult to treat. With careful surgery, however, and adherence to the strict surgical principles of treating infection, it is possible to treat sepsis associated with intramedullary nailing (Court-Brown *et al.*, 1992). Unreamed nails have been investigated by a number of authors (Whittle *et al.*, 1992; Fairbank *et al.*, 1995). The literature concerning the advantages of reamed or unreamed nails is confusing, but at this time clinical studies have not indicated that unreamed nails are superior to reamed nails and they are certainly mechanically weaker and associated with higher breakage rates.

The third method of bone fixation is external skeletal fixation. This is viewed by many surgeons as the safest method of treatment as the screws remain at a distance from the fracture site and this is thought to reduce the incidence of deep infection. In recent years there have been considerable advances in the philosophy and design of external skeletal fixators. Older external fixators tended to produce rigid fixation and often lead to unacceptably high pin site infection rates as well as delayed and non-union (Edge and Denham, 1981; Court-Brown *et al.*, 1990), although Edwards *et al.* (1988) achieved excellent results in grade III open fractures using primary external fixation but changing later to plaster cast management. As a result of the relatively poor results gained using earlier external fixators some surgeons investigated the role of initial external fixation followed by secondary intramedullary nailing (McGraw and Lim, 1988; Maurer *et al.*, 1989; Blachut *et al.*, 1990). There was debate about the use of this technique but some of the investigators had a high incidence of post-traumatic osteomyelitis which was thought to be due to seeding from pin sites and this technique is probably best reserved for the management of failed cases (Marshall *et al.*, 1991).

In recent years third generation fixators have been devised. These are bimodal external fixation devices which allow the mechanical environment to be switched from rigid to elastic (De Bastiani *et al.*, 1984). Marsh *et al.* (1991) showed that high union rates and a low infection rate could be achieved using the third generation Orthofix fixator, although malunion rates tended to be somewhat higher than with intramedullary nailing. External fixation is particularly indicated when there is doubt about tissue viability, overt infection or established shortening or significant bone loss. Ideally external fixation should be applied in such a way that it can be used for definitive fracture treatment. With the Orthofix external fixation device two or three 6 mm screws are inserted into each of two clamps, one on each side of the fracture. If the fracture is eccentric in the limb a supplementary screw may be placed in the longer bone segment for additional stability (Figure 9.2). For maximum stability the inner screw should be no more than 6 cm from the fracture site. If obese or

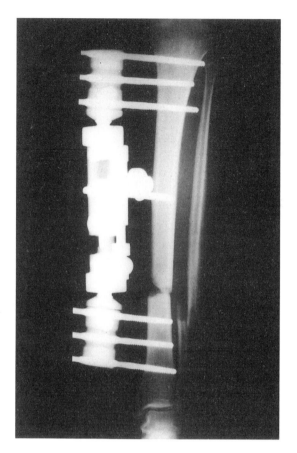

Figure 9.2   An open fracture of the distal third of the tibia with grade II bone loss. A supplementary external fixator screw has been used to provide enhanced stability

osteoporotic patients are being treated it is recommended that three screws are inserted into each clamp. As with all external fixation devices the exact placement of the screws should be discussed with the plastic surgeon if there is a large area of soft tissue loss. Recommendations have been made for safe screw placement (*BOA/BAPS, 1993*) but the exact positioning of individual pins will depend on the area of soft tissue loss and the proposed reconstructive technique. The anterior mounting, although technically demanding, is safe for all soft tissue reconstructive procedures (Figure 9.3). In some circumstances circular or hybrid constructs may be preferred since tensioned wires appear to produce superior holding power in soft and metaphyseal bone and the constructs are easily adapted to cross joints.

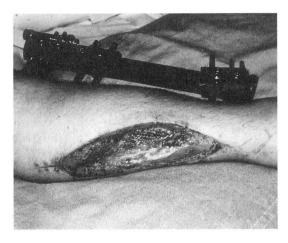

Figure 9.3 An anteriorly mounted unilateral external fixator allows good access to most soft tissue defects

Fracture stimulation

Fractures require stability and bone contact for healing. Contact areas may be improved by square osteotomy or bone grafting. Cancellous bone grafting remains the mainstay of this aspect of treatment. Smaller bone defects should be filled with cancellous autograft. If structural support is required a corticocancellous graft may be used. The iliac crest donor site is the source of significant and often understated morbidity. The incidence of donor site complications in one series was 9.4% and included chronic wound pain and hypersensitivity, buttock anaesthesia, muscle herniation, meralgia paraesthetica and even subluxation of the hip (Cockin, 1971). Meralgia paraesthetica was also described by Weikel and Habal (1977). In another series chronic donor site pain was reported in 25% of patients but this was associated particularly with tricortical grafts (Summers and Eisenstein, 1989). A limited percutaneous approach for harvesting grafts using a trephine is preferred to open techniques (Saleh, 1991) and is associated with reduced donor site morbidity (Kreibich *et al.*, 1994).

If a fracture fails to progress to union it may be due to biomechanical or vascular reasons. Biomechanically the fracture may be excessively mobile or too stable. Fractures with biomechanical instability tend to produce hypertrophic nonunions and these can either be treated by exchange nailing (Court-Brown *et al.*, 1995), plating (Müller and Thomas, 1978) or by altering the configuration of the external fixator. An unstable external fixator may be due to inadequate screws, loose screws or soft bone and stability may be increased by adding extra screws or a supplementary cast. A tight Achilles tendon should be released as this is a potent stress point. If the fixation is producing stress protection reducing the level of fracture support may be achieved with a fibula osteotomy, dynamization or progressive destabilization. Other means of stimulation include increasing vascularity and loading with exercise, weight bearing and flap surgery.

Type I bone loss

Type I bone loss represents less than 50% of the diameter of the bone (see Figure 9.1). In this situation the fracture should be reduced accurately and stabilized using either an intramedullary nail or an external fixation device. Depending on the degree of comminution the length should be easily maintained and bone contact will contribute to overall stability. Usually the nail or external fixator is not unduly stressed because of the degree of shared loading with the bone. The limb is initially elevated to allow the soft tissues to rest and monitored carefully for signs of compartment syndrome. Non-weight bearing or partial weight bearing mobilization is then commenced depending on the degree of stability achieved with the fixation system. The soft tissues are allowed to heal and autogenous cancellous bone grafting performed at 6 weeks. The surgical approach is dictated by the location of the defect and is usually mid-lateral or posteromedial. A direct anteromedial approach should be avoided since this could result in a wound problem. If flap cover has been performed, the surgical approach must be carefully planned to avoid the base or pedicle of the flap. Mobilization of a flap may require a large skin incision as the tissues are often firm and difficult to mobilize. If a fixator has been used it is recommended that the leg be elevated for 24 hours before bone grafting and that the pin sites be as clean as possible.

Surgical technique for type I bone loss

If a fixator has been used the fixator and pin sites are isolated from the operative site. The skin is prepared with an aqueous antiseptic, as are the pin sites. The convenient way of covering the fixator is with a bowel bag which has a drawstring tie at its opening. The bag ties around the screws adjacent to the skin and is covered by a 5 cm crepe bandage. The limb is covered with stockinette or a plastic leg bag and the wound area exposed by cutting into the bag and applying a clear adhesive wound dressing. A tourniquet is not usually necessary. The level of the defects is carefully marked on the skin either by transfer of a radiological measurement or X-ray screening. The approach is chosen according to soft tissue constraints and the site of the bone defect.

If the posteromedial approach is used a 5 cm incision provides direct access to the bone. Using a mid-lateral approach a 7 cm incision is usually required. The deep fascia is incised and the extensor muscles are displaced posteriorly to gain access to the lateral side of the tibia. The incision is marked on the skin and the approach continued down to the bone. The approach should permit direct access to the fracture on one surface only. Bone levers should not be used since these strip the tissues unnecessarily. Whenever possible a subperiosteal approach is made to the bone. Occasionally when working in a submuscular region the Judet technique of decortication (Judet and Patel, 1972) may be used, although in general this technique is more useful in the femur than the tibia. Even at 6 weeks the defect may be filled with fibrous tissue and the bone should be palpated with a dissector until a soft area is entered or a break in continuity is detected. Sharp dissection is then used followed by curettage with a Volkmann's spoon to expose the defect. A high speed dental burr may be used to denude the bone ends of fibrous tissue. The bed is correctly prepared when the bone edges are exposed and bleeding and the surrounding tissue is shown to be vascular. It is recommended that if a tourniquet has been used it is deflated at this stage.

Fine cancellous autograft is packed into the defect and the author's preference is to harvest this using a percutaneous approach (Saleh, 1991). Grafts may also be laid in the submuscular plane adjacent to the presenting cortex. If the presenting cortex looks avascular it may be petalled using an osteotome. The wound is then closed in layers and a drain placed in a separate layer from the graft. If, following this procedure, the bone gap is eliminated but the fracture line persists, dynamization or fibular osteotomy may be required. Occasionally a second bone graft is required for a persistent defect. The aim of this early active intervention is to ensure that shared loading is achieved as rapidly as possible and fracture healing occurs well before fixation failure.

Type II bone loss

In type II bone loss there is a loss of more than 50% of the bone diameter (see Figure 9.1). These injuries may be complicated by vascular damage and soft tissue loss. Realignment and stabilization are carried out rapidly with a view to restoring the circulation and permitting vascular repair. Since there may be little in the way of shared loading fixation, stability is much more critical than for type I injuries. If there is an extensive soft tissue defect the fixator screws should be placed well away from the fracture site providing adequate temporary support whilst the patient is on supervised bed rest. Fasciotomies are not infrequently required. Supplementary external fixator screws may be added within one or two weeks, if necessary, through the site of the flap taking care not to damage its vascular pedicle. Good quality soft tissue cover is vital to healing since at least two bone grafts will be required. Occasionally, and particularly in the elderly where soft tissue is poor, acute shortening may be used to convert the fracture line to a more stable configuration with well vascularized bone ends (Edwards, 1983). Grafting should be performed at around 6 weeks, adhering to the same careful surgical principles used in type I injuries. Often, however, the most appropriate approach is posterolateral. At 12 weeks an anterior graft is inserted using a mid-lateral or posteromedial approach (Figure 9.4). Cancellous autograft is preferred, although corticocancellous grafting may occasionally be considered where stability is a problem. This technique is less than ideal since there remain two fracture surfaces to be incorporated and typically one heals preferentially. Where there is major pelvic damage, a poor quality iliac crest or a large defect morcellized allograft mixed with the patient's own marrow has proved useful in the author's experience. In very resistant cases a repeat posterolateral approach may be used for tibiofibular grafting (Vidal *et al.*, 1982).

Surgical technique for type II bone loss

The posterolateral approach is contraindicated if the posterior tibial artery is the only blood supply to the leg. This is, however, rare and a posterolateral approach will be commonly used for type II bone loss. The procedure is best performed with the patient in the prone position, although if the patient has respiratory problems the lateral position may be chosen. Depending on the quality of the tissue a 10–15 cm incision may be required.

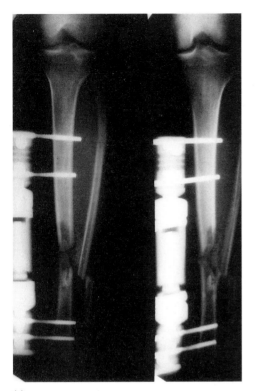

(a)

Figure 9.4 The management of a Gustilo IIIC open tibial fracture.
(a) A unilateral external fixator has been used to stabilize the fracture.
(b) Posterolateral bone grafting was undertaken at 6 weeks; the
operative approach is shown. (c) Anterolateral bone grafting was
undertaken at 14 weeks; the operative approach is illustrated. Note how
the external fixator has been isolated. (d) Radiological appearance of
graft incorporation at 13 weeks. (e) Radiological appearances of graft
incorporation at 22 weeks. (f) Radiological appearances of bone
healing at one year. (g) Clinical appearance of leg at one year after
fracture. Note the satisfactory cosmesis

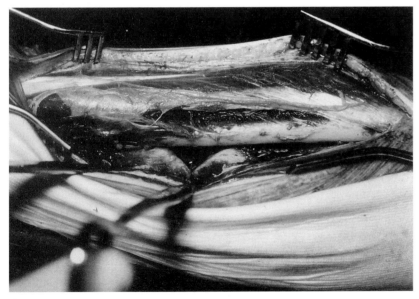

(b)

Figure 9.4   *cont.*

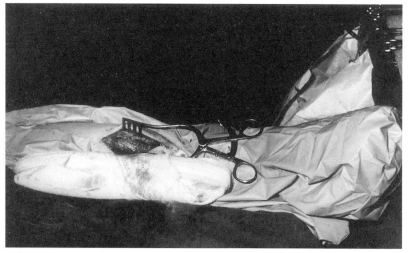

(c)

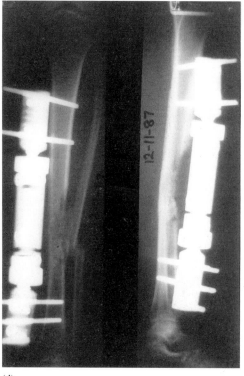

(d)

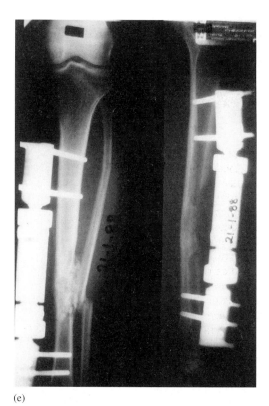

(e)

Figure 9.4 *cont.*

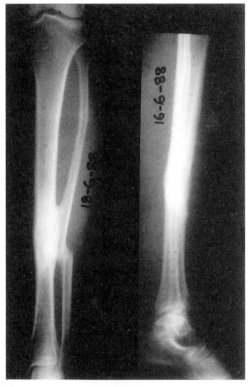

(f)

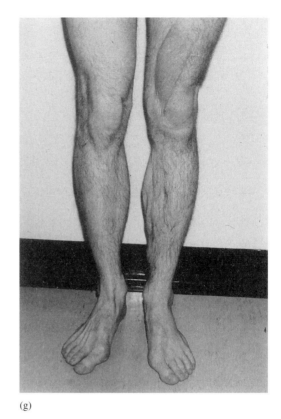

(g)

This is placed just posterior to the fibula. The deep fascia is divided and the thin posterior peroneal intermuscular septum identified. The peronei are separated from soleus and flexor hallucis longus by splitting along the septum. Branches of the peroneal artery winding around the fibula are identified and divided. The flexor surface of the fibula is exposed by stripping off the flexor hallucis longus which protects and carries the peroneal artery with it. The tibialis posterior is swept off the interosseous membrane and flexor digitorum longus is taken off the posterior surface of the tibia exposing the posterior and posterolateral aspects of the tibia. Proximally care must be taken to avoid the common peroneal nerve, and distally the surgeon may find it difficult to expose the lower quarter of the tibia. Bone is laid into the defect after appropriate preparation of the non-union site as described in the management of type I bone loss. For tibiofibular grafting more bone is harvested and laid between the posterior and lateral surfaces of the tibia and the medial and anterior surfaces of the fibula. If insufficient autograft is present allograft may be used. The wound is closed in layers over suction drains.

Type III bone loss

Type III bone loss consists of loss of the full diameter of the tibial diaphysis (see Figure 9.1). Large defects may be reconstructed with repeated massive autogenous grafting (Christian *et al.*, 1989), fibular transfer (Blauth, 1973) or vascular bone grafts (Weiland *et al.*, 1983). Significant donor site morbidity may occur with these techniques and this is particularly undesirable since it occurs at a site distant from the involved segment resulting in a second area of weakness. Microvascular procedures have a good record of reliability. They are long procedures but may be expedited by the use of two teams of surgeons, one to harvest and one to prepare the host area. Specialist training in microvascular surgery is mandatory and centralization is desirable to ensure consistent results. Particular caution is required in the traumatized limb since there may be occult vascular injury. The choice remains between transfer of the ipsilateral or contralateral fibula where a composite flap based on the deep circumflex iliac artery may be used. Such flaps may be raised with a soft tissue and skin component. In some tibial defects the ipsilateral fibula may be mobilized on its vascular pedicle and transplanted medially. Whether vascular or non-vascularized grafts are used, bone must be protected from stress for a considerable period to encourage full incorporation and hypertrophy of the imported bone. Close cooperation between plastic and orthopaedic colleagues is essential to ensure adequate re-alignment and stabilization. Microvascular techniques remain an attractive option, providing instant closure of a defect. However the replaced segment may take 2 years or more to hypertrophy.

Cortical allograft fixed with an intramedullary nail may be employed to provide immediate structural support. Incorporation occurs by local junctional fusion. Vascular ingrowth is discouraged since this will lead to a reduction in strength and is associated with a significant infection risk. Morcellized allograft and other bone substitutes may be used as a replacement for autogenous cancellous graft but clinical experience of these techniques remains limited.

In 1969 Ilizarov described a method of closing bone defects by a technique of internal movement of the bone known as bone transport (Ilizarov and Ledyaev, 1969). This is illustrated diagramatically in Figure 9.5. The technique involves a second bone division, hence the name bifocal surgery. New bone is generated by distraction at the second bone cut and the bone segment that is created is encouraged to move relative to the soft tissue envelope maintaining length but closing the gap. Another similar strategy for smaller defects is immediate or slowly progressive shortening to close a gap followed by lengthening at a healthy metaphysis, a technique known as compression–distraction (Figure 9.5). These techniques have significant advantages over conventional methods. First, the surgery is confined to the affected segment. Secondly, the metaphyseal corticotomy has been shown using technetium uptake studies to increase the blood supply to the bone (Sveshnikov *et al.*, 1984; Aronson, 1994). This has important implications when the healing of a non-union of the tibia is considered. Paley *et al.* (1989) demonstrated the value of this clinically and believed that adding a corticotomy improved union rates and lowered the incidence of atrophic non-union. The new bone is formed by the process of callus distraction, a slow but infinitely controllable process, leading to bone which is indistinguishable from normal (Saleh *et al.*, 1993). In three studies bifocal techniques have proved superior to repeated bone grafting (Marsh *et al.*, 1994; Cierny and Zorn, 1994; Green, 1994).

Bone transport and compression–distraction were compared in one series in the author's unit (Saleh and Reese, 1995). There were 8 patients with large defects treated by bone transport and 8 patients with smaller defects or deformity treated by compression–distraction. There were 5 femoral and 11 tibial cases. At a mean follow-up of 24 months all 16 patients had excellent or good results with union of the fracture, correction of deformity and restoration or near restoration of leg length without major complications. Treatment times

(a) Compression-distraction

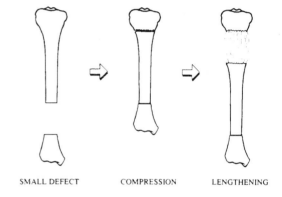

SMALL DEFECT   COMPRESSION   LENGTHENING

(b) Bone transport

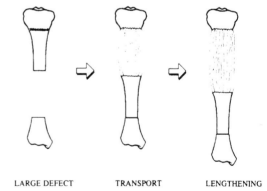

LARGE DEFECT   TRANSPORT   LENGTHENING

Figure 9.5 A management scheme for bone loss.
(a) Compression–distraction: for small defects (<3 cm tibia or <5 cm femur) compression of the defect is followed by osteotomy and lengthening at the other end of the bone.
(b) Bone transport: in larger defects, lengthening and compression occur simultaneously so the middle segment of bone is transported to fill the defect. Once the defect has been closed, further lengthening can be carried out as required. (From, with permission of the *British Journal of Bone and Joint Surgery*)

were longer (mean 16 months) for bone transport compared with compression–distraction (mean 9.8 months) and the procedure was more complicated, requiring on average 2.2 additional operative procedures compared to only one for compression–distraction. Femoral cases had shorter treatment indices than tibial cases but were associated with a less favourable outcome.

In general surgeons can choose between two types of external fixator. We have used the Orthofix monolateral fixator since it is a simple system with excellent rigidity. It is preferred to circular frames as it is less cumbersome, quicker to apply and better tolerated by the patient. However circular frames are useful in certain situations. Their use should be considered where the fracture is adjacent to a joint, the bone is osteoporotic or gradual correction of angulation or a soft tissue contracture is necessary. Where previous microvascular free flaps have been performed it may not be safe to use transfixion wires in the transported segment because of the risk of pedicle transection.

Surgical technique for Type III bone loss

Circular frames are built preoperatively from radiographs, plans and plaster casts. They are checked on the patient prior to surgery and then sterilized. Monolateral frames need little prior planning except to select the correct size and length and ensure that any special clamps that may be required are available. Final detailed planning is performed in the operating theatre and screw lengths are selected and osteotomy sites rehearsed. When the patient is asleep joint ranges are checked. The image intensifier is used to identify bony landmarks and the anatomical and mechanical axes and these are then marked on the skin. Scars are also marked out and the preoperative plan is then transferred to the skin to show screw positions and osteotomy sites.

Circular frames are designed to contour to the tibial deformity and appropriately placed hinges facilitate progressive postoperative correction whereas monolateral frames are usually applied with immediate deformity correction. Three fixation points are required. Three clamps are used in the case of a monolateral frame and three paired rings, or their equivalent, with a circular device. An alignment grid may be used in combination with an image intensifier to allow accurate immediate angular corrections (Saleh *et al.*, 1991). An example of the use of a circular frame in the man-

agement of a 15 cm length of bone loss is shown in Figure 9.6. Here the proximity of the missing segment to the knee joint necessitates the use of a circular frame.

Once the fixator is applied a bone cut is made between two of the fixation points with minimal thermal and vascular damage to avoid inhibiting the callus response. Although a medulla sparing osteotomy (corticotomy) was initially described by Ilizarov, there has been increasing evidence of early recovery of the medullary blood supply and there is no particular advantage in this technique provided a sufficient delay is allowed before lengthening (White and Kenwright, 1990). We recommend an osteotomy under tension (Saleh, 1992a), which allows precise division of the bone. The distractor unit is applied to the fixator and 3–5 mm of distraction is applied. The bone is approached in a normal way through an anteromedial longitudinal incision and the periosteum is reflected with stay stitches. A 3.2 mm drill is used to drill through the whole diameter of the bone at three or four sites. The drill holes are connected with an osteotome paying particular attention to division of the posteromedial and posterolateral corners. Once the cortex is sufficiently broken down, the osteotomy will gradually drift open under the applied tension force. Having confirmed that the osteotomy is complete, it should be closed down since contact between the bone ends is essential for callus generation. A drain should be inserted but left clamped to preserve fracture haematoma and only opened if there is significant haematoma or wound tension. A fibular osteotomy may be required if angular correction or further lengthening is planned. The bone defect or site of resection may be closed immediately (compression–distraction) or held apart for internal transport. For immediate closure appropriate fibular resection may be necessary. Lengthening is commenced on the seventh postoperative day at 0.25 mm four times per day and thereafter the rate is varied according to the rate of new bone formation. Follow-up must be meticulous in order to avoid complications (Paley, 1990; Saleh and Scott, 1992). In compression–distraction the defect site is often healed before the lengthening site. However, in bone transport docking is a much more complicated and delayed process. The fixation system is gradually destabilized once the bone is mature.

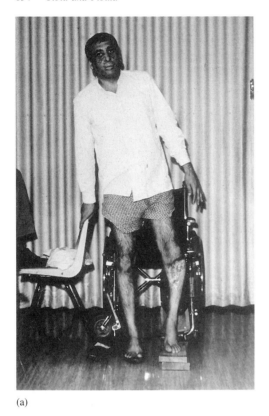

(a)

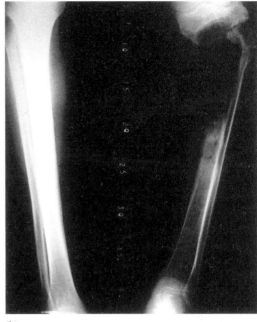

(b)

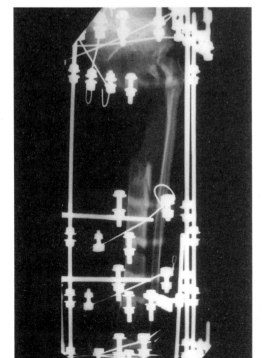

(c)

Figure 9.6 A 15 cm bone defect in the proximal tibia treated by bifocal transport using an Ilizarov frame. (a) The clinical appearance of the patient before surgery. Note the varus knee, the short leg and the eqinus foot deformity. (b) The preoperative radiological appearance showing a large segment of bone loss. (c) The radiological appearance after application of the Ilizarov device. (d) The proximal tibia has been straightened and bone transport undertaken. (e) The clinical appearance of the Ilizarov frame. It has been applied across the ankle and knee joints. The preoperative equinus deformity has been corrected. (f) The radiological appearance after bone union and cessation of treatment. (g) The final clinical appearance

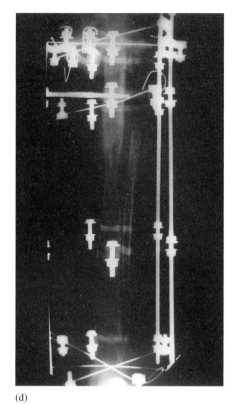

(d)

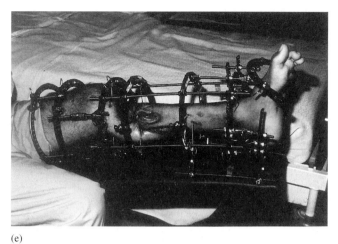

(e)

Figure 9.6 *cont.*

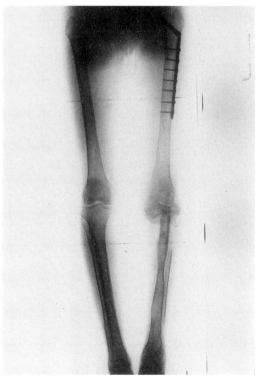

(f)

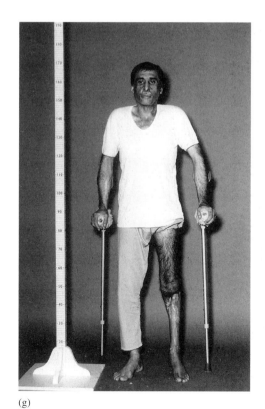

(g)

Docking

When bone transport is used soft tissue obstruction, docking site mismatch or limited contact and non-union may occur. Bone grafting, manipulation and realignment and resection may be required. Although Ilizarov originally described the procedure without bone graft or resection, and in some cases this has been adhered to (Morandi *et al.*, 1989; Paley *et al.*, 1989; Dagher and Roukoz, 1991), other authors have recommended routinely resecting bone to achieve a satisfactory docking configuration (Cattaneo *et al.*, 1992; Green *et al.*, 1992). Green also found bone grafting necessary on occasion and biopsies taken at the time of grafting showed empty lacunae at the forward end of the transported segment indicating avascular bone. Routine bone grafting does not seem to be necessary, although it is

indicated when the contact area is small. Many authors have reported high complication rates and the need for further procedures with bone transport (Paley *et al.*, 1989: Cattaneo *et al.*, 1992; Green *et al.*, 1992; Marsh *et al.*, 1994). In our series further operations were necessary at a rate consistent with the intrinsic complexity of the procedure, and although minor complications occurred, none was serious or persisted following the end of treatment. In part this may be due to careful patient selection and preparation prior to surgery.

Surgical treatment of defects of 6–10 cm

A number of options are available to the surgeon in addition to microvascular bone transfer. These are summarized in Figure 9.7. The choice of management method will, to a certain extent, depend

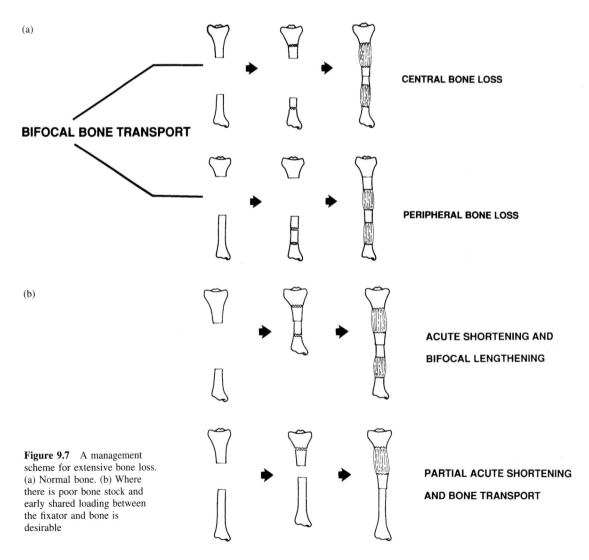

(a)

BIFOCAL BONE TRANSPORT

CENTRAL BONE LOSS

PERIPHERAL BONE LOSS

(b)

ACUTE SHORTENING AND
BIFOCAL LENGTHENING

PARTIAL ACUTE SHORTENING
AND BONE TRANSPORT

Figure 9.7 A management scheme for extensive bone loss. (a) Normal bone. (b) Where there is poor bone stock and early shared loading between the fixator and bone is desirable

on the quality of the bone stock that is left. A clinical example of the treatment of a 10 cm tibial defect is shown in Figure 9.8. It must be remembered that this type of surgery is difficult and it is suggested that patients who have large bone defects should be transferred to surgeons experienced in these techniques. No matter which method is used, the treatment time is long and the morbidity is not inconsiderable.

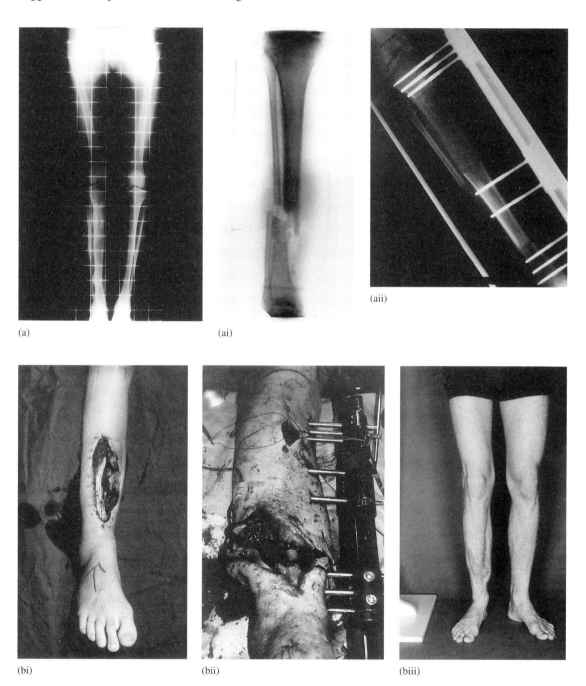

Figure 9.8 The management of a combined soft tissue and bone defect. An open tibial diaphyseal fracture was initially treated by plating and soft tissue closure. Infection ensued. After debridement there was a 10 cm bone defect. (a) Radiographs before, during and after fixation. (b) Clinical appearance before, during and after treatment

Management of bone and soft tissue loss

Acute shortening of extensive bone defects has been recommended by Giebel (1991) in order to close soft tissue and bone defects whilst length is restored by simultaneous metaphyseal osteotomy and lengthening. Using this technique major plastic surgery may be avoided. However, the safe limits of acute shortening are not yet fully understood.

Acute shortening and staged lengthening

If acute shortening is performed in the interests of rapid rehabilitation, lengthening by callotasis may be offered one year to 18 months after completion of treatment. The patient should use a temporary shoe raise. When the bone is sufficiently strong to support an external fixator lengthening by distraction osteogenesis is performed (Ilizarov, 1989a, 1989b; De Bastiani *et al.*, 1987; Saleh, 1992b). Bifocal lengthening may be used for lengthenings of over 6 cm (Saleh and Hamer, 1993).

Techniques based on callus distraction provide salvage of more difficult bone loss problems without significant donor site morbidity. They require careful planning and patient preparation and surgeons should be well versed in callus distraction techniques. Postoperative care is fairly labour-intensive and treatment times are long.

References

Aronson, J. (1994) Temporal and spatial increases in blood flow during distraction osteogenesis. *Clin. Orthop.*, **301**, 124–31

Blachut, P.A., Meek, R.N. and O'Brien, P.J. (1990) External fixation and delayed intramedullary nailing of open fractures of the tibial shaft. *J. Bone Joint Surg.*, **72A**, 729–35

British Orthopaedic Association and the British Association of Plastic Surgeons (1993). *A report by the BOA/BAPS working party on severe tibial injuries*. BOA/BAPS

Blauth, W. and Von Torne, O. (1978) Die fibula-pro-tibia-fusion (hahn-brandes-plastik) in der behandlung von knochendefekten der tibia. *Z. Orthop.*, **116**, 20–6

Cattaneo, A., Catagni, M. and Johnson, E.E. (1992) The treatment of infected non-unions and segmental defects of the tibia by the methods of Ilizarov. *Clini. Orthop.*, **280**, 143–52

Christian, E.P., Bosse, M.J. and Robb, G. (1989) Reconstruction of large diaphyseal defects, without free fibular transfer, in grade IIIB tibial fractures. *J. Bone Joint Surg.*, **71A**, 994–1004

Cierny, G. and Zorn, K.E. (1994) Segmental tibial defects: comparing conventional and Ilizarov methodologies. *Clin. Orthop.*, **301**, 118–23

Clifford, R.P., Beauchamp, C., Kellum, J.F., Webb, J.K. and Tile, M. (1988) Plate fixation of open fractures of the tibia. *J. Bone Joint Surg.*, **70B**, 644–8

Cockin, J. (1971) Autologous bone grafting: complications at the donor site. *J. Bone Joint Surg.*, **53B**, 153

Court-Brown, C.M., Wheelwright, E.F., Christie, J. and McQueen, M.M. (1990) External fixation for type III open tibial fractures. *J. Bone Joint Surg.*, **72B**, 801–4

Court-Brown, C.M., McQueen, M.M., Quaba, A.A. and Christie, J. (1991) Locked intramedullary nailing of open tibial fractures. *J. Bone Joint Surg.*, **73B**, 959–64

Court-Brown, C.M., Keating, J.F. and McQueen, M.M. (1992) Infection after intramedullary nailing of the tibia: incidence and protocol for management. *J. Bone Joint Surg.*, **74B**, 770–4

Court-Brown, C.M. and Rose, C. (1995) Reamed nailing of open tibial fractures. *Osteo. Int.*, **3**, 178–82

Court-Brown, C.N.M., Keating, J.F., Christie, J. and McQueen, M.M. (1995) Exchange intramedullary nailing. Its use in aseptic tibial nonunion. *J. Bone Joint Surg.*, **77B**, 407–11

Dagher, F. and Roukoz, S. (1991) Compound tibial fractures with bone loss treated by Ilizarov technique. *J. Bone Joint Surg.*, **73B**, 316–21

De Bastiani, G., Aldegheri, R. and Brivio, L.R. (1984) The treatment of fractures with a dynamic axial fixator. *J. Bone Joint Surg.*, **66B**, 538–45

De Bastiani, G., Aldegheri, R., Renzi Brivio, L. and Trivella, G. (1987) Limb lengthening by callus distraction (callotasis). *J. Paed. Orthop.*, **7**, 129–34

Edge, A.J. and Denham, R.A. (1981) External fixation for complicated tibial fractures. *J. Bone Joint Surg.*, **63B**, 92–7

Edwards, C.C. (1983) Staged reconstruction of complex open tibial fractures using Hoffmann external fixation: clinical decisions and dilemmas. *Clin. Orthop.*, **178**, 130–61

Edwards, C.C., Simmons, S.C., Browner, B.D. and Weigel, M.C. (1988) Severe open tibial fractures. Results treating 202 injuries with extent fixation. *Clin. Orthop.*, **230**, 98–115

Fairbank, A.C., Thomas, D., Cunningham, B., Curtis, M. and Jinnah, R.H. (1995) Stability of reamed and unreamed intramedullary tibial nails: a biomechanical study. *Injury*, **26**, 483–5

Giebel, G. (1991) Resektions debridement mit kompensatorischer kallusdistraktion. *Unfallchirurg*, **94**, 401–8

Green, S.A., Jackson, J.M., Wall, D.M., Marinow, H. and Ishkanian, J. (1992) Management of segmental defects by the Ilizarov intercalary bone transport method. *Clin. Orthop.*, **280**, 138–42

Green, S. (1994) Skeletal defects: a comparison of bone grafting and bone transport for segmental defects. *Clin. Orthop.*, **301**, 111–17

Gustilo, R.B. and Anderson, J.T. (1976) Prevention of infection in the treatment of one thousand and twenty-five open fractures of long bones: retrospective and prospective analysis. *J. Bone Joint Surg.*, **58A**, 453–8

Gustilo, R.B., Mendoza, R.M. and Williams, D.N. (1984) Problems in the management of type III (severe) open fractures: a new classification of type III open fractures. *J. Trauma*, **24**, 742–6

Gustilo, R.B. (1991) *The Fracture Classification Manual*, Mosby Year Book, St Louis

Ilizarov, G.A. (1989a) The tension-stress effect on the genesis and growth of tissues. Part 1: the influence of stability of fixation and soft tissue preservation. *Clin. Orthop.*, **238**, 249–81

Ilizarov, G.A. (1989b) The tension-stress effect on the genesis and growth of tissues. Part 2: the influence of the rate and frequency of distraction. *Clin. Orthop.*, **239**, 263–85

Ilizarov, G.A. and Ledyaev, V.I. (1992) The replacement of long tubular bone defects by lengthening by distraction osteotomy of one of the fragments. Reproduced in *Clin. Orthop.*, **280** 7–10 (Original in Russian, *Vestn. Khir.*, 1969; **102**: 77)

Judet, R. and Patel, A. (1972) Muscle pedicle bone grafting of long bones by osteoperiosteal decortication. *Clin. Orthop.*, **87**, 74–80

Keating, J.F., Kuo, R.S. and Court-Brown, C.M. (1994) Bifocal fractures of the tibia and fibula. *J. Bone Joint Surg.*, **76B**, 395–400

Kreibich, D.N., Wells, J., Scott, I.R. and Saleh, M. (1994) Donor site morbidity at the iliac crest: comparison of percutaneous and open methods. *J. Bone Joint Surg.*, **76B**, 847–8

McGraw, J.M. and Lim, E.V.A. (1988) Treatment of open tibial shaft fractures. External fixation and secondary intramedullary nailing. *J. Bone Joint Surg.*, **70A**, 900–11

Marsh, J.L., Nepola, J.V., Wuest, T.K. *et al.* (1991) Unilateral external fixation until healing with the dynamic axial fixator for severe open tibial fractures. *J. Orthop. Trauma*, **5**, 341–8

Marsh, J.L., Prokuski, L. and Biermann, S. (1994) Chronic infected tibial nonunions with bone loss: conventional techniques versus bone transport. *Clin. Orthop.*, **301**, 139–46

Marshall, P., Saleh, M. and Douglas, D.L. (1991) Intramedullary nailing following the use of external fixators: the risk of deep infection. *J.R. Coll. Surg. Edinb.*, **36**, 268–71

Maurer, D.J., Merkow, R.L. and Gustilo, R.B. (1989) Infection after intramedullary nailing of severe open tibial fractures initially treated with external fixation. *J. Bone Joint Surg.*, **71A**, 835–8

Morandi, M., Zembo, M.M. and Ciotti, M. (1989) Infected tibial pseudarthosis: a 2-year follow up on patients treated by the Ilizarov technique. *Orthopaedics*, **12**, 497–508

Müller, M.E. and Thomas, R.J. (1979) Treatment of nonunion in fractures of long bones. *Clin. Orthop.*, **138**, 141–53

Müller, M.E., Nazarian, S., Koch, P. and Schatzker, J. (1990) *The Comprehensive Classification of Fractures of Long Bones*, Springer-Verlag, Berlin

Paley, D. Catagni, M.A., Argnani, F. *et al.* (1989) Ilizarov treatment of tibial nonunions with bone loss. *Clin. Orthop.*, **241**, 146–65

Paley, D. (1990) Problems, obstacles and complications of limb lengthening by the Ilizarov technique. *Clin. Orthop.*, **250**, 81–104

Papineau, L.J., Alfageme, A., Dalcourt, J.P. *et al.* (1979) Chronic osteomyelitis: excision and open cancellous bone grafting after extensive saucerisation. *Int. Orthop.*, **3**, 165–76

Ribbans, W.J., Stubbs, D.A. and Saleh, M. (1992) Non-union surgery. Part II: the Sheffield experience – 100 consecutive cases, results and lessons. *Int. J. Orthop. Trauma*, **2**, 19–24

Saleh, M., Harriman, P. and Edwards, D.J. (1991) A radiological method for producing precise limb alignment. *J. Bone Joint Surg.*, **73B**, 515–16

Saleh, M. (1991) Bone graft harvesting. A percutaneous technique. *J. Bone Joint Surg.*, **73B**, 867–8

Saleh, M. (1992a) Technique selection in limb lengthening: the Sheffield practice. *Semin. Orthop.*, **7**, 137–51

Saleh, M. and Scott, B. (1992) Pitfalls and complications in leg lengthening: the Sheffield experience. *Semin. Orthop.*, **7**, 207–22

Saleh, M. (1992b) Non-union surgery. Part I: Basic principles of management. *Int. J. Orthop. Trauma*, **2**, 4–18

Saleh, M. and Hamer, A. (1993) Bifocal lengthening – preliminary results. *J. Paed. Orthop.*, **2**, 42–8

Saleh, M., Stubbs, D.A., Street, R.J., Lang, D.M. and Harris, S.C. (1993) Histologic analysis of human lengthened bone. *J. Paed. Orthop.*, **2**, 16–21

Saleh, M. and Reese, A.R. (1995) Bifocal surgery for deformity and bone loss – bone transport and compression–distraction compared. *J. Bone Joint Surg.*, **77B**, 429–34

Summers, B.N. and Eisenstein, S.M. (1989) Donor site pain from the ileum. *J. Bone Joint Surg.*, **71B**, 677–80

Sveshnikov, A.A., Barabash, A.P., Chepelenko, T.A., Smotrova, L.A. and Larionov, A.A. (1984) Radionuclide studies of osteogenesis and circulation in substitution of large defects of the leg bones. *Exp. Ortop. Traumatol. Protex*, **11**, 33–7

Vidal, J. Buscayret, C., Finzi, M. and Melka, J. (1982) Les greffes inter-tibio-perionières dans le traitement des retards de consolidation jambier. *Rev. Chir. Orthop.*, **68**, 123

Weikal, A.M. and Habal, M.B. (1977) Meralgia paraesthetica: a complication of iliac bone procurement. *Plast. Reconstr. Surg.*, **60**, 572–4

Weiland, A.J., Moore, J.R. and Daniel, R.K. (1983) Vascularised bone grafts. Experience with 41 cases. *Clin. Orthop.*, **174**, 87–95

White, S.H. and Kenwright, J. (1990) The timing of distraction of an osteotomy. *J. Bone Joint Surg.*, **69A**, 356–61

Whittle, A.P., Russell, T.A., Taylor, J.C. and Lavelle, D.G. (1992) Treatment of open fractures of the tibial shaft with the use of interlocking nailing without reaming. *J. Bone Joint Surg.*, **74A**, 1162–71

10

Primary and secondary soft tissue management in open tibial fractures

J. Grünert

Every fracture is accompanied by a greater or lesser degree of damage to the soft tissues. The extent of the damage depends on the fracture mechanism and the amount of kinetic energy involved (Table 10.1). If the trauma is due to a direct, external event, extensive laceration of the tissues and bacterial contamination of the fracture and the adjacent tissue is to be expected. Indirect damage to the soft tissues occurs as a result of pressure from bone fragments or the penetration of bone from the inside to the outside. This damage is not usually as severe but is not to be overlooked. Any closed fracture can become an open one if secondary soft tissue necrosis occurs or as a result of operative intervention, possibly paving the way for an infection or disturbed fracture healing. Uneventful fracture healing requires stable reduction.

An adequate blood supply is equally important in achieving fracture healing. This is the only biological way to combat bacterial contamination in an open fracture and prevent infection. In addition to the metaphyseal arteries, the main blood supply to the tibia is provided by the endosteal vessels which run longitudinally in the medullary canal. These vessels are normally ruptured in displaced shaft fractures. Under these circumstances, the periosteal blood supply will provide the main

vascular support for the bone in those areas where it has remained intact (MacNab and De Haas, 1974; Rhinelander, 1974). Since the tibia lies directly under the skin with only a minimal soft tissue covering, concomitant soft tissue injury can rapidly lead to complications. The associated soft tissue necrosis and devascularization encourages infection. If infection does not become manifest, the blood supply to the bone due to rupture of the vessels and soft tissue fibrosis will be reduced. These conditions favour delayed fracture healing and the formation of pseudarthroses.

Fracture classification

In addition to facilitating the scientific comparison of treatment strategies, the classification of open fractures aims to determine the prognosis for open fractures and aid decisions about treatment. The majority of classifications are based on the first attempts by Cauchoix et al. (1957) to describe the size of the skin defect, the degree of soft tissue contusion and the complexity of the fracture. The most widely used classifications today are those of Tscherne and Oestern (1982), which describe tissue damage in closed and open fractures (Figure 1.12, Chapter 1), and the modified and revised versions of Gustilo et al. (1976, 1984) (Table 1.1, Chapter 1). Third-degree open fractures will be referred to here on the whole: IIIA fractures with considerable soft tissue lesions but adequate coverage of the bone; IIIB fractures with extensive soft tissue loss and severe devascularization of the bone; and IIIC fractures which have additional injuries to the vascular system. This classification

Table 10.1 Energy forces dissipated in injuries

Mechanism	Level of energy (ft/lb)
Fall (off curb)	100
Skiing	300–500
Gunshot wound	2 000
Motorcycle injury	80 040
Bumper injury (20 mph)	100 000

Table 10.2   Infections and amputations in type III open fractures

Type of fracture	Infection (%)	Amputation (%)
IIIA	4.4	0
IIIB	52	16
IIIC	41.7	41.7

Source: Gustilo *et al.*, 1984

reflects the prognosis for these fractures and forms a basis for the assessment of the risk of infection and the probability of an amputation (Table 10.2).

Treatment schedule

The treatment of severe, open tibial fractures takes in four separate stages:

1 Assessment, debridement and stabilization
2 Wound management
3 Soft tissue reconstruction
4 Bony reconstruction

Assessment, debridement and stabilization

The initial assessment of an open tibial fracture involves an investigation of the whole patient (Bosse *et al.*, 1984). The tibial fracture must be considered in the context of the concomitant injuries. Edwards *et al.* (1988) reported that in 80% of cases there were associated injuries, 30% of which were life-threatening. After primary stabilization of essential functions, time should not be lost on superfluous investigations. However, assessment of the vascularization of the limbs and neurological examination is essential. Overlooking damage to the vessels following closed, blunt trauma may have catastrophic consequences. McCabe *et al.* (1983), Keeley *et al.* (1983) and Martin *et al.* (1994) demonstrated that the main determinants of successful treatment were immediate recognition and rapid restoration of the circulation. Only 82% of patients show positive clinical signs of impaired vascularity at the first assessment. Likewise, it is important to be aware that 5–10% of all open tibial fractures will be affected by compartment syndrome (DeLee, 1981; Gulli and Templeman, 1994). Even in open fractures, all the compartments are not necessarily decompressed sufficiently. Simply measuring the tissue pressure can speed up the decision to perform fasciotomy. If there is additional injury to the vessels, then fasciotomy is obligatory. If vessel damage is suspected, it is advantageous

to perform angiography which can be done as a single-shot angiography in the operating theatre to save time. This is the only way of localizing the damage, knowledge of which is essential to the plastic surgeon in planning the soft tissue coverage. Pulse oximetry and Doppler ultrasound provide additional information, and if available may be used during the primary assessment.

Operative treatment begins with debridement. Only during the operation can the extent of the injury be properly assessed. Once the leg has been washed and shaved, the wound can be irrigated. Wound contact with concentrated antiseptics or alcohol and soap solutions containing iodine should be avoided because of their toxic effects on the tissues. The wound should be irrigated with large quantities of isotonic solution. Foreign bodies and obvious dirt are removed. Jet-lavage is an advantageous method which effectively cleans the contaminated wound. Bone fragments which have become detached from the soft tissues are removed unless they form part of a joint. Initial cleansing is followed immediately by surgical debridement. This involves the radical removal of all necrotic, devitalized or inadequately perfused tissue. Debridement will not eliminate bacterial contamination completely, but will considerably reduce the multiplication of bacteria. In the case of open fractures, the administration of antibiotics is always therapeutic and never prophylactic. Antibiotics never replace surgical debridement. Only healthy, well-vascularized tissue can withstand the onslaught of infection. Insufficient debridement increases the degree of primary tissue trauma due to hypoxia which can lead to local inflammation from which secondary tissue trauma may develop. Since the true extent of the injury cannot always be exactly assessed initially, a series of regular debridements should be planned. In the case of third-degree open tibial fractures with considerable soft tissue damage, devascularization and denervation, amputation may be a treatment option and should not be interpreted as clinical resignation.

Stabilization of a fracture aims at restoring the anatomical length and alignment of the bone. Movement at the fracture gap should be avoided. Mechanical immobility is a prerequisite for the undisturbed healing of the soft tissues. Exposing large areas of bone and stripping of the periosteum will not improve the results. Plating is only indicated for intra-articular fractures. It is preferable to stabilize the fracture with an external fixator placed away from the fracture site. It is quick to apply, does not compromise vascularity further, and allows access to the soft tissues if reconstruction should be necessary (Brug *et al.*, 1987).

Wound management

If soft tissue reconstruction is not performed immediately, the dressings should be changed several times daily. The tissue must not be allowed to dry out. Vital structures, such as nerves and vessels, must be preserved. Further debridements should be carried out every 48 hours (Steinau and Germann, 1991). Swabs must be taken regularly in order to adjust the antibiotic treatment accordingly. The development of granulation tissue is not the objective of delayed soft tissue reconstruction. Granulation tissue forms a barrier, reduces vascularity, develops into scar tissue and leads to contractures, therefore it should be resected before definitive soft tissue reconstruction. The right time for definitive reconstruction of the soft tissues is dictated by local factors as well as the general condition of the patient. The situation must be individually assessed and timed. The aim is to intervene within the first 5–8 days and achieve definitive wound closure before secondary colonization appears. Numerous studies have emphasized the advantages of early closure (Cierny *et al.*, 1983; Ketterl *et al.*, 1990) (Table 10.3). Godina (1986) demonstrated that early reconstruction of the soft tissues, i.e. within the first 72 hours, is associated with a very low infection rate (1.5%). If reconstruction is delayed and carried out after 9 days, the infection rate increases to 17.5%. For soft tissue closure after 3 months, the infection rate is 14%. Complications such as flap necrosis, secondary amputations, pseudoarthrosis and osteomyelitis increase as would be expected the longer the delay. Furthermore, the costs of treatment escalate with every new delay and every relapse and this may be associated with personal and social difficulties for the patient.

Table 10.3 Benefits of aggressive debridement and early soft tissue coverage in type III open tibial fractures

Osteomyelitis	30% versus 12%
Pseudoarthrosis	16% versus 6%
Amputation rate	18% versus 6%
Fracture healing	30 versus 23 weeks
Hospitalization	137 versus 74 days

Source: Ketterl *et al.*, 1990

Soft tissue reconstruction

The significance of early definitive soft tissue reconstruction of an open tibial fracture cannot be overestimated. The restoration of an intact soft tissue covering is essential for healing in general since the deep structures will not heal better than the surface covering (Cannon *et al.*, 1977). Conventional reconstruction procedure (classic reconstructive ladder) involving direct suture, skin graft, local flap, distant pedicled graft and finally free microsurgical flap transfer, need not always be strictly adhered to. Since microsurgical methods are so reliable (the success rate is approximately 95%), it is no longer obligatory to commence with the simplest reconstruction stages and find that when they have all failed a free flap transfer is indeed needed.

Uncomplicated wounds due to low velocity trauma can be closed immediately or with very little delay once debridement has been completed provided that injury to the tissue is limited, that there is no devitalized tissue and that the wound has not been seriously contaminated. All superficial wounds with good capillary circulation of the wound bed, for example, subcutaneous fatty tissue, exposed muscle, can be reconstructed with a split-skin graft from the lateral thigh. Exposed bone and tendons with intact periosteum and paratenon will also accept a skin graft, but in the mid- and long term this will lead to the formation of scar tissue. Unstable scars with fistula formation, adhesions and restriction of movement are generally the result. More complex wounds with exposed bone should only be treated with local flaps if they are due to low velocity trauma. In the case of high velocity trauma, the area of injury is larger and the soft tissue more badly affected, which means the vascularity of the existing tissue is impaired. The vitality of fasciocutaneous and muscle flaps which can be applied locally is then endangered. Local muscle flaps are also unlikely to be adequate to cover such defects. A combination of several muscle flaps is required. This, however, only leads to an additional, unacceptable loss of function of the already injured limb. Traditionally, the possibilities for soft tissue reconstruction of the tibia are expressed in terms of thirds (Figure 10.1). The pedicled gastrocnemius flap is the treatment of choice for soft tissue reconstruction in the proximal third. The reservations regarding soft tissue reconstruction in the mid-third by transposition of the local muscles have been mentioned above. The main indication for the free micro-

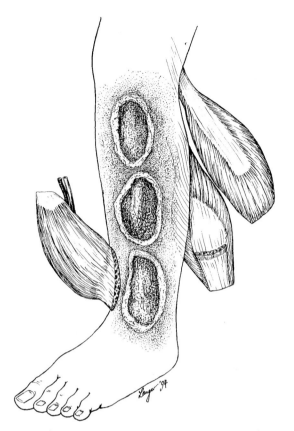

Figure 10.1 For a strategical approach to soft tissue coverage, the leg is divided into three zones. Defects of the proximal third and popliteal fossa can be closed with a pedicled gastrocnemius flap. Those in the middle third with a soleus or free flap, while in the distal third there is a clear indication for free flaps

surgical flap is clearly soft tissue defects in the distal third (Figures 10.2–10.4). Only 30–40% of all third-degree open tibial fractures require extensive grafting (Behrens *et al.*, 1983; Edwards *et al.*, 1988). Muscle flaps are best applied with immediate split-skin graft. The advantage of the muscle flap is not only its good vascularity but also its accessibility. This is particularly true for the latissimus dorsi flap. The muscle flap is highly resistant to infection and when covered with a split-skin graft best restores the contours of the tibia. Primary wound healing can be achieved by applying a microsurgical flap and this is more likely to lead to success than the alternative techniques.

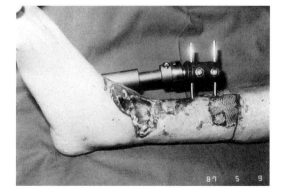

Figure 10.2 This 44-year-old male sustained a type IIIB open fracture in the distal third of the tibia with extensive skin defect, periosteal stipping and signs of infection due to delay in soft tissue coverage

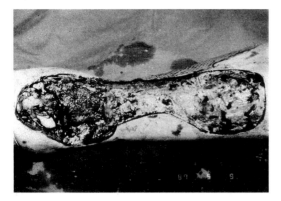

Figure 10.3 A thorough and aggressive debridement is mandatory to combat infection

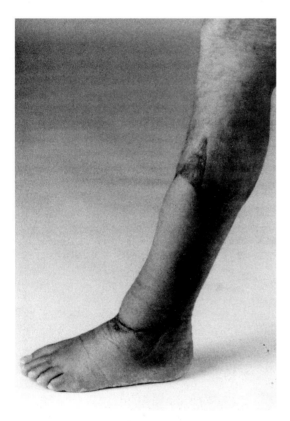

Figure 10.4 Two months after soft tissue reconstruction with a free musculocutaneous latissimus dorsi flap. Further atrophy of the muscle will improve the contour of the leg

Bony reconstruction

The microsurgical reconstruction of large bone defects is only justifiable if infection is definitely absent. Rarely there is a primary indication to transfer the free contralateral fibula with a latissimus dorsi flap. Bone defects *up to 8 cm* can be treated just as successfully with the conventional technique of cancellous bone grafting or segmental transport. Free microsurgical bone transplants have proved more advantageous for larger defects (Stock and Hierner, 1994). Remodelling and healing occur more rapidly and functional hypertrophy is more pronounced compared with conventional cancellous bone grafting. Callus distraction now offers an alternative to microsurgical bone reconstruction in cases of large defects (Ilizarov, 1992). In selecting the bone reconstruction technique to match the indication, the predicted time to healing, the estimated success, the risk of the particular technique and possible alternative procedures must be considered.

Technical aspects

Certain technical considerations have proved helpful for microsurgical soft tissue reconstruction. Nowadays almost any soft tissue defect can be closed by plastic surgery. This fact must be taken into account during initial treatment and debridement. A plastic surgeon should be consulted as early as possible, preferably on the day of the accident. Many infections have developed from the original contamination of the open tibial fracture because of too much reliance on antibiotics and subsequent neglect of wound management. Prerequisites for microsurgical flap transfer are training in the technique of microvascular anastomosis, a detailed knowledge of anatomy and the special techniques of raising and transferring different free flaps and a knowledge of alternative procedures. If one particular flap proves impossible or if a method fails, the surgeon must be able to switch to another procedure or be able to retreat successfully. Preoperative angiography to plan a large flap transfer is desirable. The anastomoses should always be placed at intact, unscarred sites. In terms of blood flow, the end-to-side anastomosis has proved beneficial (Godina, 1979). It is not unusual to be forced to use this procedure if only one main vessel is still functioning. This technique can be expected not to further compromise distal perfusion. The posterior approach is appropriate to access uninjured large calibre vessels (Godina *et al.*, 1991). The anterior tibia can easily be reached by tunnelling for a short distance and the flap can be securely attached.

This is best done with the patient in the lateral

Table 10.4   Characteristics of cutaneous flaps

Flap	Pedicle length (cm)	Pedicle size (mm)	Maximum size (cm)	Sensory innervation
Groin	6–7	A: 1–1.5 V: 1–2	10 × 25	No
Dorsalis pedis	5–10	A: 2–3 V: 2–3	8 × 15	Yes
Scapular	4–15	A: 2–3 V: 3–4	12 × 24	No
Parascapular	6–15	A: 2–3 V: 3–4	12 × 30	No
Lateral arm	6–7	A: 1–1.5 V: 1.5–2	6(14) × 20	Yes
Radial forearm	5–10	A: 1.6–2.6 V: 1–1.5	10 × 20	Yes
Posterior interossseus	3–5	A: 0.8–1.2 V: 0.6–1	4(6) × 10	Yes

A, Artery; V, vein

decubitus position. The tibia can be accessed from the ventral and the dorsal sides and a latissimus dorsi flap can be raised by a team of two surgeons simultaneously.

The main characteristics of the most widely used flaps will now be described. These are summarized in Tables 10.4 and 10.5. The type of flap (muscle or cutaneous), the maximal area of the flap, the length of the vascular pedicle, the size of the vessels, the possible anatomical variations and the donor site morbidity must all be considered.

Preferred flaps

Local flaps are only of limited use in soft tissue reconstruction of the tibia. Free flaps are used in most cases of large defects. Depending on the required size, the surgeon may wish to select free cutaneous and fasciocutaneous flaps, such as the groin flap, the scapular flap (Figures 10.5 and 10.6),

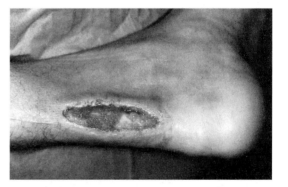

Figure 10.5   After suture of a ruptured Achilles tendon, wound breakdown revealed a partially necrotic tendon in this 38-year-old female

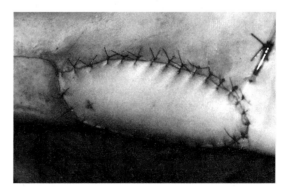

Figure 10.6   Soft tissue coverage was achieved by transfer of a free scapular flap, only leaving a horizontal scar at the donor site. The X marks the point of emergence of the circumflex scapular artery which is best identified preoperatively by Doppler sonography

Table 10.5   Characteristics of muscle flaps

Flap	Pedicle length (cm)	Pedicle size (mm)	Maximum size (cm)
Latissimus dorsi	7–10	A: 2–3 V: 3–4	30 × 40
Serratus anterior	7–10	A: 2–3 V: 3–4	4(6) × 10–12
Rectus abdominis	8–12	A: 2–3 V: 2–3.5	8 × 30
Gracilis	6–8	A: 2 V: 2–2.5	6 × 24
Tensor fascia lata	4–10	A: 1.1–2 V: 1.3–2.5	8(20) × 30
Greater omentum	10–15	A: 1.8–2.8 V: 2–3.2	15(20) × 20(45)

the parascapular flap, the lateral upper arm flap and the radial forearm flap (Thorne *et al.*, 1990). The particular advantages of the muscle flap have already been described. The pedicled gastrocnemius flap has proved useful for the proximal third of the tibia. For the majority of defects the latissiumus dorsi flap is standard procedure. It can be used to cover almost any defect because of its size (30 × 40 cm). The intramuscular blood supply is constant throughout so that the flap can be tailored to fit any defect and is well suited to filling cavities. The constant pedicle is long (7–9 cm) and the thoracodorsal artery is large (2–3 mm) so that an anastomosis can be carried out away from the injury in healthy tissue.

Alternatives for smaller defects are the serratus anterior flap, the gracilis flap or the rectus abdominis flap. A latissimus dorsi flap covered with a split-skin graft is, however, often preferable since it can be safely raised and the donor site morbidity is minimal. After muscle removal, shoulder function is impaired by only 2%, which very rarely disturbs the patient.

Tissue expansion

If there is no infection but an unstable area of scar tissue in the tibia, the insertion of a tissue expander under the skin makes it possible to pre-extend the skin and then to transfer it after excision of the scar tissue. The areas of scarring are surrounded by one or usually two long rectangular or croissant-shaped expanders. These are inserted via radially oriented incisions to avoid tension in the scars during expansion. The expansion phase during which the expander is filled with saline at weekly intervals lasts for at least 3–4 months. A frequent error is the premature interruption of expansion, although volume is still too low. Once the expansion phase has been completed, the skin must rest for at least 3–4 weeks before the scar can be excised and the expanded skin transferred. The functional and cosmetic results are very promising.

Sequelae of incomplete primary management in tibial fracture

Chronic infection of the tibia is frequently the result of inadequate or incomplete primary treatment of open tibial fractures. The treatment of these conditions by conventional means is generally associated with a high failure rate in which there may be a 20% to 60% incidence of recurrent infection (Hall *et al.*, 1983). Chronic osteomyelitis of the tibia is typical. There are areas of accumulated pus in the bone, infectious granulation tissue, sequester, formation of fistulae, and chronic inflammatory infiltrations. These inflammatory foci are often encapsulated by sclerotic bone, perfusion is poor, the soft tissue coverage consists of scarred periosteum, the muscles are fibrotic and cicatrized and the skin is less resistant. Conservative measures (e.g. antibiotics) often do not reach the infected areas.

In 1946, Stark demonstrated the positive effects of local muscle flaps grafted on to sites of chronic infection. The advantageous influence of muscle flaps as compared with cutaneous flaps was proved in numerous experimental studies. A muscle flap reacts to infection by increasing the blood supply; a cutaneous flap does not. The leucocyte count increases, which is a clear sign of a defence reaction (Chang and Mathes, 1982; Feng *et al.*, 1990). Necrosis of a muscle flap is very rare, and if it occurs at all, is only partial, whereas cutaneous flaps are regularly affected by necrosis. Muscle flaps eliminate bacteria efficiently. The adequate elimination of bacteria when there is increased macrophage activity can only be expected under conditions of physiological oxygen concentrations in the tissue. These advantages only apply to the muscle flap. The revascularization of the bone can be observed from 4 weeks in cases of muscle flap transplant which is not the case for cutaneous flaps (Fisher and Wood, 1987).

The conclusions to be drawn are similar to those for acute open fractures – radical and aggressive debridement of all infected and necrotic tissue and adequate muscle flap transfer to fill all cavities and to improve the vascularity (Mathes, 1982; Steinau and Germann, 1991; Winckler and Grünert, 1993). Numerous clinical observations confirm the value of these procedures.

References

Behrens, F., Searls, K., Comfort, T., Denis, F. and Young, T. (1983) Treatment of severe open tibial fractures: prospective evaluation. *J. Bone Joint Surg. Orthop. Trans.*, **7**, 528

Bosse, M.J., Burgess, A.R. and Brumback, R.J. (1984) Evaluation and treatment of the high-energy open tibia fracture. *Adv. Orthop. Surg.*, **8**, 3–17

Brug, E., Klein, W. and Grünert, J. (1987) Die Behandlung der offenen Frakturen mit dem Fixateur externe – unter Berücksichtigung der dynamischen-axialen Fixation 'Orthofix'. *Chirurg.*, **58**, 699–705

Cannon, B., Constable, J.D., Furlaw, L.T. *et al.* (1977) Reconstructive surgery of the lower extremity. In *Reconstructive Plastic Surgery* (ed. J.M. Converse), 2nd edn, W.B. Saunders, Philadelphia, p. 3521

Cauchoix, J., Duparc, J. and Boulez, P. (1957) Traitment des fractures ouvertes de jambe. *Med. Acta Chir.*, **83**, 811–22

Chang, N. and Mathes, S.J. (1982) Comparison of the effect of bacterial inoculation in musculocutaneous and random-pattern flaps. *Plast. Reconstr. Surg.*, **70**, 1–9

Cierny, G., Byrd, H.S. and Jones, R.E. (1983) Primary versus delayed soft tissue coverage for severe open tibial fractures. *Clin. Orthop.*, **178**, 54–63

DeLee, J.C. and Stiehl, J.B. (1981) Open tibia fracture with compartment syndrome. *Clin. Orthop.*, **180**, 175–84

Edwards, C.C., Simmons, S.C., Browner, B.D. and Weigel, M.C. (1988) Severe open tibial fractures: results treating 202 injuries with external fixation. *Clin. Orthop.*, **230**, 98–115

Feng, L.J., Price, D.C., Mathes, S.J. and Hohn, D. (1990) Dynamic properties of blood flow and leukocyte mobilisation in infected flaps. *World J. Surg.* **14**, 796–803

Fisher, J. and Wood, M.B. (1987) Experimental comparison of bone revascularization by musculocutaneous and cutaneous flaps. *Plast. Reconstr. Surg.*, **79**, 81–90

Godina, M. (1986) Microsurgical reconstruction of complex trauma of the extremities. *Plast. Reconstr. Surg.*, **78**, 285–92

Godina, M. (1979) Preferential use of end-to-side arterial anastomoses in free flap transfers. *Plast. Reconstr. Surg.*, **64**, 673–82

Godina, M. Arnez, Z.M. and Lister, G.D. (1991) Preferential use of the posterior approach to blood vessels of the lower leg in microvascular surgery. *Plast. Reconstr. Surg.*, **88**, 287–91

Gulli, B. and Templeman, D. (1994) Compartment syndrome of the lower extremity. *Orthop. Clin. North Am.*, **25**, 677–84

Gustilo, R.B. and Anderson, J.T. (1976) Prevention of infection in the treatment of one thousand and twenty-five open fractures of long bones. *J. Bone Joint Surg.*, **58A**, 453–8

Gustilo, R.B. Mendoza, R.M. and Williams, D.N. (1984) Problems in the management of type III (severe) open fractures: a new classification of type III open fractures. *J. Trauma*, **24**, 742–6

Hall, B.B., Fitzgerald, R.H. and Rosenblatt, J.E. (1983) Anaerobic osteomyelitis. *J. Bone Joint Surg.*, **65A**, 30–5

Ilizarov, G.A. (1992) *Transosseous Osteosynthesis*. Springer, Heidelberg

Keeley, S.B., Snyder, W.H. and Weigelt J.A. (1983) Arterial injuries below the knee: fifty-one patients with 82 injuries. *J. Trauma*, **23**, 285–92

Ketterl, R.L., Steinau, H.U., Feller, A.M., Stübinger, B. and Claudi, B.F. (1990) Aggressives Debridement und frühzeitige Weichteildeckung bei drittgradig offenen Tibiafrakturen. *Zentralbl. Chir.*, **115**, 209–18

MacNab, I. and De Haas, W.G. (1974) The role of periosteal blood supply in the healing of fractures of the tibia. *Clin. Orthop.*, **105**, 27–33

Martin, L.C., McKenney, M.G., Sosa, J.L. *et al.* (1994) Management of lower extremity arterial trauma. *J. Trauma*, **37**, 591–9

Mathes, S.J. (1982) The muscle flap for management of osteomyelitis. *N. Engl. J. Med.*, **306**, 294–5

McCabe, C.J., Ferguson, C.M. and Ottinger, L.W. (1983) Improved limb salvage in popliteal artery injuries. *J. Trauma*, **23**, 982–5

Rhinelander, F.W. (1974) Tibial blood supply in relation to fracture healing. *Clin. Orthop.*, **105**, 34–81

Stark, W.J. (1946) The use of pedicled muscle flaps in the surgical treatment of chronic osteomyelitis resulting from compound fractures. *J. Bone Joint Surg.*, **28**, 343–50

Steinau, H.U. and Germann, G. (1991) Plastisch-rekonstruktive Mikrochirurgie zur posttraumatischen Infektionsprophylaxe und-therapie. *Chirurg.*, **62**, 852–60

Stock, W. and Hierner, R. (1994) Vascularized bone transfer. *Injury*, **25** (Suppl. 1), 33–45

Thorne, C.H.M., Siebert, J.W., Grotting, J.C., *et al.*, (1990) Reconstructive surgery of the lower extremity. In *Plastic Surgery* (ed. J.G. McCarthy), W.B. Sanders, Philadelphia, pp. 4029–92

Tscherne, H. and Oestern, H.J. (1982) Die Klassifizierung des Weichteilschadens bei offenen und geschlossenen Frakturen. *Unfallheilkunde*, **85**, 111–15

Winckler, S. and Grünert, J. (1993) Posttraumatische postoperative Osteitis. In *Die dynamisch-axiale externe Fixation* (eds H. Neumann, W. Klein and E. Brug), Hans Marseille Verlag, Munich, pp. 65–74

11

The management of non-union

D. Pennig

Introduction

One of the first surgeons to study non-union was John Hunter (1728–93). He observed that the ends of bones that had not united were eburnated and smooth. He also observed that they formed pseudoarthroses and he understood that the non-union process converted bone into an almost hyalin-like material which would prevent union. From these observations a treatment method consisting of removal of the eburnated bone, 'irrigation' of the surfaces and bringing the bone ends into contact was formulated. The non-union was then immobilized until union occurred (Hunter, 1837).

This method remained the operation of choice until bone grafting became popular in the twentieth century (Phemister, 1931; Campbell, 1932; Key, 1937; Henderson, 1938). Hunter himself had performed the earliest experiments on bone transplantation during his studies on bone growth. He transplanted the spurs of a chicken to its head and also reinserted a tooth into its socket from which it had recently been extruded. The tooth remained firmly held by new bone laid about its roots (Hunter, 1937).

There are about 2 000 000 long-bone fractures treated annually in the United States and Heppenstall has estimated that about 5% will result in non-union and even more in delayed union. While operative treatment of acute fractures has lowered the incidence of non-union and delayed union in some bones some authors suggest that in the tibia the incidence has increased (Taylor, 1992).

Definition of pseudoarthrosis

Treatment of non-union requires a thorough understanding of the biology of bone and fracture repair (Bier, 1923; Pennig, 1990). The normal evolution of a fracture is to progress to union provided the fracture is stabilized adequately for an appropriate period. Several factors may contribute to delay in union. These being periosteal stripping in open fractures, high velocity injuries with soft tissue and bone loss and infection after an open fracture or an open reduction (Rosenthal et al., 1977).

With the exception of congenital pseudoarthrosis of the tibia non-union usually occurs after operative fracture management. The tibial diaphysis appears to be the most commonly affected bone (Taylor, 1992).

The exact causes of non-union in the tibia remain obscure. Boyd and Lipinski (1960) reported on a large number of long bone non-unions and suggested that non-union was more common when the fractures were open, infected, segmental, associated with impaired blood supply, located in the middle fragment, associated with major comminution, poorly fixed, immobilized for an insufficient time, treated by a technically incorrect open reduction or distracted by traction or plating. It has also been suggested that an intact fibula, a fracture in the distal third of the tibia and the development of infection after primary wound closure in open fractures are important factors in the development of non-union (Albert, 1944; Heppenstall et al., 1984).

Dickson and Catzman (1994) examined a series of 114 patients with open tibial fractures. Sixty-two patients had a normal arteriogram whereas 52 demonstrated occlusion of one, two or all three

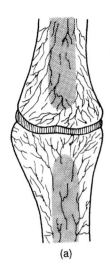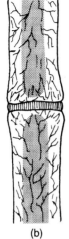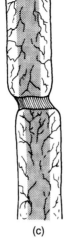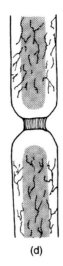

(a) (b) (c) (d)

Figure 11.1 (a) Hypertrophic non-union (b) Oligotrophic non-union (c) Atrophic non-union (d) Pseudoarthrosis The hypertrophic and oligotrophic non-unions show adequate vascularity, the atrophic non-union shows impaired vascularity. (After Weber and Cech, 1976)

arteries that supply the lower leg. In this latter group of patients the incidence of delayed union or non-union was 46% compared to 16% in the patients with normal arteriograms. The incidence of osteomyelitis was also higher in the patients with poor arterial supply.

The failure to weight bear early has been suggested as a cause of non-union and Taylor (1992) demonstrated that in a group of 185 tibial non-unions 92.4% had an initial delay in weight bearing of more than 6 weeks. De Souza (1987) studied a group of Ugandan Africans who had closed and open tibial fractures treated with immediate unrestricted weight bearing in a cast. The incidence of non-union was 0.8% with an average time to union of 10 weeks.

Most tibial fractures can usually be expected to unite within 6 months although clearly the time to union will depend on the amount of soft tissue injury. By 6 months however either a delay in union or an established non-union has to be suspected. However some fractures are slow to unite. If there is still progress radiologically and an improvement in the clinical stability then a non-union has not as yet been established. It is always important to understand the personality of the fracture to predict its eventual outcome and to understand its development.

In 1986 a panel of the FDA defined non-union as 'established when a minimum of 9 months has elapsed since injury and the fracture has shown no visible progressive signs of healing for 3 months' (Taylor, 1992). This definition is not applicable to every fracture and the lack of clinical progress is probably more important than the exact time elapsed after a fracture.

Three different types of non-union exist, these are hypertrophic, oligotrophic and atrophic. The final state of non-union is probably best referred to as a pseudoarthrosis (Weber and Cech, 1976; Weber and Brunner, 1975) (Figure 11.1).

Diagnosis of pseudoarthrosis (Table 11.1)

The clinical presentation of a delayed union or a non-union is usually characterized by pain and motion at the former fracture site. There may be swelling and the area may feel warmer than the opposite side. The vascular status of the affected limb should be recorded and the state of the peripheral pulses rated (Dickson *et al.*, 1994). General disorders such as diabetes mellitus and peripheral neuropathy should be identified.

Radiological studies indicate that bridging callus

Table 11.1 Diagnosis of pseudoarthrosis

Clinical sign
  Pain
  Swelling
  Skin temperature elevated
  Motion at fracture site
  Vascular status
  Absent peripheral pulses

Radiological sign
Standard (tomograms)
  Persisting fracture lines
  'Irritation' callus
  Three cortices not bridged (in two planes)
  Active technetium or leucocyte scan
  Mobility under image intensifier

is absent and fracture lines persist. Tomograms in both the anteroposterior and lateral planes are frequently useful in assessing the non-union in detail. For a proper analysis of the non-union the surgeon must carefully consider the original treatment as well as any subsequent therapy and a thorough radiological analysis of the current situation.

The most important decision for the surgeon to make is whether he or she is dealing with an aseptic or septic non-union. Standard tests such as the ESR and CRP should be performed. A bone scan may be helpful to assess the activity at the non-union site (Esterhai *et al.*, 1984) and if necessary a leucocyte scintigram is performed. An aspiration biopsy from the area of the non-union may be sent for laboratory testing to assist in distinguishing septic from aseptic non-union. CAT scanning and MRI do not have an established role in the assessment of non-union. However CAT scans with three-dimensional reconstruction may be useful in analysing an intra-articular malunion (Schatzker, 1990).

No matter how many tests are performed the identification of a low grade sepsis may be difficult. It is highly unlikely that a non-operatively treated closed procedure will be septic and virtually all non-union under these circumstances will be aseptic. Repeated interventions carry a higher risk of a low grade sepsis and it is always safer to assume this and plan the treatment accordingly.

Treatment of pseudoarthrosis

When treating a pseudoarthrosis it is important to undertake a careful assessment of the patient as a whole. The psychological profile may show severe abnormalities and this is important when planning treatment (Rehn and Lies, 1981). Smoking is known to have a deleterious effect on bone healing and it is important to ask the patient to stop before any treatment is instituted. The majority of patients are young males and may well have been unemployed for a considerable length of time prior to treatment. This may have serious implications and it is as important to consider the social, psychological and professional circumstances of the patient as it is to consider the clinical outcome for the fracture.

Treatment should not be undertaken without a thorough understanding of the personality of the pseudoarthrosis. An important distinction to be made at the beginning of the treatment regime is whether there is any potential for union and

instability is the problem, or whether the pseudoarthrosis has occurred because of insufficiency of the osteoinductive power of the bone ends. If instability is the primary cause the treatment focuses on providing the required skeletal stabilization. If the healing potential has been disturbed skeletal stabilization has to be supplemented by osteoinductive bone grafting.

There are a number of methods of managing non-unions and it is advisable that when choosing an appropriate treatment regime it be the simplest and most easily tolerated technique possible. The technique should be discussed in full with the patient and any potential risks explained. Preoperative planning is mandatory (Mast, 1983) and it is suggested that preoperative plans are drawn on transparencies overlying the X-rays. If possible it is worthwhile arranging for the patient to meet another patient who has already undergone this type of treatment.

All techniques for treating non-unions demand good reduction, adequate stabilization of the fractures and sufficient induction of healing. A combination of techniques is often required. Prophylactic antibiotic cover using a second generation cephalosporin is started the night before surgery and it is suggested that the antibiotic regime be continued for 5 days.

Aseptic non-union without malalignment

Intramedullary nailing

The details of the use of reamed interlocked intramedullary nails in the management of tibial fractures are described in Chapter 6. As with all operative techniques the successful use of nailing requires familiarity with the procedure (Figure 11.2). The intramedullary nailing of non-unions is more difficult than the intramedullary nailing of primary fractures and most authorities would suggest that it would be ill advised for an inexperienced surgeon to nail a non-union without prior practice (Kempf *et al.*, 1986; Baranowski and Pennig, 1988a, b; Brug and Pennig, 1988, 1990; Sledge *et al.*, 1989; Mayo and Benirschke, 1990; Tornquist, 1990; McLaren and Blokker 1991; Brug *et al.*, 1992; Pennig, 1994).

The patient is set up on a traction table. Usually a tourniquet is not required. The intramedullary canal of the tibia is opened through a standard approach. Frequently the bone is osteoporotic and penetration of the guidewire through the posterior tibial cortex is possible and must be avoided. Initially an olive tipped guidewire is placed into

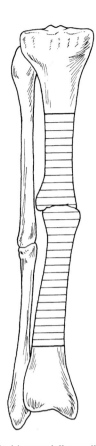

Figure 11.2 Locked intramedullary nailing in the tibia is suitable for the highlighted area

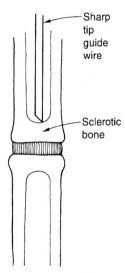

Figure 11.3 Penetration of sclerotic bone with an olive tip guidewire is impossible. A sharp tip guidewire is used which can be hammered or drilled through the sclerotic bone

the canal and advanced down to the level of the non-union. If there is only a little intramedullary sclerosis the guidewire may be held with a bundle nail clamp which not only provides for good grip on the guidewire but allows the guidewire to be rotated if necessary (Pennig, 1994). However it is often impossible to penetrate the non-union site with the olive tipped guidewire, this often being predictable by an examination of preoperative X-rays which will show a quantity of sclerotic bone at the non-union site. If this is the case one should change to a sharp tipped guidewire (Figure 11.3). This guidewire should be straight. With the assistance of the bundle nail clamp the sharp guidewire is hammered centrally through the non-union site. If there are difficulties in centralizing the guidewire at the site of the non-union one can avoid eccentric penetration by reaming down to the non-union site and inserting a nail of either 10 or 11 mm diameter. The nail is advanced down to the non-union (Figure 11.4). The sharp tipped guidewire is

now placed through the nail and as it is now centralized it can be advanced through the non-union. An alternative to hammering the guidewire through the sclerotic non-union site is to use a drill and drill the wire through.

If the sharp guidewire cannot be passed through a particularly sclerotic non-union the guidewire is advanced as far as possible into the non-union and the proximal fragment is reamed 12 or 13 mm using the standard flexible reamer. The guidewire is then removed under image intensifier control and the rigid Küntscher type hand reamers are used (Figure 11.4c). The non-union site is traversed by hammering and turning the reamer alternately. Once the non-union site is crossed the olive tipped guidewire is reinserted. It is necessary to use an olive tipped guidewire to retrieve a flexible reamer should it get stuck at or below the site of the non-union.

It is recommended that the flexible reamers be passed slowly across the non-union site and that

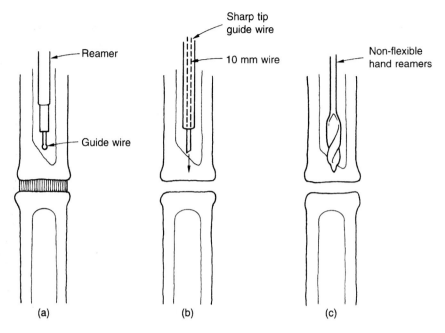

Figure 11.4 (a) If the guidewire cannot be centralized over the non-union to enter the distal fragment centrally, the proximal medullary canal is reamed to 12 mm. (b) A 10 mm nail is inserted and the sharp tip guidewire advanced through this nail for better guidance. (c) Non-flexible hand reamers can be used in very hard sclerotic bone. The hand reamers are advanced by hammering and turning

one should always start with an 8 or 9 mm reamer which cuts both at the tip and the sides. Slow reaming serves as a precaution against heat generation which may further devitalize the bone. When choosing the appropriate nail size the surgeon should be aware of the prolonged time to union and the different biomechanical requirements of non-unions compared to fresh fractures. It is recommended that a 12 mm tibial nail is used.

Reaming the intramedullary canal results in bone fragments being pushed into the non-union site and these act as a centromedullary bone graft (Tydings *et al.*, 1986; Sim *et al.*, 1993). This alone will stimulate healing and the insertion of the nail provides stability. In non-unions of the middle third unlocked nailing may be sufficient (Clancey *et al.*, 1992), but in more proximal non-unions proximal locking in two planes should be performed (Figure 11.5) (Kempf *et al.*, 1986), and in more distal non-unions distal locking with two screws is required (Figure 11.6) (Pennig *et al.*, 1988; Pennig and Brug, 1989). Statically locked nailing with screws above and below the non-union site is not advisable since weight bearing should lead to loading of the fracture site which helps to achieve union and bone remodelling (Pennig, 1994).

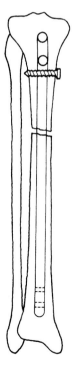

Figure 11.5 Placement of an intramedullary locking nail in a proximal tibial non-union. Locking in two planes is carried out proximally

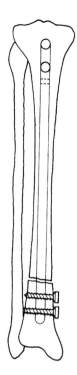

Figure 11.6 Locking nail in a distal tibial non-union. Distal locking with two screws

Aseptic non-union without malalignment

External fixation

External skeletal fixation may be used for compression of the non-union in cases without malalignment and, in conjunction with a partial fibulectomy, for stimulation of healing by gradual distraction and recompression (Ilizarov, 1971, 1990; De Bastiani *et al.*, 1990; Ribbons *et al.*, 1992; Saleh, 1992; Catagni *et al.*, 1994). The advantage of external fixation is that it is relatively non-invasive and the soft tissues around the non-union are not disturbed as they are in reamed nailing or plate fixation. Modern unilateral external fixators are stable enough to be used for the management of non-unions (Broekhuizen *et al.*, 1990).

In hypertrophic and oligotrophic non-unions without axial malalignment the unilateral, standard or LRS fixator as discussed in Chapter 9 is applied. It is recommended that the innermost pins should be about 3 cm from the non-union site. Three pins per clamp are used as the bone is almost always osteoporotic. A partial fibulectomy at the level of the non-union is performed (Sorensen, 1969;

Ternandez-Palazzi, 1969). In hypertrophic non-unions it is usually sufficient merely to compress the non-union site (Figure 11.7). It is recommended that the non-union be recompressed after one week but care should be taken not to overstrain the fixator pin. The patient can bear about 15 kg of weight as soon as the soft tissues have healed. After 4 weeks the fixator is dynamized and the patient is allowed to weight bear fully within a further 2 weeks. It is important that the fixator body is aligned with the axis of the tibia for weigh bearing to be effective (Figure 11.8).

In oligotrophic non-unions a partial fibulectomy should also be performed and the fixator applied in the same manner (Figure 11.9*a*). Oligotrophic non-unions require some stimulation of callus formation and a period of distraction of 1 mm per day for 7–10 days (Figure 11.9*b*) followed by recompression at the same speed of 1 mm per day is performed (Figure 11.9*c*). This was shown to stimulate callus formation by Yamagishi and Yoshimura (1955) and it has also been shown to promote bone union (Ilisarov, 1971; Ribbons *et al.*, 1992; Catagni *et al.*, 1994). It is particularly important to align the fixator body with the long axis of the tibia in order to avoid shear forces at the non-union site while undertaking distraction and compression.

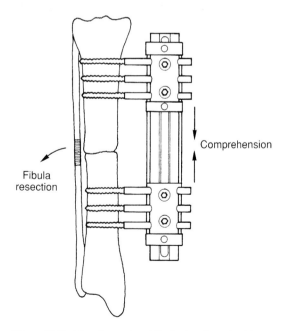

Figure 11.7 Use of an external fixator in a hypertrophic non-union. After fibular resection the non-union site is compressed during surgery and recompressed after 1–2 weeks

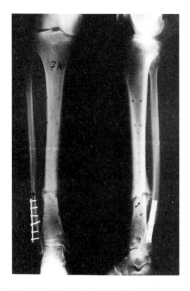

Figure 11.8 (a) Distal tibial non-union after plating with no progress for 7 months and intermittent infection

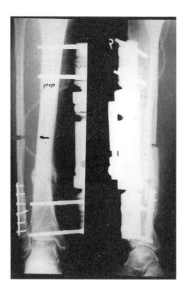

Figure 11.8 (b) Partial fibulectomy and fixator application

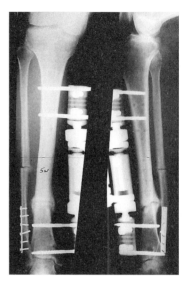

Figure 11.8 (c) After 5 weeks signs of bridging callus formation are present. The non-union site had been compressed mechanically

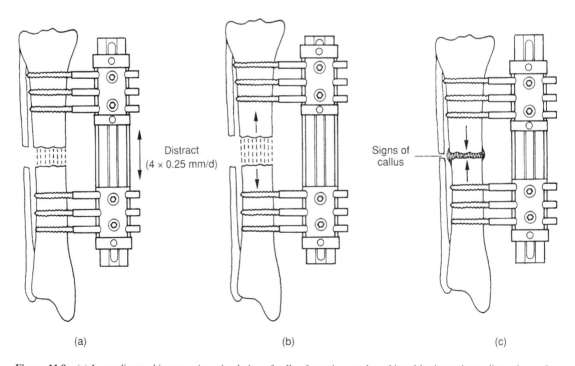

(a)   (b)   (c)

Figure 11.9 (a) In an oligotrophic non-union stimulation of callus formation can be achieved by intermittent distraction and compression. The limb reconstruction system (LRS) fixator is used in cases with no malalignment. (b) The non-union site distracted for 7–10 days at 1 mm per day. (c) Recompression results in formation of callus

In atrophic non-unions there is usually bone loss and the bone ends have to be squared off. The techniques applicable in these circumstances are described in Chapter 9 (De Bastiani *et al.*, 1987; Aldegheri *et al.*, 1989; Alonso and Regazzoni, 1990; Ilisarov, 1990; Johnson, 1994).

Aseptic non-union with malalignment

Intramedullary nailing: closed reduction

As in primary fracture treatment, it is mandatory to reduce the non-union prior to insertion of the nail. Closed reduction of the tibia after fibular osteotomy or partial fibulectomy lowers the risk of infection and should always be attempted.

The patient is placed on a traction table. If there is a valgus deformity the first step consists of undertaking a fibular osteotomy at the level of the non-union. If the deformity is varus a partial fibulectomy of between 15 and 20 mm is required. This again should be undertaken at the site of the non-union. An attempt is then made to reduce the mal-positioned tibia.

If the tibia can be reduced the assistant should maintain the reduction while the guidewire is advanced through the non-union site as described previously. The tip of the guidewire has to be placed exactly in the centre of the distal fragment of the tibia in both the anteroposterior and lateral planes to avoid a residual varus or valgus deformity (Pennig, 1994). During reaming the assistant must maintain the reduction. If this is impossible temporary external fixation may be used to maintain reduction. Correction of the axis is easier if the fixator is applied in the plane of the malalignment. In varus or valgus deformity one pin of the fixator is inserted from the medial side in the frontal plane parallel to the joint line at a distance of about 10 mm from the joint line. The second pin is inserted distally, again parallel with the joint line, so that sufficient space is available for the nail to be inserted and advanced (Figure 11.10*a*). The non-union is then reduced and the fixator used to maintain reduction (Figure 11.10*b*). The nail is then inserted (Figure 11.10*c*) and the fixator is removed after the nail and locking screws have been inserted.

Intramedullary nailing: open reduction

If it is impossible to align the non-union using closed means an open procedure must be performed. Usually small incisions are sufficient

(Saleh, 1991) as the stabilization is achieved by the nail insertion. Thus only the non-union site needs to be exposed.

In bayonet malalignments with an overlap of the fracture fragments the non-union site has to be mobilized with an osteotome. The overlap is reduced by distraction with a fixator and this may be quite difficult (Figure 11.11). Fibular osteotomy is necessary. Over-distraction is advisable to facilitate the reduction of the fragments. If the overlap is more than 1 cm a fixator may be applied over several days gradually to restore the length. Again over-distraction is necessary to facilitate reduction of the fragments. The surgeon may then choose either to carry on with external fixation or remove the fixator after intramedullary nailing.

It is important that when correcting valgus or varus deformities the soft tissues are given due consideration. A fibular osteotomy at the level of the non-union is initially performed. A closing wedge resection of the non-union is advisable if a valgus deformity is present as this reduces the soft tissue tension. If there is a varus deformity a medially based opening wedge osteotomy increases soft tissue tension. Instead of using a temporary external fixator it is possible to use a pelvic clamp for compression or distraction closing wedge and opening wedge osteotomies. This is illustrated in Figure 11.12. This method is particularly useful in those cases of non-union where plates have to be removed prior to nailing (Figure 11.13*a*). In cases where there is no plate the technique can be applied through a 4 to 5 cm incision. Prior to carrying out an opening wedge osteotomy a short 4.5 mm or 6.5 mm screw is inserted 15 to 20 mm proximal and distal to the base of the osteotomy (Figure 11.13*b*). For optimal purchase these screws are inserted through both cortices. After the correction has been achieved the screw has to be loosened such that it is unicortical in order to prevent obstruction of the intramedullary canal. In valgus deformities a wedge resection of the non-union site is carried out, the required angle having been calculated pre-operatively. The cortical screws are now tightened over the pelvic clamp and closing the pelvic clamp with the built-in compression device will lead to axial alignment (Figure 11.13*c*). Any small residual gap at the bone ends can be accepted as reaming is osteogenic and the reaming products will fill the gap (Tydings *et al.*, 1986; Pennig, 1994). The guidewire is now inserted centrally into the distal fragment (Figure 11.13*d*). The medullary canal is reamed to the level of the proximal screw and it is recommended that it is reamed 1–1.5 mm more

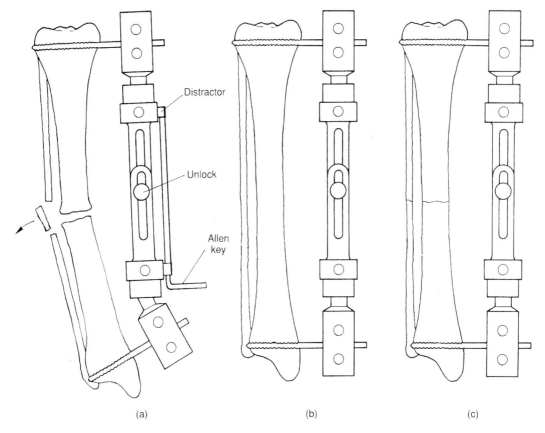

(a)   (b)   (c)

Figure 11.10   (a) Use of an unilateral external fixator (Orthofix) for correction of a varus deformity. Step one consists of a partial fibulectomy, and while distracting the distal ball joint is left unlocked. The reduction is assisted manually. (b) After correction of the varus deformity the fixator is locked. (c) Through using the standard technique an olive tip guidewire is inserted into the medullary canal. If penetration of the non-union is impossible, follow the steps outlined in Figure 11.4 and Figure 11.5 (a–c)

than the selected nail size. The screws are then backed out so that the reamer can pass (Figure 11.13*e*). Retightening of the pelvic clamp may be necessary at this point because of the increased leverage on the screws. The nail is inserted as described previously (Figure 11.13*f*). Distal or proximal locking is then performed. Finally the pelvic clamp and screws are removed (Figure 11.13*g*). Opening wedge osteotomies are performed in the same way and the resulting gap is packed with material collected from the reamer head. Usually the non-union will consolidate although some cases may require bone grafting of the gap. The alternative of a laterally based closing wedge osteotomy is technically more difficult and more traumatic to the adjacent soft tissue (Figure 11.14*h*).

This technique has the advantage of being more easy to control than the use of the external fixator

with the pins being placed at a distance from the osteotomy site. The osteotomy should always be subtotal leaving the lateral cortex intact. This acts as a hinge (Figure 11.12) and provides more stability and better control of the correction.

Intramedullary nailing in non-unions has the added benefit of restoring the morphology of the intramedullary canal. This reduces the likelihood of refracture compared with non-unions where the intramedullary nail is obliterated (Figure 11.14). The use of grafting techniques alone (Simon *et al.*, 1992; Rijnberg and van Linge, 1993) or in conjunction with internal fixation using a plate tend to obliterate the canal (Meyer *et al.*, 1975; Wiss *et al.*, 1992) and for this reason nailing techniques should be employed wherever possible.

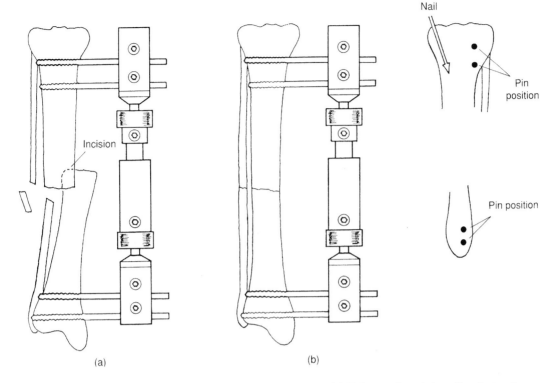

Figure 11.11 (a) Overlap in the tibial non-union with shortening. First a partial fibulectomy is carried out. Two fixator pins proximally and distally are inserted. The non-union site is mobilized and slow distraction over 20–30 minutes is carried out. *Insert*: the lateral view shows the position of the two proximal and two distal pins. (b) After slow distraction and overdistraction for about 5–10 mm the position is corrected. If this proves to be impossible, shortening of the fragments is required with an open approach

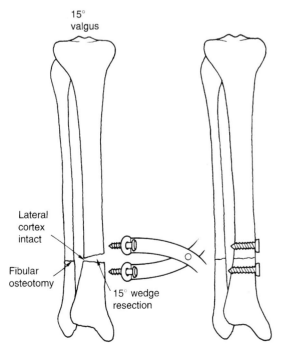

Figure 11.12 (a) Use of the pelvic clamp in correction of a valgus deformity in the distal tibia. An axial malalignment of 15° is corrected with the pelvic clamp after a fibular osteotomy. Note that the lateral cortex after wedge resection is intact. The reduction is manually assisted. (b) After the correct alignment has been achieved the pelvic clamp is locked

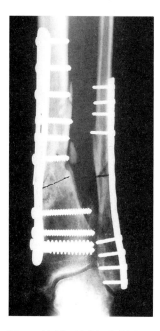

Figure 11.13   (a) Distal tibial non-union, fatigue fracture of the plate and malalignment with 20° valgus

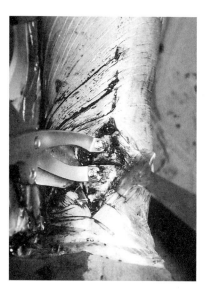

Figure 11.13   (c) With the assistance of the pelvic clamp the malalignment is corrected

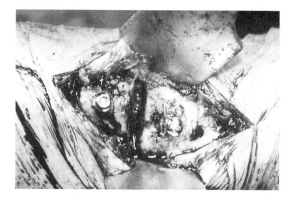

Figure 11.13   (b) Intraoperative photograph showing the resected area as well as the position of the proximal and the distal screw

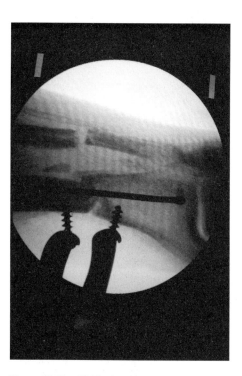

Figure 11.13   (d) The image intensifier view shows correct axial alignment. The guidewire has penetrated the non-union and is centralized in the distal fragment

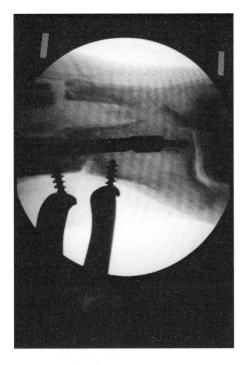

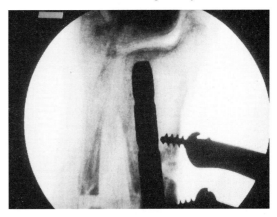

Figure 11.13   (f) The nail is inserted into the distal fragment

Figure 11.13   (e) It may be necessary to back out the screws to allow passage of the flexible reamer

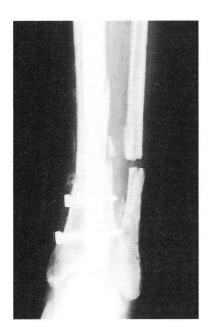

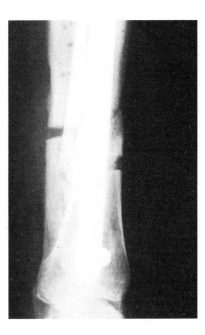

Figure 11.13   (g) AP and lateral film of the nail in place with two distal locking screws

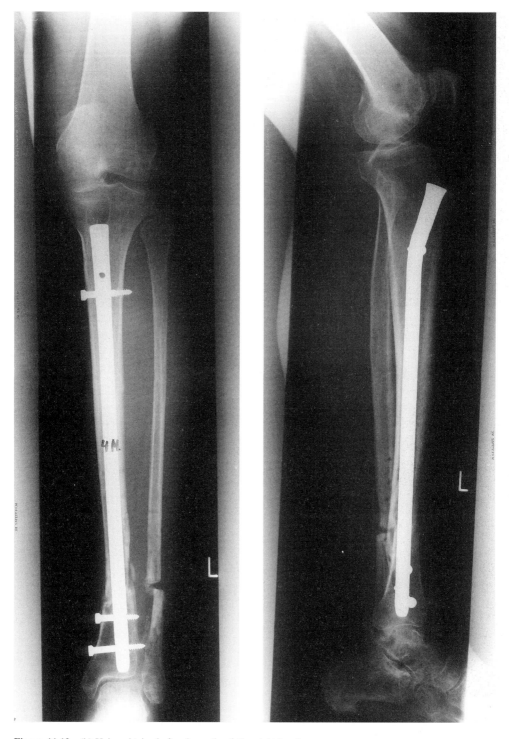

Figure 11.13   (h) Union obtained after 4 months; full weight bearing

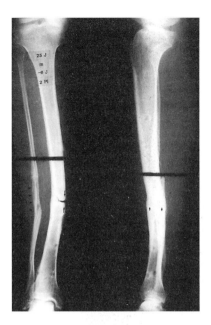

Figure 11.14 (a) Malalignment and sclerotic bone after plate fixation leading to fatigue fracture/non-union 6 years after the initial operation

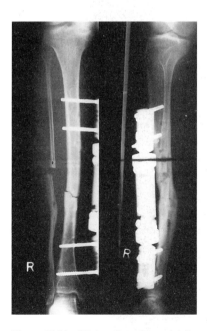

Figure 11.14 (b) A unilateral external fixator is used after a fibular osteotomy to achieve anatomical alignment which is a prerequisite for axial loading of the tibia

Aseptic non-union with malalignment

External fixation

In cases of non-union with axial malalignment a fibular osteotomy is required if the malalignment is valgus in direction and a partial fibulectomy is necessary should there be a varus malalignment.

Closed reduction of the non-union is initially attempted but if this is unsuccessful the non-union site must be mobilized with an osteotome if the non-union is hypertrophic or oligotrophic. An additional soft tissue release may be required. If the deformity is valgus the incision through which the soft tissue release is undertaken is placed over the lateral aspect of the tibia. With a varus deformity the incision is placed over the anteromedial aspect of the bone.

Once the non-union has been mobilized the malalignment is corrected and anatomical reduction achieved. It is important not to overlook any residual antecurvatum or recurvatum deformity persisting after the varus or valgus deformity has been corrected. Only correct axial alignment will lead to the diminution of the shear forces that are known to contribute to the development on non-union (Pauwels, 1965). In cases with axial malalignment it is important to insert the fixator pins at right angles to the long axis of the proximal and distal fragments. This will improve the alignment of the fixator body once the correction has been performed. If rotational correction is required this can also be dealt with by appropriate placement of the fixator pins. The same protocol for dynamization and full weight bearing as has already been described is followed after operative treatment.

The external fixation device can be expected to stay in position for about 4–6 months. Attention to pin care is important and adherence to a firm protocol is required. Radiological examination is performed twice during the first month and monthly thereafter. Union can be assumed when three cortices in both planes are bridged. If in doubt tomography may be helpful. As a routine practice it is recommended that the body of the fixator be removed and the fixator pins and clamps left in place. It is then possible to perform a clinical examination to assess the stiffness of the non-union. In addition the patient can be allowed to walk with unrestricted weight bearing. If no sequelae are reported by the patient he or she can be sent home with the fixator pins in position for a week and told to report back to the hospital if any problems are noted. Prior to the removal of the fixator pins a control X-ray should be taken and if the patient does not complain of any tenderness at the non-union site the pins can be removed. The patient should be protected with a brace for another 2–3 months.

In proximal and distal diaphyseal non-unions with or without malalignment the previously described technique can also be used. It is important to obtain good purchase in the shorter proximal or distal fragment and a three-dimensional pin placement using a metaphyseal clamp provides better fixation than the standard unilateral configuration. This is described in Chapter 7.

Varus malunions of the proximal tibia are almost invariably hypertrophic. Correction of such a malunion involves partial fibulectomy at the site of the non-union and care must be taken not to damage the peroneal nerve. The fixator pins are inserted parallel to the articular surface of the tibia

(Figure 11.15*a*) and a hemicallotasis hinge is employed (Figure 11.15*b*) (Baranowski *et al.*, 1989; Pennig and Baranowski, 1989; O'Dwyer *et al.*, 1991; A.G. MacEachern, personal communication). The non-union site is mobilized with an osteotome through a small medial incision. The lateral part of the non-union should be left intact to act as a hinge (Figure 11.15*b*). After a period of 10 days the non-union is asymmetrically distracted at a rate of 1 mm per day (Figure 11.15*e*, 11.15*f*). The asymmetrical distraction has been shown to promote callus formation (Ilizarov, 1971; Catagni *et al.*, 1994). During the distraction period X-rays should be taken weekly. These should be taken so that the axes of both the femur and the tibia can be assessed (Figure 11.15*g*, 11.15*h*). Care must be taken to apply an overcorrection of 8° valgus if there are degenerative changes present in the medial compartment of the knee (Coventry, 1985, 1987). During this asymmetrical distraction, or

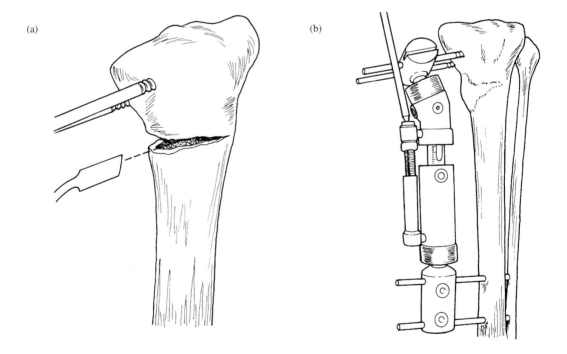

(a)

(b)

Figure 11.15 Asymmetrical distraction in proximal and distal varus non-union of the tibia. (a) The proximal horizontal pins are inserted parallel to the articular surface at a distance of 15–20 mm. The non-union is penetrated by an osteotome leaving the lateral cortex intact. Partial fibulectomy. (b) Gradual distraction of the hinged fixator corrects the varus deformity and promotes callus formation at the non-union site. (c) In varus deformities of the distal tibia a similar approach is used, with the pins being inserted parallel to the articular surface. (d) Gradual distraction corrects the malalignment and promotes callus formation in the non-union site. (e) Use of a hinged type unilateral external fixator for asymmetrical callus distraction (hemicallotasis) in a varus deformity. (f) Postoperative film showing the partial fibulectomy and the fixator in place. (g) Gradual distraction at 1 mm per day results in correction of the varus deformity as well as callus formation after 68 days. (h) Postoperative film after 4 months showing union

(c)

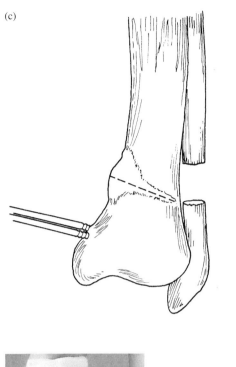

(d)

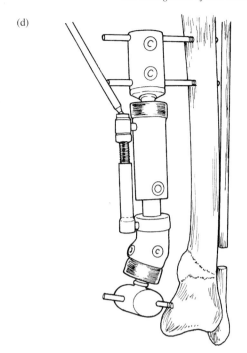

(e)

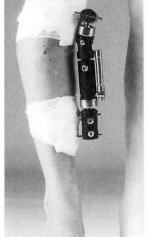

(f)

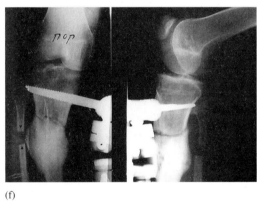

(g)

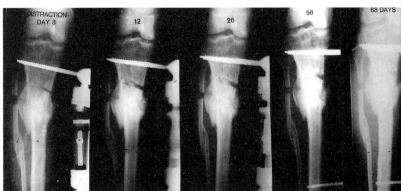

Figure 11.15 *cont.*

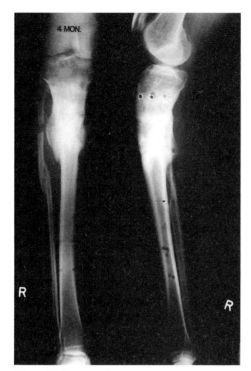

Figure 11.15 *cont.*   (h)

hemicallotasis, the surgeon should look for callus. If callus does not appear intermittent recompression at the rate of 1 mm per day is performed followed by redistraction. Once the desired fracture orientation has been achieved the fixator is adjusted to allow dynamization without shortening. This is described in Chapter 7. The patient should achieve full weight bearing within 4 weeks after controlled dynamization is initiated. In varus deformities of the distal tibia opening wedge osteotomies with the lateral cortex intact are performed in a similar fashion (Figure 11.15c, 11.15d). Again a partial fibulectomy of 15–20 mm in length is carried out to avoid any undue strain on the lateral malleolus. If there is a proximal or distal valgus deformity a closing wedge-osteotomy can be performed as has previously been described.

Bone grafting of tibial non-union

There are three main types of bone graft. These are cancellous grafts, corticocancellous grafts and bi-cortical or tricortical grafts (Figure 11.16). In tibial non-union cancellous and corticocancellous grafts are more commonly used (Weber and Cech,

1976; Weber and Brunner, 1981). The incidence of donor site morbidity is considerable if bicortical and tricortical grafts are harvested and alternative methods should be considered as up to 25% of patients report chronic pain after graft harvesting (Summer and Eisenstein, 1989). When bone grafting is required it is often helpful to estimate exactly how much bone can be harvested before exploring the non-union site.

The patient is positioned with a sandbag under the ipsilateral buttock as this not only permits access to the iliac crest but also facilitates the posterolateral approach to the tibia (Hanson and Eppright, 1966; Lamb, 1969; Simon *et al.*, 1992). A standard incision 1 cm below and parallel to the iliac crest is used. The incision should not extend as far as the anterior superior iliac spine to avoid any risk of injury to the lateral cutaneous nerve of the thigh (Figure 11.17a). The deep fascia is identified and divided close to the supero-medial edge of the wing of the ilium. A strip of muscle is left attached to the iliac crest to facilitate later repair. The oblique muscles are divided and the periosteum detached from the inner table of the wing of the ilium (Figure 11.17b). Corticocancellous chips can now be obtained from the inner table of the ilium (Figure 11.17c). It is suggested that the iliac crest be left intact if at all possible. If part of the iliac crest has to be elevated it is best to elevate it from the medial to the lateral side and leave the soft tissue attachment of the outer table intact (Figure 11.17c). It is always useful to harvest both corticocancellous strips and cancellous bone. The wound is closed over a suction drain. The harvesting of a bicortical graft is shown in Figure 11.17d and a tricortical graft in Figure 11.17e.

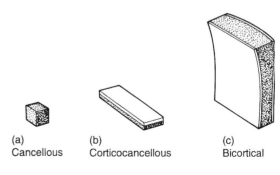

Figure 11.16 Types of bone graft. (a) Cancellous; (b) corticocancellous; (c) bicortical

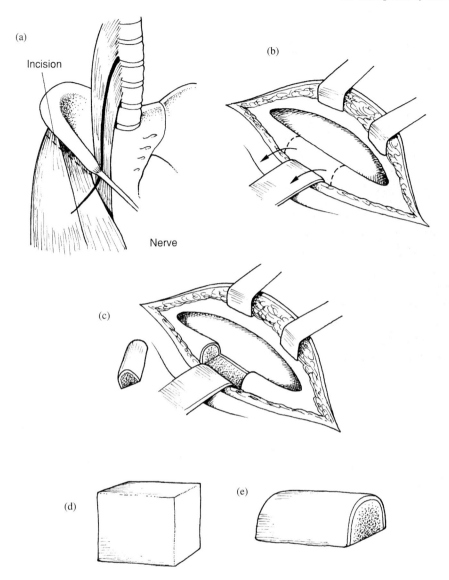

Figure 11.17 (a) Incision for open bone grafting 1 cm below the iliac crest. Observe the lateral femoral cutaneous nerve. (b) The iliac crest is exposed and the deep fascia detached from the medial side. After incision of the oblique muscles the inner table is exposed. The periosteum is detached from the iliac crest 3–5 cm distally from the inner table. After insertion of two Hohmann retractors, a lid of iliac crest may be lifted based laterally. (c) Corticocancellous chips from the inner table may be harvested with a suitable osteotome together with cancellous bone. (d) A bicortical block underneath the intact iliac crest may be elevated. (e) A tricortical block taken from the iliac crest

Percutaneous bone grafting

If smaller amounts of corticocancellous bone are required a percutaneous technique can be used (Saleh, 1991). A Meunier needle is inserted through a 2 cm incision which is made 5 cm from the anterior superior iliac spine. At this point the iliac crest is wide and permits the safe passage of the needle. The deep fascia is incised and dissected down to the bone. The Meunier needle is advanced with rotary movements between the inner and outer table and bicortical cones with a 7 mm diameter can be obtained (Figure 11.18*a*).

This technique may also be used through the

(a)

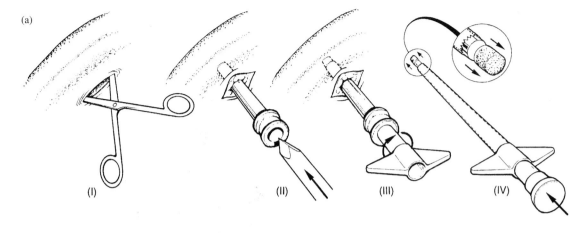

(b)

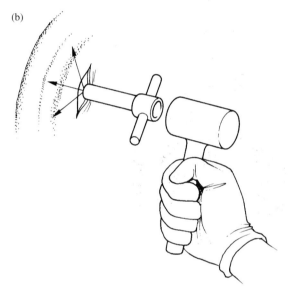

Figure 11.18   (a) Percutaneous bone grafting as described by Saleh (1991). 7 mm cones are obtained with a trephine. (b) A direct approach through the iliac crest allows two or three long cylinders to be harvested

iliac crest if more cancellous bone is desired. The iliac crest is thicker and more difficult to penetrate and assistance from an osteotome may be required. A 7–10 mm bone trephine can then be directed downwards and inserted almost parallel to the iliac crest. Long cylinders of cancellous bone can be obtained in this way (Figure 11.18*b*). Wound closure is undertaken in the usual fashion and it is recommended that a drain be used prior to closure. The fascia should also be sutured. Postoperative use of ice packs is recommended as in all bone harvesting procedures.

On-lay bone grafting

On-lay bone grafting was originally described by Henderson (1938) and Campbell (1932) but it is however rarely performed nowadays (Heppenstall, 1984). The technique involves considerable dissection and periosteal stripping. Shavings are removed from a small portion of the shaft forming a flat surface which extends 5 cm onto both bone fragments after non-union resection (Figure 11.19*a*). All soft tissues between the fragments must be removed.

The bone ends must be shaped so that their contact is good and the medullary canal of each fragment is opened until normal marrow is encoun-

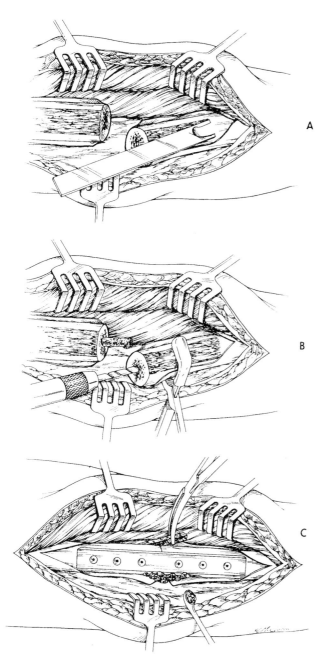

Figure 11.19 (a) Technique of on-lay bone grafting. Decortication is carried out on a small portion of the shaft. (b) The medullary canal of the proximal and distal fragment is opened by a drill. An endosteal graft is placed in the medullary canal. (c) Completion of on-lay bone grafting by screw fixation and cancellous bone chips

tered (Figure 11.19*b*). A full thickness cortical graft of sufficient length and width is removed from another part of the tibia. The graft is split longitudinally with a saw leaving an outer plate of solid cortical bone and an inner part consisting of endosteum. The cortical part should be as thick as possible. Prior to reduction fragments of the endosteum are inserted into the medullary canal. The strong cortical part of the graft is then placed across the non-union and held in place with two clamps. It is subsequently screwed into position using 3.5 or 4.5 mm cortical screws. Three screws proximal and distal to the non-union are required. Cancellous bone chips are then packed on both sides of the on-lay graft (Figure 11.19*c*). Postoperatively a cast is applied and once the swelling has subsided this can be changed to a walking cast which is kept in position for as long as required for consolidation to take place.

The major drawbacks of this technique are the large exposure that is required and the invasiveness of the harvesting technique. Nowadays this technique is rarely performed and its use is infrequently justified. The Phemister technique (1931) is not dissimilar but there is required dissection at the non-union site. One of the major problems of both these grafting techniques is that they invariably result in dense bone which is mechanically less efficient than the tubular bone that is produced after nailing of a non-union.

Electrical stimulation of tibial non-unions

Several methods of electrical stimulation have been devised to promote healing of tibial non-unions (Brighton, 1981; Day, 1981; Bassett, 1984). These are either invasive requiring the implantation of electrodes, semi-invasive requiring the percutaneous application of multiple electrodes, or non-invasive utilizing inductive coupling. The devices have to be used for several hours a day and are always used in conjunction with adequate cast immobilization. With the capacitive or inductive coupling devices several signals exist but clear scientific evidence is not as yet available despite the fact that the use of these devices dates back more than 20 years. The use of inductively coupled electromagnetic fields was first described in 1974 and was later used in the treatment of fracture non-unions (Bassett, 1984).

Sharrad (1990) published the results of a double-blind trial of the use of pulsed electromagnetic fields in delayed union of the tibia using fractures which did not all meet the criteria for established non-union. The series consisted of a very selective group of patients but was double-blind and randomized. Forty-five patients were treated, 20 of whom have active treatment with the remaining 25 having dummy units. There was a statistically significant difference in favour of the active group with $P = 0.02$. With the exception of this double-blind trial, no other trials of a similar design exist for established tibial non-union and therefore no firm recommendation can be made on the use of electronic stimulation.

Septic non-union

Low grade sepsis

Whenever low grade sepsis is present with clinical signs such as intermittent reddening or swelling or a history of drainage from the fracture site, the surgeon should bear in mind the potentially disastrous effects of an internal implant that becomes infected (Morandi *et al.*, 1989). A bone scan is performed and tomograms should be scrutinized for any sequestrum. The use of external fixation is advocated in these cases since no implant should be used at the non-union site. Antibiotic coverage should start the day before surgery and be administered for 2 weeks intravenously. A second generation cephalosporin is recommended. The principles described for aseptic non-unions should be followed in low grade sepsis and Ilizarov (1971, 1990) observed that the infection settles after union has been achieved. If the non-union site has been quiescent for some time it is best left undisturbed. If axial malalignment is present an attempt at a closed correction should be made. A fibular osteotomy or partial fibulectomy is required. If mobilization of the non-union site is necessary one has to avoid the thin vulnerable skin on the anteromedial surface of the tibia. A postero-medial or a lateral approach is more advisable.

Weight bearing and dynamization of the fixator frame should be started after the soft tissue situation has improved and healing of the soft tissues has been achieved.

Bone grafting in these cases should be avoided since the larger incision required may cause the infection to accelerate. If necessary, a posterolateral approach is advantageous. One has to bear in mind, however, that the grafted material initially is avascular, and as with all avascular material, is prone to being invaded by bacterial organisms. Therefore the indications for bone grafting should be questioned and alternative treatments should be sought.

Infected tibial non-union

In frank infection a combination of local bacterial sinuses and mechanical instability usually exists. The mechanical instability can be resolved with a unilateral or circular external fixator. The use of the circular fixator is described in Chapter 9. Technetium bone scans and tomograms as well as a complete study of the fracture X-rays and the evolution are necessary to understand the personality of the non-union. With an infected non-union the soft tissue situation is often less than ideal and after several attempts at surgical debridement one has to consider segmental resection of the whole non-union site and acute shortening of the tibia with an external fixator (see Chapter 9 for details). A partial fibulectomy (1 cm more than the tibial segment) is required and is the first step of the operation. This shortening has the added advantage of releasing the soft tissue tension and may allow excision of unstable scars and poor soft tissue areas which are adherent to the antero-medial aspect of the tibia. After consolidation has been obtained the tibia may be lengthened or the lengthening can be planned along with acute shortening (see Chapter 9 for details).

If acute shortening is not an option, skin cover remains the most serious problem. The first stage of the treatment consists of stabilization of the non-union. This is best carried out with a uni-lateral fixator using three pins per clamp since osteoporosis will be present and the fixator will stay on for a long period. The infected skin is excised and the avital and infected bone removed. Gentamicin beads are placed in the non-union site to release antibiotics into the infected area. Bacteriological testing should be carried out prior to insertion of the beads. Parenteral antibiotic administration is also used and the antibiotic chosen depends on the results of the bacteriological testing. Immediate definitive skin cover is unnecessary but a temporary split-thickness skin graft can be used. The split-thickness skin graft may be replaced by a fasciocutaneous flap some weeks after the initial operation. Clinical and laboratory signs of infection must be monitored. As the ESR and CRP improve, the second stage of the treatment can be started. This consists of adequate soft tissue coverage. The gentamicin beads are removed and the bone is re-explored. A fasciocutaneous flap is raised and it is important to avoid any tension when suturing it into place. Gentamicin beads are used again and a Ch 14 or 16 drain is mandatory. The gentamicin beads should be positioned in such a way that stepwise removal is possible. One bead is left protruding from the wound. If a fasciocutaneous flap is not sufficient, a local muscle flap, especially in the proximal tibia (gastrocnemic muscle), may be used. Alternatively custom tailored muscle flaps like the rectus abdominus or latissimus dorsi are employed (see Chapter 10). It is important to understand that the infection will not settle unless the soft tissue coverage is adequate and the importance of a good soft tissue envelope cannot be overemphasized. Two weeks after the operation the gentamicin beads are removed one or two a day, thereby allowing the soft tissues to form granulative tissue to fill the gap left by removal of the beads. If the gentamicin beads were removed all at once, too a large cavity would result.

Papineau grafting

In cases with problematic soft tissues and co-existing vascular problems prohibiting the use of free vascularized flaps the Papineau technique may be used (Ribbons *et al.*, 1992; Saleh, 1992). The non-union site is cleared of all fibrous tissue and infected bone. Gentamicin beads are used and the wound is left open and kept moist for conditioning (Figure 11.20*a*). Parenteral antibiotics are required and 1–2 weeks after the initial operation a second look is carried out. A bone decortication is carried out until bleeding bone is reached and the cavity, which by then should look healthy and granular, is packed with small diameter cancellous bone (Figure 11.20*b*). It is important to fill the cavity to the level of the skin and keep the graft moist from the outside. Temporary cover using artificial skin is not required since the wound should not be occluded. With a successful application of this technique about one-third of the graft can be expected to be resorbed but granulation of the skin from the edges is expected to take place. A split-thickness skin graft is used as soon as a granulating surface is apparent (Figure 11.20*c*).

The bone requires stabilization with an external fixator while this treatment is carried out and weight bearing is not allowed. We temporarily immobilize the ankle joint to avoid mechanical irritation caused by muscle moving at the non-union site.

With longstanding septic non-union amputation has to be discussed with the patient as an alternative. Invariably with further surgery to preserve the leg the treatment will be lengthy and in most cases last for more than a year. A higher proportion of patients with infected non-unions also have scarring of the deep calf muscles, and the function of the knee, the ankle and foot has to be carefully assessed. Patients should be allowed to consider their position, and should ideally be brought into contact with patients having had a successful reconstruction as well as those who opted for amputation. Amputation for the surgeon should not be seen as a defeat, but in some cases the better choice for the patient (Ribbons *et al.*, 1992).

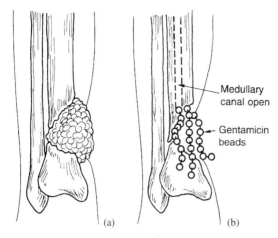

Medullary
canal open

Gentamicin
beads

(a)   (b)

Figure 11.20   (a) After thorough debridement and opening of the medullary canal gentamicin beads are inserted in a distal tibial non-union defect. The cavity has to be kept moist with an aseptic betadine solution. (b) Removal of gentamicin beads and further decortication. The cavity is filled with cancellous bone which is lightly packed until it reaches the skin level

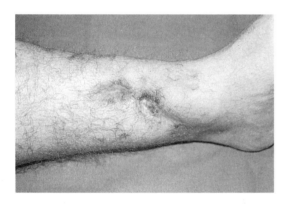

Figure 11.20   (c) Clinical photograph after Papineau grafting

Results

Non-unions tend to be very different in personality and therefore a comparison of different techniques is difficult.

Fifteen non-unions of the tibia in 49 patients after external fixation and immobilization in a cast treated by compression plating resulted in a non-union rate of 92%. Deep infection occurred in 6%, a fatigue fracture of the plate in 8%, necessitating replating or external fixation. The incidence of bone grafting in these series was 78% (Wiss *et al.*, 1992).

Twenty-five non-unions of tibial fractures treated with a GK locked intramedullary nail without bone grafting resulted in a union rate of 100% (Alho *et*

al., 1993). There were 3 postoperative infections, 2 showed persistent drainage. All patients had a fibular osteotomy or resection in addition to the nailing procedure. In 15 tibial non-unions locked intramedullary nailing resulted in a 93% non-union rate (Warren and Brooker, 1992). There was one refracture after nail removal. Rosson and Simonis (1992) treated 24 patients with established non-union of tibial shaft fractures with locked intramedullary nailing and achieved union in 22 patients. Two failures were in patients developing active infection. The principle of distraction osteogenesis in the treatment of stiff hypertrophic non-unions was applied by Catagni *et al.* (1994): 21 hypertrophic non-unions in 19 patients were treated and remained 4–12 months in the frame. Stable union was achieved in all patients and angular axial and translational deformities were corrected.

De Bastiani *et al.* (1990) treated 85 cases of non-union, of which 51 were atrophic, 21 were hypertrophic and 13 septic, with their unilateral fixator. Forty-four cases were in the tibia. Treatment included decortication in septic cases and application of the fixator under compression and hypertrophic cases. The average healing time in aseptic non-union was 150 days (in septic, 270 days). Six non-unions persisted (7%) and there were 5 cases of pin site osteolysis in 340 screws (1.5%).

Marsh *et al.* (1992) treated 25 long bone non-unions with a dynamic axial fixator of which 17 cases were culture-positive; 10 had open draining wounds. The additional treatment consisted of debridement, soft tissue repair and bone grafting. It is worth noting that 9 of the 10 hypertrophic cases healed without grafting and further intervention at an average of 18.1 weeks. There was no treatment failure.

Other techniques included autologous marrow in percutaneous injection (Bier, 1905) resulting in union in all cases, which was achieved after an average of 10 weeks clinically (range 4–23 weeks), and radiologically after 17 weeks (range 9–29 weeks). (Sim *et al.*, 1993). Central grafting for persistent non-union of the tibia was used by Rijnberg and van Linge (1993) in 48 tibias. Union was obtained in 45 out of 48 after one operation only. There was one failure which required amputation.

The treatment of non-union remains a challenge. There are many aspects which merit consideration, starting with the individual patient, the surgeon's personal experience and the familiarity with the technique to be used. For optimal treatment the management of these patients is best concentrated in specialized units.

References

Albert, M. (1944) Delayed union in fractures of the tibia and fibula. *J. Bone Joint Surg.*, **26**, 566

Aldegheri, R., Renzi-Brivio, L. and Agostini, S. (1989) The callotasis method of limb lengthening. *Clin. Orthop. Rel. Res.*, **241**, 137

Alho, A., Ekeland, A., Stromsoe, K. *et al.* (1993) Nonunion of tibial shaft fractures treated with locked intramedullary nailing without bone grafting. *J. Trauma*, **34** (1), 62

Alonso, J.E. and Regazzoni, P. (1990) The use of the Ilizarov concepts with the AO/ASIF tubular fixateur in the treatment of segmental defects. *Orthop. Clin. North Am.*, **21**, 655

Baranowski, D. and Pennig, D. (1988a) Grenzindikationen der Verriegelungsnagelung. in *Osteosynthèse International* (eds H.C. Nonnemann, V. Vécsei and R. Lindholm), Schnetztor-Verlag, Konstanz, p. 402

Baranowski, D. and Pennig, D. (1988b) Zum Zeitpunkt des Verfahrenswechsel Verplattung/Verriegelungsnagelung. In *Osteosynthèse International* (eds H.C. Nonnemann, V. Vécsei, R. Lindholm), Schnetztor-Verlag, Konstanz, p. 419

Baranowski, D., Pennig, D. and Klein, W. (1989) Posttraumatische Varusdeformität der Tibia – Korrektur durch Osteoklasie und Kallotaxis. *Zentralbl. Chir.*, **114**, 1427

Bassett, C.A.L. (1984) The development and application of pulsed electromagnetic fields (PEMFs) for ununited fractures and arthrodeses. *Orthop. Clin. North Am.*, **15**, 61

Bier, A. (1905) Die Bedeutung des Blutergusses für die Heilung des Knochenbruches. Heilung von Pseudarthrosen und von verspäteter Callusbildung durch Bluteinspritzung. *Medizin. Klin.*, 1, 6

Bier, A. (1923) Knochenregeneration, Pseudarthrosen und Knochentransplatation. *Arch. Klin. Chir.*, **127**, 1

Boyd, H.B. and Lipinski, S.W. (1960) Causes and treatment of nonunions of the shafts of the long bones, with a review of 741 patients. *AAOS Instr. Course Lect.*, **17**, 165

Brighton, C.T. (1981) Treatment of nonunion of the tibia with constant direct current. *J. Trauma*, **21**, 189

Broekhuizen, A.H., Boxma, H., van der Meulen, P.A. *et al.* (1990) Performance of external fixation devices in femoral fractures; the ultimate challenge? *Injury*, **21**, 145

Brug, E. and Pennig, D. (1988) Standortbestimmung der Verriegelungsnagelung. In *Jahrbuch der Chirurgie* (ed. H. Bünte), Regensberg & Biermann, Münster, p. 145

Brug, E. and Pennig, D. (1990) Indikation zur Verriegelungsnagelung. *Unfallchirurg*, **93**, 492

Brug, E., Pennig, D. and Baranowski, D. (1992) Verriegelungsnagelung nach aseptischen Komplikationen an Femur und Tibia. In *Osteosynthèse International* (eds V. Vécsei and H.C. Nonnemann), Schnetztor-Verlag, Konstanz, p. 357

Campbell, W.C. (1932) Ununited fractures. *Arch. Surg.*, **24**, 990

Catagni, M.A., Guerreschi, F. and Holman, J.A. *et al.* (1994) Distraction osteogenesis in the treatment of stiff hypertrophic nonunions using the Ilizarov apparatus. *Clin. Orthop. Rel. Res.*, **301**, 159

Clancey, G.J., Winquist, R.A. and Hansen, S.T. Jr (1982) Nonunion of the tibia treated with Küntscher intramedullary nailing. *Clin. Orthop.*, **167**, 191

Coventry, M.B. (1985) Current concepts review: Upper tibial osteotomy for osteoarthritis. *J. Bone Joint Surg.*, **67A**, 1136

Coventry, M.B. (1987) Proximal tibial varus osteotomy for osteoarthritis of the lateral compartment of the knee. *J. Bone Joint Surg.*, **69A**, 32

Day, L. (1981) Electrical stimulation in the treatment of ununited fractures. *Clin. Orthop.*, **161**, 54

De Bastiani, G., Agostini, S. and Leso, P. *et al.* (1990) Trattamento delle pseudartrosi con fissatore esterno assiale. *Atti della Societa Eliliana Romagnola Triveneta di Ortopedia e Traumatologia*, vol. **XXXII**, fascicolo I, p. 17

De Bastiani, G., Aldegheri, R. and Renzi-Brivio, L. *et al.* (1987) Limb lengthening by callus distraction (callotasis). *J. Pediatr. Orthop.*, **7**, 129

De Souza, L.J. (1987) Healing time of tibial fractures in Ugandan Africans. *J. Bone Joint Surg.*, **69B**, 56

Dickson, K., Katzman, S. and Delgado, J. *et al.* (1994) Delayed nonunions of open tibial fractures. *Clin. Orthop. Rel. Res.*, **302**, 189

Esterhai, J.L. Jr, Brighton, C.T. and Heppenstall, R.B. *et al.* (1984) Technetium and gallium scintigraphic evaluation of patients with long-bone fracture nonunion. *Orthop. Clin. North Am.*, **15**, 125

Hanson, L.W. and Eppright, R.H. (1966) Posterior bone-grafting of the tibia for nonunions: a review of twenty-four cases. *J. Bone Joint Surg.*, **48A**, 27

Henderson, M.S. (1938) Bone graft in ununited fractures. *J. Bone Joint Surg.*, **20**, 635

Heppenstall, R.B. (1984) The present role of bone graft surgery in treating nonunion. *Orthop. Clin. North Am.*, **15**, 113

Heppenstall, R.B., Brighton, C.T. and Esterhai, J.L. Jr *et al.* (1984) Prognostic fractors in non union of the tibia. *J. Trauma*, **24**, 790

Hunter, J. (1837) *Collected Works* (ed. by J.F. Palmer), 4 vols, London

Ilizarov, G.A. (1971) Basic principles of transosseous compression and distraction osteosynthesis (Russian). *Orthop. Traumatol. Protez*, **32**(11), 7

Ilizarov, G.A. (1990) Clinical application of the tension-stress effect for limb lengthening. *Clin. Orthop.*, **250**, 8

Johnson, E.E. (1994) Acute lengthening of shortened lower extremities after malunion or non-union of a fracture. *J. Bone Joint Surg.*, **76A**, 379

Kempf, I., Grosse, A. and Rigaut, P. (1986) The treatment of noninfected pseudarthrosis of the femur and tibia with locked intramedullary nailing. *Clin. Orthop.*, **121**, 142

Key, J.A. (1937) Treatment of nonunion of fractures. *Surgery*, **1**, 730

Lamb, R.H. (1969) Posterolateral bone graft for nonunion of the tibia. *Clin. Orthop.*, **64**, 114

Marsh, J.L., Nepola, J.V. and Meffert, R. (1992) Dynamic external fixation for stabilization of nonunions. *Clin. Orthop. Rel. Res.*, **278**, 200

Mast, J. (1983) Preoperative planning in the surgical correction of tibial nonunions and malunions. *Clin. Orthop.*, **178**, 26

Mayo, K.A. and Benirschke, S.K. (1990) Treatment of tibial malunions and nonunions with reamed intramedullary nails. *Orthop. Clin. North Am.*, **21**, 715

McLaren, A.C. and Blokker, C.P. (1991) Locked intramedullary fixation for metaphyseal malunion and nonunion. *Clin. Orthop. Rel. Res.*, **265**, 253

Meyer, S., Weiland, A.J. and Willenegger, H. (1975) The treatment of infected non-union of fractures of long bones: study of 64 cases with a 5 to 21 year follow-up. *J. Bone Joint Surg.*, **57A**, 836

Morandi, M., Zembo, M.M. and Ciotti, M. (1989) Infected tibial pseudarthrosis: a 2-year follow-up on patients treated by the Ilizarov technique. *Orthopedics*, **12**, 497

O'Dwyer, K.J., MacEachern, A.G. and Pennig, D. (1991) Corrective tibial osteotomy for genu recurvatum by callus distraction using an external fixator. *Chirugia degli Organi de Movimentto*, **76**(4), 355

Paley, D., Chaludray, M. and Pirone, M. *et al.* (1990) Treatment of malunions and mal-nonunions of the femur and tibia by detailed preoperative planning and the Ilizarov techniques. *Orthop. Clin. North Am.*, **21**, 667

Pauwels, F. (1965) *Gesammelte Abhandlungen zur funktionellen Anatomie des Bewegungsapparates.* Springer-Verlag, Berlin

Pennig, D. (1990) Zur Biologie des Knochens und der Knochenbruchheilung. *Unfallchirurg*, 23, 488

Pennig, D. (1994) Current use of the intramedullary nail. In *Current practice of Fracture Treatment* (ed. P.C. Leung), Springer-Verlag, Berlin, p. 119

Pennig, D. and Baranowski, D. (1989) Genu recurvatum due to partial growth arrest in the proximal tibial physis: correction by callus distraction. *Arch. Orthop. Trauma Surg.*, **108**, 119

Pennig, D. and Brug, E. (1989) Das Einbringen der distalen Bolzen bei der Verriegelungsnagelung mit einem neuen Freihand-Zielgeräte. *Unfallchirurg*, **92**, 331

Pennig, D., Brug, E. and Kronholz, H.L. (1988) A new distal aiming device for locking nail fixation. *Orthopedics*, **11**, 1725

Phemister, D.B. (1931) Splint grafts in the treatment of delayed and non-union of fractures. *Surg. Gynecol. Obstet.*, **52**, 376

Rehn, J. and Lies, A. (1981) Die Pathogenese der Pseudarthrose, ihre Diagnostik und Therapie. *Unfallheilkunde*, **84**, 1

Ribbans, W.J., Stubbs, D.A. and Saleh, M. (1992) Non-union surgery. Part II: The Sheffield experience – one hundred consecutive cases. Results and lessons. *Int. J. Orthop. Trauma*, **2**, 19

Rijnberg, W.J. and van Linge, B. (1993) Central grafting for persistent nonunion of the tibia. *J. Bone Joint Surg.*, **75B**, 926

Rosenthal, R.E., MacPhail, J.A. and Ortiz, J.E. (1977) Nonunions in open tibial fractures. *J. Bone Joint Surg.*, **59A**, 244

Rosson, J.W. and Simonis, R.B. (1992) Locked nailing for nonunion of the tibia. *J. Bone Joint Surg.*, **74B**, 358

Schatzker, J. (1990) Intraarticular malunions and nonunions. *Orthop. Clin. North Am.*, **21**, 743

Saleh, M. (1991) Bone graft harvesting: a percutaneous technique. *J. Bone Joint Surg.*, **73B**, 867

Saleh, M. (1992) Non-union surgery. Part I: Basic principles of management. *Int. J. Orthop. Trauma*, **2**, 4

Sharrad, W.J.W. (1990) A double-blind trial of pulsed electromagnetic stimulation. *J. Bone Joint Surg.*, **72B**, 347

Sim, R., Liang, T.S., Tay, B.K. (1993) Autologous marrow injection in the treatment of delayed and non-union in long bones. *Singapore Med. J.*, **34**(5), 412

Simon, J.P., Stuyck, J., Hoogmartens, M. *et al.* (1992) Posterolateral bone grafting for nonunion of the tibia. *Acta Orthop. Belg.*, **58**(3), 308

Sledge, S.L., Johnson, K.D., Henley, M.B. *et al.* (1989) Intramedullary nailing with reaming to treat non-union of the tibia. *J. Bone Joint Surg.*, **71A**, 1004

Sorensen, K.H. (1969) Treatment of delayed union and nonunion of the tibia by fibular resection. *Acta Orthop. Scand.*, **40**, 92

Summer, B.N. and Eisenstein, S.M. (1989) Donor site pain from the ilium; a complication of lumbar spinal fusion. *J. Bone Joint Surg.*, **71B**, 677

Taylor, J.C. (1992) Delayed union and nonunion of fractures. In *Campbells Operative Orthopaedics* (ed. A.H. Crenshaw), 8th edn., vol. II, Mosby-Year Book, St Louis, p. 1287

Ternandez-Palazzi, F. (1969) Fibular resection in delayed union of tibial fractures. *Acta Orthop. Scand.*, **40**, 105

Tornqvist, H. (1990) Tibia nonunions treated by interlocking nailing: increased risk of infection after previous external fixation. *J. Orthop. Trauma*, **4**, 109

Tydings, D., Leon, J., Martino, J. *et al.* (1986) The osteoinductive potential of intramedullary canal bone reamings. *Curr. Surg.*, **43**, 121

Warren, S.B. and Brooker, A.F. Jr (1992) Intramedullary nailing of tibial nonunions. *Clin. Orthop. Rel. Res.*, **285**, 236

Weber, B.G. and Brunner, C. (1981) The treatment of nonunions without electrical stimulation. *Clin. Orthop.*, **161**, 24

Weber, B.G. and Cech, O. (1976) *Pseudarthrosis: Pathology, Biomechanics, Therapy, Results*, Hans Huber, Berne

Wiss, D.A., Johnson, D.L. and Miao, M. (1992) Compression plating for non-union after failed external fixation of open tibial fractures. *J. Bone Joint Surg.*, **74A**, 1279

Yamagishi, M. and Yoshiyuki, Y. (1955) The biomechanics of fracture healing. *J. Bone Joint. Surg.*, **37A**, 1035

12

Post-traumatic amputation

D. Pennig

Introduction

The sudden unexpected loss of part or all of a limb is obviously very upsetting to a patient. In addition the surgeon who has to carry out an amputation in a seriously injured extremity often perceives the amputation as representing failure (Shah *et al.*, 1987; Heatley, 1988).

A review of the history of amputation surgery shows that it dates back to prehistoric times. Hippocrates, Galen and others discussed amputation surgery at length. It used to be a brutal affair performed without anaesthesia and usually associated with significant mortality. In the 16th century Paré used ligation of major blood vessels for the first time and thereby avoided the torture of cauterization (Harris, 1944). Subsequent progress in amputation technique has usually come about as a result of wars with their attendant casualties. Dominique Jean Larrey, the surgeon in chief of the 'Grande Armée' under Napoleon Boneparte developed amputation techniques further and was able to improve survival rates (Harris, 1944). Amputation surgery was also very important in both World War I and World War II. The incidence of amputation rose in the Second World War to 5.3% compared with an incidence of between 2–3% in the First World War, the rise being due to the use of more powerful and sophisticated weaponry.

Until recently the objective of all amputation surgery was to conserve limb length at all costs. However within the past five to six decades it has become recognized that an efficient artificial prosthesis may be more desirable than a poorly covered stump encased in a device which cannot be effectively used (Baumgartner, 1983). It has also become recognized that a well-fashioned below-knee end bearing stump providing a number of pressure sensitive areas around which a weight-bearing prosthesis can be moulded (Figure 12.1) is the best amputation after many serious injuries.

The development of amputation surgery was mainly related to trauma, usually from the battlefield. Other indications for amputation such as peripheral vascular disease, malignant tumours or sepsis were less common (De Bakey and Simeone, 1946; American Medical Association, 1989). Post-traumatic amputation mainly occurs in younger patients and fortunately therefore the surgeon can usually rely on an adequate blood supply to the

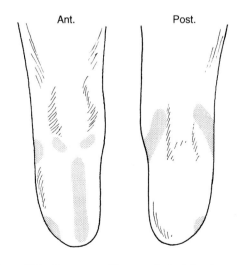

Figure 12.1 Pressure-sensitive areas in the below-knee stump

tissues proximal to the amputation site (Conkle *et al.*, 1975; Flint and Richardson, 1983; Caudle and Stern, 1987; Edwards *et al.*, 1988).

Recently there has been a change in the epidemiology of amputation. Currently between 20 000 and 30 000 new amputees are recorded in the United States of America each year. These are now mainly the result of an ageing population with high incidences of amputations being recorded secondary to diabetes mellitus and peripheral vascular disease (Tooms, 1992a,b). However in younger patients amputations are still usually post-traumatic in origin (Gustilo and Anderson, 1976; Gustilo *et al.*, 1984; Georgiadis *et al.*, 1993). About 75% of all new amputees are men and approximately 85% of amputations occur in the lower limbs with an equal distribution of right and left legs (Tooms, 1992b).

Indications for amputation

Trauma remains the second most common cause of amputation and is the principal indication in adults under 50 years of age (Tooms, 1992b). In burns and frostbite potentially viable tissue may be saved by allowing time for a clear demarcation line to appear. This will assist in the decision as to the amputation level. Electrical burns are often more difficult to assess as frequently the deep tissues are involved and a superficial inspection of the wound does not suggest the severity of deep tissue damage. Thus frequently the required amputation is performed at a higher level than initially anticipated (Tooms, 1992b).

Most commonly, however, it will be blunt or penetrating trauma that will be the reason for consideration of amputation of the lower leg (Hicks, 1964; Seiler and Richardson, 1986; Hansen, 1987; Herve *et al.*, 1987; Helfet *et al.*, 1990). In these cases a decision has to be made as to whether reconstruction offers a reasonable chance of restoring function or whether primary amputation should be performed (Hutchins, 1981; Rojczyk, 1983; Mellissinos and Parks, 1985; Lancaster *et al.*, 1986; Herve *et al.*, 1987; Howe *et al.*, 1987; Lange, 1989).

Preoperative assessment

The vascular and neurological status of the limb is of paramount importance (McNamara *et al.*, 1973; Sher, 1975; Peacock and Proctor, 1977; Snyder, 1982; Keeley *et al.*, 1983; Lange *et al.*, 1985).

Arteriography will not provide sufficient information as to the adequacy of tissue perfusion and therefore percutaneous oximetry together with Doppler ultrasound may be used. Before a decision is made regarding the necessity of amputation the affected limb should be explored (Gustilo and Anderson, 1976; Gustilo *et al.*, 1984). A tourniquet should be used and the wound cleaned. This should be followed by a thorough surgical debridement with all contaminated and devitalized tissues being removed. At this stage it is important to assess the neurological status of the limb (Johansen *et al.*, 1983; Kemp *et al.*, 1993). If limb function is to be adequate it is important that the posterior tibial and peroneal nerves are intact. If the posterior tibial nerve has been transected the usefulness of the limb is questionable and consideration should be given to amputation (Gregory *et al.*, 1985).

There are a number of other factors to consider when considering amputation. Surgeons often concentrate on the damage to arteries or veins. However reconstruction of both arteries and veins is technically possible even if the defect is large. It is important to assess adequately the state of the skin and its perfusion. In addition it should be remembered that viable muscle is necessary if there is to be useful function in the limb and if most of the muscle mass on the dorsal and anterolateral aspects of the limb has been extensively damaged then, even in the presence of intact nerves, the function will be very limited. Lastly the extent of any coexisting fractures and soft-tissue injuries to the knee, ankle and foot play an important part in the decision as to whether to attempt salvage or to amputate the limb (Gregory *et al.*, 1985). Two level injuries with vascular and neurological impairment are almost impossible to reconstruct (Keeley *et al.*, 1983) and amputation is generally the best choice. The Mangled Extremity Severity Score (Johansen *et al.*, 1983) is useful in summarizing the different factors that may lead to a decision about salvage or amputation (Hutchins, 1981; Clarke and Mollan, 1994). Often the indications for salvage or amputation are borderline and it is strongly advised that senior expertise be sought to assess the extent of the injury and to relate these findings to the eventual functional outcome (Fairhurst, 1994). If possible the decision to amputate should be agreed by two surgeons.

There are a number of other considerations when making a decision about amputation, not least of these is the surgeon's experience with the management of the severely injured extremity and the first decision to be made is whether to refer the patient to a specialist trauma centre. In addition the age and physical state of the patient will also determine his or her suitability for amputation. A young patient may have sufficient time to get used to a prosthetic limb but in elderly patients this is not always the case. However if the decision to amputate is delayed in an elderly patient an above knee amputation may be required rather than a below knee amputation which might have been possible had a decision been taken earlier. It is important to bear in mind that elderly patients will rarely use an above knee prosthesis and if an above knee amputation is performed the patient will probably be confined to a wheelchair (Tooms, 1992b).

In the presence of multiple life-threatening injuries reconstruction of a limb is usually impossible and attempts to do so many compromise the patient (Goris, 1983). In addition coexisting disorders such as peripheral vascular disease, hemiplegia affecting the injured side or paraplegia affect the decision as to whether amputation or reconstruction be performed. The social background of the patient should be assessed if this is possible. If limb reconstruction is undertaken this will involve the patient in a prolonged rehabilitation time and while this may save the limb it may well have a deleterious effect on the social and professional life of the patient (Bondurant *et al.*, 1988). In adults any delay of more than 6 hours in restoring tissue perfusion makes successful restoration of muscle function unlikely (McQuillan and Nolan, 1968). Under these conditions muscle has been devitalized for too long a period and this may lead to myonecrosis, renal failure and death of the patient.

Technical aspects of amputation

Once a decision to amputate the limb has been made it should be performed as early as possible. Although the patient will be understandably upset about having had an amputation performed after a major injury it is important that those cases that are obviously unreconstructable should be amputated immediately. It has been shown that the earlier the decision is made to amputate the easier it is to salvage most tissue and the longer the amputation stump will be (Bondurant *et al.*, 1988).

In post-traumatic amputations the local tissues may be very oedematous rendering skin closure difficult. The skin flaps will have to be designed depending on the area and location of the traumatized tissues and atypical skin flaps may therefore

be required. Poor skin coverage may be tolerated more readily than in amputations carried out for peripheral vascular disease as perfusion in this younger age group can be expected to be better. The surgeon should remember that skin grafts can be harvested from the amputated leg.

In those cases where there is excessive swelling or severe contamination a guillotine amputation should be considered or if a standard amputation is performed the skin flaps should be left open (Saleh, 1993). This assists in identifying viable tissues and eventually may lead to a longer stump. It is usually dangerous to wait for demarcation of damaged tissue as myonecrosis may lead to hypoxaemia, renal damage and death. It is therefore safer to err on the cautious side when planning the amputation level.

Operative techniques

Knee disarticulation

The main advantage of a knee disarticulation (Tooms, 1992b; Saleh, 1993) compared with an above knee amputation is that it provides a robust stump capable of full weight bearing. In addition it often allows the prosthesis to be stabilized without a supplementary waistband. The disadvantages include a higher incidence of partial flap necrosis with impaired wound healing and the fact that a slightly bulkier prosthesis will be required. As a general rule the skin flaps should never be sutured even under the slightest tension. Despite these advantages of knee disarticulation the surgeon should always remember that even a short below knee amputation stump is preferable to a knee disarticulation.

The operation is performed with the patient in the prone position. A tourniquet should be used and the knee flexed to 90°. The skin flaps should be designed bearing in mind that the aim is to raise medial and lateral flaps and suture them in the midline at the end of the operation. Preoperatively skin flaps are marked with methylene blue or a marker pen. Since there is no bone transection less bleeding is encountered. This is particularly important in the multiply injured patient. In addition there is a decreased risk of infection.

The incision is started mid-way between the inferior pole of the patella and the tibial tuberosity. The lateral incision is curved 5 cm down from the level of the tibial tubercle. The incision then curves proximally to the mid-line of the popliteal fossa 2 cm above the joint line with the knee in extension. The medial flap should be 2 cm longer than the lateral flap since the medial condyle is larger (Figures 12.2, 12.3).

The patella tendon is then identified anteriorly and divided from the tibial tuberosity (Figure 12.4). The medial flap is elevated with the surgeon staying close to the knee joint capsule and preserving the whole length of the pes anserinus (Figure 12.5). The dissection of the medial flap is then continued posteriorly and the medial head of the gastrocnemius is divided leaving a muscular stump (Figure 12.6).

The lateral flap is elevated anteriorly dividing the anterolateral muscles. The vessels are then identified and a sharp dissection of the soft tissues attached to the lateral tibial plateau is performed. The knee is then extended and the biceps tendon and the lateral head of the gastrocnemius are both divided, the biceps tendon being divided from the fibula head. The posterior aspect of the knee, with the neurovascular structures, is then approached. The popliteal artery and vein are identified and divided as are the tibial, peroneal and sural nerves

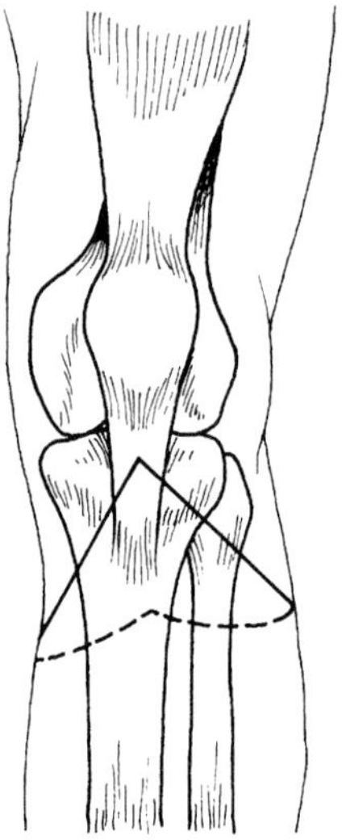

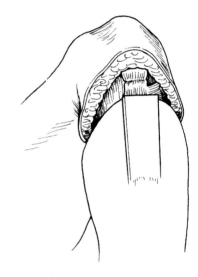

Figure 12.4 Division of the patellar tendon close to its insertion

Figure 12.2 Flap incisions for knee exarticulation

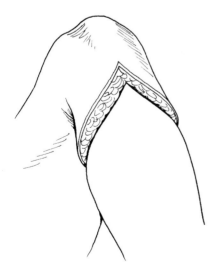

Figure 12.3 With the knee in flexion, the anterior incision is carried out

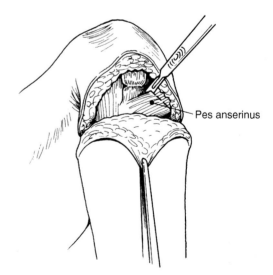

Pes anserinus

Figure 12.5 The pes anserinus is divided and the knee entered from the medial side

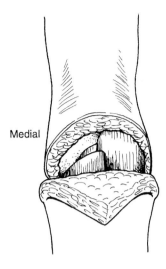

Medial

Figure 12.6   The gastrocnemius is divided

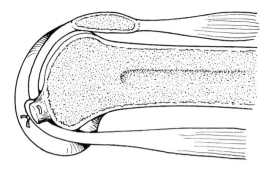

Figure 12.8   The patellar tendon is sutured to the anterior cruciate ligament; pulling down of the patella is avoided. Posterior cruciate ligament, hamstring tendons and gastrocnemic muscles are sutured together

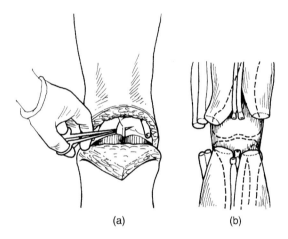

(a)   (b)

Figure 12.7   The neurovascular structures in the popliteal fossa are identified (a) and divided (b)

(Figure 12.7). The nerves are allowed to retract proximally. The posterior capsule is incised and the cruciate ligaments transected. This completes the dissection.

The patella tendon is sutured to the anterior cruciate ligament without pulling the patella down beyond the distal border of the femur. The posterior cruciate ligament, hamstring tendons and gastrocnemius muscles are sutured and the pes anserinus is brought over and fixed to the lateral muscles (Figure 12.8). Two deep drains should be inserted at the most dependent point. The wound is closed using subcutaneous and skin sutures and

adhesive skin tapes may be of assistance. A soft dressing is subsequently applied. The drains should be left in place for about 48 hours and it is suggested that the operation is performed under antibiotic cover.

Below knee amputations (Tooms, 1992b; Saleh, 1993)

Under ideal circumstances a below knee amputation is preferable to a knee disarticulation. The minimum stump length to allow for adequate prosthetic fitting is 5–6 cm.

In post-traumatic amputations it is important that the operative wound should be as clean as possible. It is recommended that antibiotics be given preoperatively and continued into the postoperative period. If at all possible the contaminated areas should be sealed off with an absorbent dressing.

The following operative technique is suitable for both ischaemic and non-ischaemic limbs. In post-traumatic below knee amputations the surgeon may have to use atypical skin flaps. As with knee disarticulations the skin flaps should be marked and the length of the stump measured from the anterior joint line of the knee. The anterior skin flap should start 2 cm below the level of bone transection at right angles to the long axis of the limb and should be extended around approximately 60% of the anterior circumference. The posterior skin flaps should extend 12.5 cm to 15 cm distal to the level of bone transection and comprise of about 40% of the calf circumference (Figure 12.9). The initial incision is made through the skin and deep fascia. The saphenous veins need to be identified and ligated. The saphenous nerve should be cut and allowed to retract. When preparing the anterior

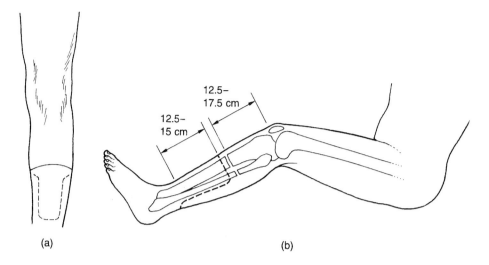

(a)   (b)

Figure 12.9   Skin flaps in below-knee amputation for ischaemic and non-ischaemic limbs

skin flap it is important not to detach it from the underlying tissues and in particular it is important to preserve its attachment to the deep fascia.

The posterior flap is raised by cutting through skin and deep fascia. The periosteum is incised 3 cm distal to the planned level of bone transection. A periosteal flap, based on the anterior and lateral surfaces of the tibia, is now raised. This flap is mobilized 2 cm proximal to the bone transection level. This helps to elevate the pressure sensitive anterior flap together with the deep structures.

The superficial peroneal nerve situated between extensor digitorum and peroneus brevis is identified and cut. The muscles of the anterior and lateral compartments are cut 3 cm distal to the level of bone transection. The muscles should be cut transversely and any muscular bleeding should be coagulated. The anterior tibial vessels should be tied off and the deep peroneal nerve cut and allowed to retract.

The fibula is exposed and the periosteum stripped to a level of 1.5 cm proximal to the planned tibial transection level. The fibula is then divided with a gigli or an oscillating saw (Figure 12.10). The gastrocnemius muscle is divided at the edge of the posterior skin flap down to its attachment to the soleus. The tibia is now cut at an angle of 45° to the proximal shaft from a point 1 cm above the planned transection level (Figure 12.11). After the anterior one third of the tibia has been cut the saw is redirected perpendicular to complete the dissection. The cut should be perpendicular to the axis of the tibia in both planes. The anterior

bevel should be slightly shorter as a long bevel would increase the pressure sensitive area.

After gaining access to the posterior compartment the muscles are stripped back and the vessels and nerves individually ligated. The larger vessels should be sutured twice for additional security. The transected tibial and peroneal nerves should be allowed to retract into the soft tissues.

At this point the tourniquet is released to identify any bleeding points. Cauterization should be reserved for small bleeding points only with larger vessels being ligated. The edges of the tibia and fibula are then smoothed with a rasp and the posterior skin flap is checked for length. If this is

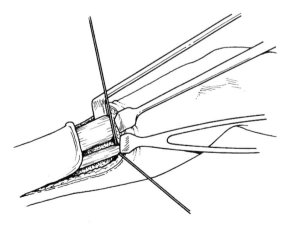

Figure 12.10   The fibula is exposed and divided with a gigli saw; a little lateral bevel is made

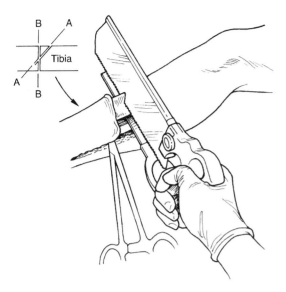

Figure 12.11 The anterior border of the tibia is bevelled

Alternatively the sagittal flap operation may be used (Tooms, 1992b) (Figure 12.15). In this amputation the length of each flap is shorter. The medial flap should be about 2 cm wider and skewed laterally from the mid-line to avoid the incision being placed at the tip of the tibia.

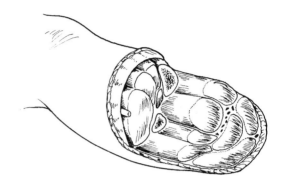

Figure 12.12 The posterior muscle flap is checked for adequate length

adequate four 2 mm holes are drilled in the tibia 5–10 mm from the end of the bone. Two holes are drilled anteroposteriorly and two further holes through the lateral cortex. The periosteum is pulled distally and secured over the end of the tibia by passing sutures through these holes. A tension myodesis, with the hip and knee in flexion, is now performed suturing the deep flexor muscles to the posterior pair of drill holes. The anterior muscles are pulled down and sutured through the lateral drill holes. The periosteal flap is then sutured over the end of the tibia onto the inner muscle layer. The inner layer of the gastrocnemius is subsequently fixed to the anterior border of the tibia through the appropriate drill holes. Following this the anterior muscles are sutured to the lateral side of the gastrocnemius aponeurosis and the edge of the gastrocnemius sutured to the anterior deep fascia (Figures 12.12 and 12.13). The skin is brought over the end of the stump and checked for tension. If necessary the skin can be trimmed at this time. If the tension is unacceptable the bone has to be shortened and the soft tissues reconstructed. Two drains should be used, one being placed deeply and one into the superficial layer. The end result should be a well padded stump (Figure 12.14). Postoperatively a soft dressing is applied and a conforming plaster may be used to prevent the formation of a knee flexion contracture. The patient should rest in bed for about one week and isometric quadriceps exercises are advised.

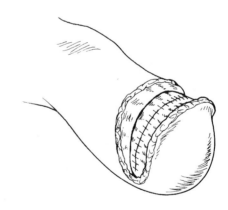

Figure 12.13 Suturing of deep fascia muscles and periosteum

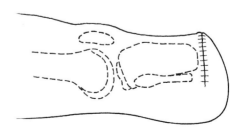

Figure 12.14 Closure of skin flap

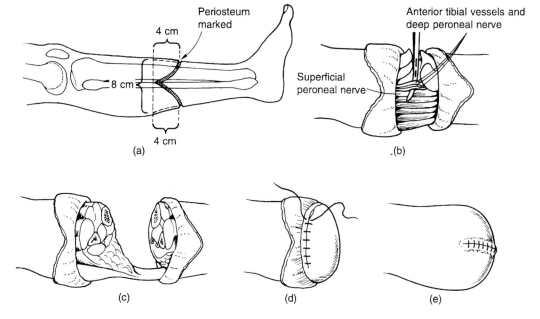

Figure 12.15 Middle third amputation for non-ischaemic limbs. (a) Equal anterior and posterior flaps are planned. (b) Identification and ligation of anterior tibial vessels and division of the deep peroneal nerve. (c) Preparation of the posterior myofascial flap. (d) The myofascial flap is sutured to the periosteum anteriorly. (e) Closure of skin flaps

Amputation criteria in lower limb injuries

In recent years several attempts have been made to identify criteria for amputation as it is well understood that unsuccessful attempts at limb salvage result in significantly increased morbidity and mortality. Bondurant *et al.* (1988) compared the outcome of patients who had primary amputations to those who had delayed amputations. They found that the hospitalization time, number of operative procedures, incidence of sepsis and mortality were increased in those patients who had delayed amputation. In addition the cost was significantly higher and the resulting stump length shorter when the amputation was delayed. The results are shown in Table 12.1.

Table 12.1 Cost of failed limb salvage in open tibial fractures

	Primary amputation (n = 14)	Delayed amputation (n = 29)
Hospitalization (days)	24.3	49.8
Operative procedures	1.6	6.7
Average hospital cost	$30,093	$48,690

Source: Bondurant *et al.*, 1988

It seems obvious that there is a group of patients with severe tibial injuries who will benefit from an early amputation. However the difficult problem is identifying which patients can be expected to have a successful limb reconstruction and which would benefit from early amputation. This is particularly true in Gustilo type IIIC fractures which have a poor prognosis with amputation rates as high as 42% (Gustilo *et al.*, 1984). Understandably patients will usually ask for limb salvage and it would be useful to predict accurately which patients should have an amputation to assist both patients and medical staff in coming to terms with the procedure.

Substantive data regarding the prognosis of Gustilo IIIB and IIIC open tibial fractures is difficult to find because of the relatively scarcity of these difficult injuries. Multi-centred trials have not been performed because of the difficulty of quantifying the degree of soft tissue and bony injury and because of the difficulty in applying the classification system in a uniform manner. In addition there are no good outcome criteria for measuring the success of amputation or limb salvage procedures.

In 1983 Johannsen *et al.* described the Mangled Extremity Severity Score (MESS) (Table 12.2). Four variables were examined taking into account

Table 12.2 Mangled extremity severity score (MES) index variables

	Points
A Skeletal/soft tissue injury	
Low energy (stab; simple fracture; 'civilian' gunshot wound)	1
Medium energy (open or multiple fractures, dislocation)	2
High energy (close-range shotgun or 'military' shot wound, crush injury)	3
Very high energy (above + gross contamination, soft tissue avulsion)	4
B Limb ischaemia	
Pulse reduced or absent but perfusion normal	1
Pulseless; paraesthesias; diminished capillary refill	2
Cool, paralysed, insensate, numb	3
(Score doubled for ischaemia > 6 h)	
C Shock	
Systolic BP always > 90 mmHg	0
Transient hypotension	1
Persistent hypotension	2
D Age (years)	
< 30	0
30–50	1
> 50	2
Borderline: 6 or less → salvage	
7 or more → amputation	

Source: Johansen *et al.*, 1983

the degree of skeletal and soft tissue injury, the presence and duration of limb ischaemia, shock and age. A retrospective and prospective trial were combined in this study and the authors found that 31 limbs which were successfully reconstructed had scores ranging from 3 to 6. All 21 patients who subsequently underwent secondary amputation had scores between 7 and 12. The advantage of this scoring system is its inherent simplicity as there are only four variables to be assessed. In this study the Mangled Extremity Severity Score had 100% sensitivity and specificity in predicting the outcome of an injured limb.

The mangled extremity syndrome grading system was described by Gregory *et al.* (1985) (Table 12.3). Sixty consecutive patients with open fractures were included to set up this index. The injury severity is taken into account as well as a more general assessment of the patient's overall condition and associated injuries. The type of skin lesion, nerve damage and vascular injury is examined in a more specific way and the bony injury is examined in more detail. Using this system the authors found that a score of 20 presented a clear dividing line between limb salvage and amputation. The mangled extremity syndrome index highlights that a thorough initial evaluation by senior members of staff is necessary to identify those patients who would benefit from amputation.

A similar protocol was devised by Lange *et al.* (1985). They had a number of absolute indications for amputation including complete disruption to the posterior tibial nerve in adults as well as crush injuries with an ischaemia time of greater than 6 hours. Their relative indications included the degree of associated injury, severe ipsilateral foot injuries and an anticipated protracted course to obtain soft tissue cover and tibial bone reconstruction. Primary amputation was indicated if one absolute indicator or two or more relative indicators were present.

Conclusion

In deciding between limb salvage and amputation it is important to assess the patient's overall social history as well as the extent of his or her injury. In addition one should be aware of one's own experience of handling severe tibial fractures and be prepared to seek help from other colleagues. The decision between limb salvage and amputation is a difficult one. Lange (1989) has drawn our attention to the kernel of their problem in that it is not intuitively obvious which is the greater disaster; a protracted salvage attempt of a limb with little realistic functional potential or the immediate amputation of a limb with reasonable functional potential that could have been salvaged.

Table 12.3   The mangled extremity syndrome grading system

	Points
Injury severity score	
0–25	1
25–50	2
> 50	3
Integument injury	
Guillotine	1
Crush/burn	2
Avulsion/degloving	3
Nerve injury	
Contusion	1
Transection	2
Avulsion	3
Vascular injury	
Artery transected	1
Artery thrombosed	2
Artery avulsed	3
Venous injury	4
Bony injury	
Simple fracture	1
Segmental fracture	2
Segmental-comminuted fracture	3
Segmental-comminuted fracture with bone loss < 6 cm	4
Segmental fracture: intra/extra-articular	5
Segmental fracture: intra/extra-articular with bone loss > 6 cm	6
Bone loss greater than 6 cm, add 1 point	
Lag time (1 point for every hour > 6)	
Age	
40–50 years	1
50–60 years	2
60–70 years	3
Pre-existing disease	1
Shock (systolic BP > 90 mmHg)	2
Borderline: 19 or less → salvage	
20 or more → amputation	

Source: Gregory *et al.*, 1985

References

American Medical Association (1989) *Guides to the Evaluation of Permanent Impairment*, 3rd edn, American Medical Association, Chicago

Baumgartner, R. (1983) *Amputation und Prothesenversorgung bei Durchblutungsstörung der unteren Extremität. Therapiewoche 33 (Sonderdruck)*. Verlag G. Braun, Karlsruhe

Bondurant, F., Cotler, H., Buckle, R. *et al.* (1988) The medical and economic impact of severely injured lower extremities. *J. Trauma*, **28**, 1270

Caudle, R.J. and Stern, P.J. (1987) Severe open fractures of the tibia. *J. Bone Joint Surg.*, **69A**, 801

Clarke, P. and Mollan, R.A.B. (1994) The criteria for amputation in severe lower limb injury. *Injury*, **25**, 139

Conkle, D.M., Richie, R.E., Sawyers, J.L. *et al.* (1975) Surgical treatment of popliteal artery injuries. *Arch. Surg.*, **110**, 1351

DeBakey, M.E. and Simeone, F.A. (1946) Battle injuries of the arteries in World War Two: an analysis of 2471 cases. *Ann. Surg.*, **123**, 534

Edwards, C.C., Simmons, S.C., Browner, B.D. *et al.* (1988) Severe open tibial fracture results treating 202 injuries with external fixation. *Clin. Orthop.*, **230**, 98

Fairhurst, M.J. (1994) The function of below-knee amputee versus the patient with salvaged garde III tibial fracture. *Clin. Orthop. Rel. Res.*, **301**, 227

Flint, L.M. and Richardson, J.D. (1983) Arterial injuries with lower extremity fracture. *Surgery*, **93**, 5

Georgiadis, G.M., Behrens, F.F., Joyce, M.J. *et al.* (1993) Open tibial fractures with severe soft-tissue loss. Limb salvage compared with below-knee amputation. *J. Bone Joint Surg.*, **75A**, 1431

Goris, R.J.A. (1983) The injury severity score. *World J. Surg.*, **7**, 12

Gregory, R.T., Gould, R.J., Pecle, M. *et al.* (1985) The mangled extremity syndrome (MES): a severity grading system for multisystem injury of the extremity. *J. Trauma*, **25**, 1147

Gustilo, R.B. and Anderson, J.T. (1976) Prevention of infection in the treatment of one thousand and twenty-five open fractures of long bones. *J. Bone Joint Surg.*, **58A**, 453

Gustilo, R.B., Mendoza, R.M. and Williams, D.N. (1984) Problems in the management of Type 3 (severe) open fractures: a new classification of Type 3 open fractures. *J. Trauma*, **24**, 742

Harris, R.I. (1944) Amputations. *J. Bone Joint Surg.*, **26**, 626

Hansen, S.T. Jr (1987) Type 3C tibial fracture. Salvage or amputation (Editorial). *J. Bone Joint Surg.*, **69A**, 799

Heatley, F.W. (1988) Severe open fractures of the tibia: the courage to amputate. *Br. Med. J.*, **296**, 229

Helfet, D.L., Howey, T., Sanders, R. *et al.* (1990) Limb salvage versus amputation. *Clin. Orthop.*, **256**, 80

Herve, C., Gaillard, M., Andrivet, P. *et al.* (1987) Treatment in serious lower limb injuries: amputation versus prevention. *Injury*, **18**, 21

Hicks, J.H. (1964) Amputations in fractures of the tibia. *J. Bone Joint Surg.*, **46B**, 388

Howe, H.R., Poole, G.V., Hansen, K.J. *et al.* (1987) Salvage of lower extremities following combined orthopaedic and vascular trauma. A predictive salvage index. *Am. Surg.*, **53**, 205

Hutchins, P.M. (1981) The outcome of severe tibial injury. *Injury*, **13**, 216

Johansen, K., Daines, M., Howey, T. *et al.* (1983) Objective criteria accurately predict amputation following lower extremity trauma. *J. Trauma*, **23**, 568

Keeley, S.B., Snyder, W.H. and Weigelt, J.A. (1983) Arterial injury below the knee: fifty-one patients with eighty-two arterial injuries. *J. Trauma*, **23**, 285

Kemp, A.G., van Niekerk, J.L. and van Meurs, P.A. (1993) Impairment scores of type III open tibial fractures. *Injury*, **24**, 161

Lancaster, S.J., Horowitz, M. and Alonso, J. (1986) Open tibial fractures: management and results. *South. Med. J.*, **79**, 39

Lange, R.H. (1989) Limb reconstruction versus amputation: decision making in massive lower extremity trauma. *Clin. Orthop.*, **243**, 92

Lange, R.H., Bach, A.W., Hansen, S.T. Jr *et al.* (1985) Open tibial fractures with associated vascular injuries prognosis for limb salvage. *J. Trauma*, **25**, 203

McNamara, J.J., Brief, D.K., Stremple, J.F. *et al.* (1973) Management of fractures with associated arterial injuries in combat casualties. *J. Trauma*, **13**, 17

McQuillan, W.M. and Nolan, B. (1968) Ischaemia complicating injury: a report of thirty-seven cases. *J. Bone Joint Surg.*, **50B**, 482

Mellissinos, E.G. and Parks, D.H. (1985) Post-trauma reconstruction with free tissue transfer: analysis of 442 consecutive cass. *J. Trauma*, **29**, 1095

Peacock, J.B. and Proctor, H.J. (1977) Factors limiting extremity function following vascular injury. *J. Trauma*, **17**, 532

Rojczyck, M. (1983) Behandlungsergebenisse bei offenen Frakturen. Aspekte der Antibiotika-Therapie. *Unfallheilkd.*, **162**, 33

Saleh, M. (1993) *Amputation Surgery. Techniques in Orthopaedic Surgery* (ed. D. Evans), Blackwell Scientific Publications, Oxford, p. 420

Seiler, J.G. and Richardson, J.D. (1986) Amputation after extremity injury. *Am. J. Surg.*, **152**, 260

Shah, P.M., Ivatury, R.R., Babu, S.C. *et al.* (1987) Is limb loss avoidable in civilian vascular injuries? *Am. J. Surg.*, **154**, 202

Sher, M.H. (1975) Principles in the management of arterial injuries associated with fracture/dislocation. *Ann. Surg.*, **182**, 630

Snyder, W.H. (1982) Vascular injuries near the knee: an updated series and overview of the problem. *Surgery*, **91**, 502

Tooms, R.E. (1992a) General principles of amputations. In *Campbell's Operative Orthopedics* (ed. A.H. Crenshaw), 8th edn, vol. 2, Mosby Year Book, St Louis, p. 677

Tooms, R.E. (1992b) Amputations of the lower extremity. In *Campbell's Operative Orthopedics* (ed. A.H. Crenshaw), 8th edn, vol. 2, Mosby Year Book, St Louis, p. 689

13

Tibial plafond fractures

J.L. Marsh and S. Bonar

Introduction

High energy intra-articular fractures of the distal tibia are uncommon and pose difficult management problems. The classification, treatment, and expected outcome are controversial. Associated soft tissue injuries play a prominent role. Complications are unfortunately frequent, difficult to manage, and may lead to devastating consequences. The treatment of these fractures is rapidly changing, and some principles learned in the 1970s and 1980s may well need to be abandoned.

Terminology

The terminology associated with articular fractures of the distal tibia has been confusing. In the literature, the terms pilon, pylon and plafond fractures have all been used. The term 'pilon' was coined by Destot in 1911. He likened the distal tibia to a pestle and mortar, and called it the pilon. However, the term pilon does not appear either in Webster's Dictionary (1980) or in Dorland's *Illustrated Medical Dictionary* (ed. Friel, 1974). The term 'pylon', according to Webster, is from the Greek word *pylè*, and refers to a gate. Current usage is: a gateway in a pyramidal form, a projection on an airplane course, a conical marker on a road, or a structure to fix onto an aircraft. Dorland's defines a pylon as a temporary artificial leg. Therefore, neither the definition of pilon nor pylon relates generally to the distal tibia or specifically to fractures in this area.

According to Webster, 'plafond' is French, from middle French with *plat* meaning flat and *fond* meaning bottom. It is typically used in English to refer to an elaborate ceiling. Since the articular surface of the bottom of the tibia indeed forms a ceiling over the ankle joint, plafond bears some relationship to the local anatomy in this region. A fracture of the tibial plafond is a fracture of the ceiling of the ankle joint. Therefore, this terminology is the most logical of the three and will be used throughout this chapter.

Classification, mechanism and incidence

The incidence of fractures of the tibial plafond is said to vary between 1 and 10% of lower extremity fractures (Meale and Seligson, 1980; Mast *et al.*, 1988). In the Edinburgh series (see Chapter 2), plafond fractures occurred in 3.2% of all tibia fractures. The wide variation in incidence depends on which injuries are included as tibial plafond fractures. Therefore, the mechanism of injury, classification of fractures and incidence all interrelate.

Lauge-Hansen (1948) classified rotational injuries of the ankle joint into five types based on mechanism. These rotational injuries may be associated with fractures of the tibial plafond. He specifically noted a type V pronation dorsiflexion fracture, which involved a significant portion of the articular surface. Giachino and Hammond (1987) described the combination of an oblique fracture of the medial malleolus with an anterolateral plafond fracture, and noted that the mechanism was external rotation, dorsiflexion and abduction. These rotational injuries are all relatively low energy, dissipate little forces to the soft tissues, and with appropriate management have an excellent prognosis. They are more appropriately classified with ankle fractures than with plafond fractures.

The far end of the spectrum is the high energy explosion fracture of the distal tibia secondary to axial compressive forces caused by a fall from a height, motor vehicle accident, or other vertical loading injury (Kellam and Waddell, 1979). Axial compressive fractures shatter all or part of the articular surface depending on the direction of impact of the talus against the tibial plafond. They dissipate large forces into the soft tissues. This axial compressive fracture has typically been called the 'pilon fracture' in the English literature.

There is a wide range between these two extremes, from low energy, mostly rotational, to high energy axial compressive. The low energy rotational fractures, when associated with some axial compressive force, will produce significant articular surface compressive damage and increased injury to the soft tissues. Alternatively, axial compressive fractures may be associated with a degree of rotation causing dislocation of the talus medially, laterally, or posteriorly as occurs with rotational injuries. The prognosis for a satisfactory outcome depends on where an injury falls on this spectrum. Unfortunately, most classifications do not adequately substratify these fractures. This has led to errors in treatment, uncertainty about prognosis, and difficulty in evaluating the literature.

Maale and Seligson (1980) described another variant of plafond fractures in which rotational tibial shaft fractures were associated with extension into the ankle joint. They termed these 'spiral extension fractures'. In addition to rotational shaft fractures, high energy predominantly transverse fractures of the metaphyseal diaphyseal junction from bending forces may have a plafond extension. The associated soft tissue injury in these two variants depends more on the shaft/metaphyseal component than on the plafond fracture itself.

The most accepted classification has been that of Rüedi and Allgöwer (1979), in which plafond injuries are divided into type I, type II and type III based on the size and displacement of articular fragments. As described in Chapter 1, type Is are cleavage fractures of the joint surface without displacement of articular fragments; type IIs have significant displacement of the articular surface without comminution; and type IIIs are associated with metaphyseal and epiphyseal comminution, and are the true high energy explosion fracture of the distal tibia. This classification is widely used in the literature, but it unfortunately does not provide enough detail to predict outcomes accurately.

A wide range of fractures with different prognosis fit between the definition of type II and type III.

The AO classification is the most useful classification currently available to define subtypes of fractures of the tibial plafond. It is an anatomical classification which includes the full spectrum from simple rotational fractures with a plafond component (B1) to high energy axial compressive fractures (B3, C2 and C3). The details of this classification are described in Chapter 1. When considered in conjunction with the soft tissue injury, this classification permits prognostication and comparison between groups. However, comminuted partial articular fractures (B3) may be more damaging to the articular surface than total articular fractures (C1, C2, C3) and, therefore, have a worse prognosis (Figure 13.1).

Finally, for this fracture more than any other extremity injury, the soft tissues must be considered, not only in the classification, but in planning treatment and determining outcome. Open fractures are appropriately classified by the method of Gustilo and Anderson (1976) as type I, type II and type III depending on the size of the open wound. The incidence of open wounds associated with tibial plafond fractures in the Edinburgh series was 9.1% (Chapter 1), which is similar to the Iowa experience of 12% (Bonar and Marsh, 1993). Therefore, the majority of these fractures are closed.

The associated soft tissue injury is significantly underestimated by only considering the size of open wounds. A large number of plafond fractures with closed soft tissue envelopes have severe soft tissue injuries. Tscherne and Goetzen's classification (1984) of soft tissue injuries associated with closed fractures applies well to high energy fractures of the tibial plafond. Soft tissue injuries are graded from grade 0 to grade 3. Closed fractures with no appreciable soft tissue injury are graded 0. Grade 1 soft tissue injuries have significant abrasion or contusion of skin and subcutaneous tissue. Grade 2 have a deep abrasion with local contused skin and some muscle involvement and grade 3 injuries have extensive contusion or crush with subcutaneous avulsion and severe muscle damage. Compartment syndrome and arterial rupture are included in this grade. The at-risk area of the subcutaneous surface on the anteromedial side of the tibia was described by these authors.

A significant proportion of the soft tissue injury is caused by the fracture itself. The energy stored in the distal tibia during an axial compressive injury is dissipated to the soft tissues as the force exceeds the yield point and the distal tibia shatters. It is this release of energy in an area without

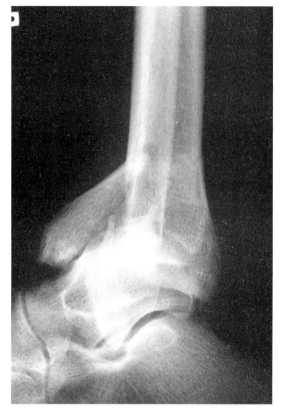

Figure 13.1   (a) A lateral radiograph of a type B3 fracture with partial articular involvement and comminution

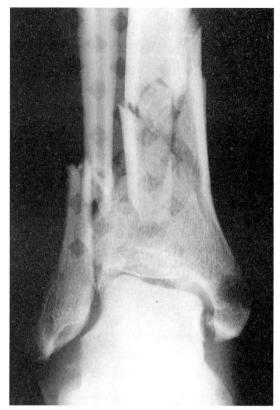

Figure 13.1   (b) An AP radiograph of a type C3 fracture with severe metaphyseal and articular comminution

muscle cover that injures the skin and subcutaneous tissues (see Figure 13.4*b*).

However, the extent of soft tissue injury does not necessarily vary directly with the AO fracture classification. It depends not only on comminution of the fracture, but on external forces such as direct abrasions or contusions, variations in the local circulatory status, and other incompletely understood factors. The treatment of the limb in the early post-injury period (dependence vs. elevation) may also make a difference. It is typical for C3 fractures with epiphyseal and metaphyseal comminution to have a severe soft tissue injury. However, it is also common for other fracture patterns such as A3, B3 and C2 to have significant associated soft tissue injury. In addition, lower energy fracture patterns from rotational injuries such as a B1 fracture may be accompanied by talar dislocation. When left unreduced for several hours, this may lead to soft tissue compromise. Finally, even simple fracture patterns such as an A1 may occasionally be accompanied by soft tissue injury and even produce compartment syndrome. Therefore, the underlying

fracture type may provide a clue to the amount of soft tissue injury, however it is important to evaluate and classify the soft tissue injury separately.

Treatment: review of the literature

Background

Prior to the 1970s, tibial plafond fractures were treated by a variety of techniques, including traction and casting with or without limited fixation, primary arthrodesis and even amputation (Scheck, 1965; Williams *et al.*, 1967; Ruoff and Snider, 1971; Etter and Ganz, 1991). The philosophy and teaching of the AO group, in conjunction with the publications of Rüedi and Allgöwer and others started a rapid evolution toward aggressive treatment in the 1970s. The principles were that anatomical reduction could and should be obtained with a wide operative approach, and that with sufficient internal fixation early joint movements were possible. Early movement was said to enhance cartilage nutrition, decrease osteoporosis, rehabilitate surrounding muscles, lead to a better final range of motion, avoid plaster disease and decrease arthrosis. Excellent results were published in European and North American literature (Rüedi and Allgöwer, 1969; Rüedi, 1973; Kellam and Waddell, 1979; Rüedi and Allgöwer, 1979; Ovadia and Beals, 1986; Ayeni, 1988; Etter and Ganz, 1991).

However, reports of the devastating complications of internal fixation in several large series have increased awareness of the potential problems of aggressive internal fixation approaches (Pierce and Heinrich, 1979; Bourne *et al.*, 1983; Dillin and Slabaugh, 1986; Teeny *et al.*, 1990; Bonar *et al.*, 1992; McFerran *et al.*, 1992; Bonar and Marsh, 1993). New techniques of treatment such as external fixation have been reported for articular fractures, including plafond fractures. Cross-ankle distracting fixators and tensioned wired ring fixators have both been used. These fixators are applied as part of a comprehensive approach permitting reduction, limited internal fixation and early motion.

The following section will review the results of treatment of tibial plafond fractures under three headings: conservative, internal fixation and external fixation. Internal fixation refers to any technique where the primary goal is to obtain rigid enough internal fixation to permit early motion; external fixation includes any technique where an external fixator is utilized as the primary method of stabilization; and conservative treatment applies to any other treatment techniques.

There are major difficulties in interpreting these results because of shortcomings in the current literature. These include:

1 The fracture classifications vary in different reports.
2 The grading systems for objective, subjective and radiographic results are different, which markedly limits comparison, i.e. a fair result in one series may correspond to a poor result in another.
3 All but one study were retrospective, which influences the interpretation of complications, i.e. postoperative wound complications may not be remembered or documented clearly.
4 All reported series lack information on the severity of soft tissue injury for closed fractures.
5 Some series do not report results in relation to the mechanism of injury, i.e. low energy rotation vs. high energy axial compression.
6 Many series comprise only a small numbers of cases.
7 Follow-up for most series is short.

With these shortcomings in mind, the current literature is reviewed and highlighted. Throughout the following discussion, fracture type refers to the Rüedi and Allgöwer classification unless otherwise specified. Summaries of the data with the critical injury and outcome data as available from the literature are presented in Table 13.1 in each of the three categories discussed for comparative analysis.

Table 13.1   Results of treatment of tibial plafond fractures

Author	Length of follow-up	No. of cases	No. of open fractures	No. R&A type III	No. of wound problems	No. of ankle fusion	No. of non-union delayed union	No. of satisfactory results
Conservative treatment								
Ruoff and Snider (1971)	6 wk–4 yr	4	2	NA	0	0	0	4
Williams *et al.* (1967)	4 yr	5	3	NA	NA	NA	NA	4
Scheck (1965)	1.5–12 yr	5	2	NA	0	0	NA	5
ORIF								
Rüedi and Allgöwer (1969)	9 yr	78	5	18	10	7	1	58
Rüedi and Allgöwer (1979)	6 yr	73	3	34	6	4	1	58
Kellam and Waddell (1979)	18 mth	21	3	NA	2	3	2	12
Teeny *et al.* (1990)	2.5 yr	60	12	30	11/30	11	8	NA
Etter and Ganz (1991)	10 yr	41	5	20	1	0	6	27
McFerran *et al.* (1992)	67 wk	46	11	21	25	1	6	NA
External fixation								
Bone *et al.* (1990)	18 mth	20	12	NA	0	2	3	15
Murphy *et al.* (1992)	6 wk–24 mth	5	1	5	0	NA	0	3
Bonar and Marsh (1993)	21 mth	16	7	12	0	0	0	NA
Marsh *et al.* (1991)	10.5 mth	25	5	13	0	0	1	NA

R&A, Rüedi and Allgöwer classification; NA, data not available.

Conservative

The least information is available concerning the results of conservative treatment. Etter and Ganz (1991) summarized the non-English literature from Europe on conservative treatment as follows: 'Management of these fractures by application of a cast, calcaneal traction with pins in plaster, percutaneous pinning of large fragments and casting, fibular stabilization alone, limited open reduction of key fragments or immediate motion with the foot in traction, has been described as difficult and often discouraging. Good functional results were achieved in less than 55% of cases.'

The English literature contains only reviews of small numbers of cases from which it is difficult to draw any conclusions. Ruoff and Snider in 1971 reported on 4 cases of 'explosion fractures' of the distal tibia. Two were treated with pins in plaster, one with a rush pin in the fibula, and one with a patellar osteochondral autograft. All patients did well without pain at follow-up, ranging from 6 weeks to 4 years. Williams *et al.*, in 1967, reported on 5 comminuted distal tibia fractures, 3 open, treated with a combination of traction and immediate ankle range of motion, followed by pins in plaster. At 4-year follow-up, all patients had returned to their usual work, which required standing and walking at least 8 hours a day. Scheck, in 1965, reported 5 cases of intra-articular distal tibia fractures treated by a combination of traction with dual pin fixation and limited open fixation of a 'key fragment'. These patients had only mild or occasional ache at follow-up from 1.5 to 12 years.

Recent reports include fractures that were treated conservatively as part of larger series. Generally, these conservatively treated cases had less favourable outcomes. Kellam and Waddell (1979) treated 4 fractures with casts alone. Three patients with rotational injuries did well, and one with a compressive injury had a poor result. Pierce and Heinrich (1979) included 9 cases treated in casts. Of the four type I fractures, 2 had good and 2 had poor results, the latter due to loss of reduction in the cast. Two type II fractures and 3 type III fractures all had poor results. Ayeni (1988) found that non-operative treatment produced good functional results in all type I fractures, poor results in type II and was not applicable to type III. Similarly, Ovadia and Beals (1986) found that type I fractures did well with conservative treatment, while all other fracture types benefited from open reduction and internal fixation (ORIF).

In summary, the literature on the conservative treatment of tibial plafond fractures is incomplete and only rough conclusions can be drawn. Type I fractures had generally favourable results, although occasional loss of reduction was reported. In the older literature, good results were obtained in more comminuted type II and type III fractures, when traction was a significant part of treatment. Casting alone was not successful for type II and III fractures. Complications occurred with conservative treatment, but were not frequent. In series where conservative treatment and internal fixation were both reported conservative treatment was generally considered by the authors to lead to poorer results, although the data supporting this were inconclusive.

Internal fixation

The publications of Rüedi and Allgöwer were the first to attract widespread attention to open reduction and internal fixation. They reported on 84 fractures followed for an average of 4 years (Rüedi and Allgöwer, 1969), and in a later publication extended their follow-up to an average of 9 years for 54 of these patients (Rüedi, 1973). The majority were skiing accidents, relatively low energy rotational injuries. In 10 patients there were problems with wound healing: 4 superficial wound infections, 2 small necrotic skin lesions, one extensive skin necrosis, and one open fracture and 2 closed fractures which developed osteomyelitis. Arthrodesis was performed in 4 for post-traumatic arthritis. They classified their results as good or excellent in 74%. The ankle range of motion was reduced in 40% and the subtalar in 32%. Most patients who developed traumatic arthritis had symptoms within the first year, and most had not deteriorated at the time of 9-year follow-up. They felt the functional result was associated with the success of articular reduction, although their definitions of functional result and articular reduction were not specified.

In 1979, Rüedi and Allgöwer reviewed 73 plafond fractures treated at a large city university hospital to see if their good results were reproducible at a teaching hospital 'far from the ski slopes'. However, 47% of these fractures were still due to sporting activities, including skiing, 34% were road or work accidents, and 19% occurred at home. Six patients had wound problems, but none developed osteomyelitis.

Kellam and Waddell, in 1979, reported on 26 distal tibial explosion fractures which they separated into two types: type A, a rotational pattern, in 7 patients, and type B, a compressive pattern, in 19 patients. Only two fractures were from skiing injuries. Acceptable results were attained in 84% of type A fractures and 53% of type B fractures. They noted that pain, stiffness and arthrosis were more related to the ability to obtain anatomical articular reduction than the initial injury severity.

Ovadia and Beals (1986) compared internal fixation in 79 patients to treatment by other methods in 65 patients (see above under Conservative treatment). Twenty-one patients subsequently required ankle arthrodesis, arthroplasty or amputation. Type I fractures generally did well regardless of treatment method, while all other types fared better after open reduction and internal fixation. They noted, like many other authors, that several patients with only a fair or poor objective result had a satisfactory clinical result. They also found that the quality of the reduction correlated well with the clinical result. Soft tissue procedures for skin coverage were required in 16 patients, but these were not specified as to fracture type or treatment category.

Etter and Ganz (1991) retrospectively reviewed a series of 41 plafond fractures treated by ORIF. Anatomical reduction was achieved in 60% of type II fractures and 50% of type III fractures. Ten-year average follow-up showed 66% good and 24% fair objective results overall. Only 50% of the type III fractures, however, were high velocity injuries. They noted no correlation between radiographic arthrosis and subjective results. Reoperation was required in 3 patients. These authors stressed the use of semitubular plates, multiple screws, or K-wires to avoid putting bulky plates under tenuous soft tissue. They used a spoon plate in 14 cases, which is placed anteriorly on the distal tibia to avoid the more compromised medial tissues. They also stated that since writing, it had become their standard practice to use an external fixator initially if there was any question about soft tissue viability.

Unfortunately, many authors have not reproduced these generally favourable results and have experienced a high incidence of complications associated with internal fixation. Pierce and Heinrich (1979) retrospectively reviewed 21 patients with severe vertical compressive plafond fractures. Seven patients developed skin loss and infection occurred in 3, one of whom required a below-knee amputation. Varus angulation occurred in 6 and erosion of metal fixation devices through skin in 5. Secondary procedures were required in 42%. The overall evaluation revealed no good, 6 fair and 15 poor results.

Bourne *et al.* (1983) reviewed 33 plafond fractures treated by ORIF. Type I and II fractures achieved good or fair results in 14 of 17 cases. ORIF was attempted in 16 type III fractures, but anatomical reduction and stable fixation were achieved in only 2. In these 16 fractures there were 4 good, 3 fair and 9 poor results. Four of these developed non-union and 2 became infected. Six of the type III fractures (32%) required arthrodesis.

Dillin and Slabaugh (1986) reported on 11 patients with vertical compression fractures treated by resident surgeons under staff supervision. Five were treated by interfragmentary screws alone and all had wound problems. Three patients were treated with plating and bone grafting. One developed osteomyelitis and a non-union, and one closed fracture required below-knee amputation for intractable infection. A third developed chronic wound drainage and required early removal of hardware. Overall, these authors found a 55% incidence of osteomyelitis and a 36% incidence of delayed wound healing or superficial infection.

McFerran *et al.* (1992) retrospectively reviewed 52 plafond fractures to define the complication rate after treatment. Eighty-nine per cent were treated by ORIF. The local complication rate was 54%. A total of 21 (40%) had major local complications requiring 77 additional surgeries. There were 18 flaps performed on 13 patients. There were 9 deep infections and 6 additional patients with wound breakdown.

We retrospectively reviewed our own experience with ORIF in 20 consecutive severe plafond fractures (Bonar *et al.*, 1992). Sixteen were Müller grade B3 or C3 fractures. Anatomical reductions were achieved in 11. There were 4 early deep infections around the tibial plate, 2 lateral plate infections and 3 wounds with chronic drainage. Thirty-one additional operative procedures and 8 readmissions were required. When just the cases with complications of the tibial wound were considered, these 6 cases accounted for 24 additional procedures.

Several highlights can be drawn from the review of results of open reduction and internal fixation presented above.

1 A distinction should be made between vertical compression injuries and the less severe rotational injuries. High energy fractures occurred in motor vehicle accidents or falls from a height, while lower energy fractures were associated with sporting accidents or falls at ground level. Most of the series reporting favourable results after ORIF include a high percentage of low energy fractures.

2 All papers that separately report or include only high energy fractures have an alarming rate of complications in those fractures treated with ORIF.

3 Even authors reporting generally favourable results have a significant number of wound complications. The cost of these complications is high.

4 Poor objective or radiographic results did not correlate well with subjective or clinical results. The results do not significantly deteriorate with time. If complications are avoided, the long-term prognosis is satisfactory.

External fixation

Few reports exist on the results of treatment with external fixation, but they are generally favourable. Murphy *et al.* (1992) reported using the Monticelli–Spinelli small wire circular external fixator in 5 cases. There were no complications related to the fractures although a good reduction was not achieved in one patient with poor bone stock. They still 'strongly favour' ORIF, however, when soft tissues permit.

Tornetta *et al.* (1992) and Chau and Catagni (1992) presented results of tensioned wire ring fixation for plafond fractures. Both felt that their techniques decreased the complications of treatment seen with ORIF, and that their follow-up results were satisfactory.

Bone *et al.* (1990) reported on cross-ankle rigid monolateral external fixation. Sixteen patients with 13 type II and III plafond fractures were treated with a delta frame external fixator. All fractures additionally had ORIF with either screws or small plates with minimal dissection. All fractures healed, but 2 delayed unions required bone graft. There were no infections. Ten were originally open fractures. Results were excellent or good in 11 at an average of 18 months.

Bonar and Marsh (1993) retrospectively reviewed 16 fractures that were treated with monolateral external fixation combined with limited internal fixation. There were nine type II and 12 type III. Articular surface reduction was anatomical in 11 and fair in 5. Two patients developed shaft angulation after fixator removal. The length of external fixation averaged 15 weeks. All tibial fractures healed and there were no cases of wound infection, skin slough or osteomyelitis. This technique was not associated with significant early or late complications.

We have also reported on a multicentre trial of a prospective protocol utilizing an articulated unilateral external fixator with limited internal fixation for 25 consecutive fractures followed for a minimum of 6 months (Marsh *et al.*, 1991). Thirteen were Müller grade C3 fractures. The articular surface reduction was good in 19, fair in 5 and poor in one. The duration of external fixation averaged 12.6 weeks. All tibial fractures healed and one had a delayed union, which was bone grafted at 3 months. There were no wound breakdowns or infections. There were 7 minor screw tract infections and no cases of screw tract osteomyelitis. Saleh *et al.* (1993) reported on a similar technique for 9 patients with one non-union but no infections.

Although the number of reported cases is small, there is a lower wound complication rate reported with external fixation compared to ORIF. The decreased rates of infection and wound problems in external fixation compared to ORIF are illustrated in Table 13.1. Considering the devastating nature of this complication, this is an important difference. In addition, the need for bone grafting and the non-union rate may both be decreased. Enough data are not available to compare the accuracy of reduction obtained with the two techniques. However, in our experience, reductions were more accurate with external fixation when compared to our own results with internal fixation. In our hands, wide open approaches were not the optimal way to obtain exact reductions.

It is not yet possible to compare long-term outcomes. However, to the extent that outcome is affected by complications, external fixation may have a considerable advantage.

Treatment: current strategies

Conservative

The complications that have been reported from wide operative approaches for tibial plafond fractures should make us once again consider the role of conservative management. Conservative treatments include casting and traction, with or without minimal internal fixation and, in rare instances, primary arthrodesis.

Casting on its own is usually reserved for fractures where articular displacement is minimal, and a satisfactory position can be maintained with an external plaster. In the AO classification, this treatment applies to A1, B1 or C1 fractures where the articular displacement is judged to be 2 mm or less. CT scans or tomograms aid in judging articular incongruity. Weight bearing should be restricted for 4–6 weeks. The prognosis is good for these minimally displaced injuries.

Casting may be supplemented by minimal internal fixation used to aid in either stability or reduction. For instance, fibular plating or rodding to obtain length and alignment in conjunction with casting for the tibia may be satisfactory in some A2, A3 or C1 fractures. Occasionally a carefully placed screw will reduce an articular displacement without using a wide operative approach, such as for a B1 fracture. Unfortunately, most fractures have a degree of instability, which requires more support than limited internal fixation and plaster casting, and, therefore, these methods have limited applications.

Traction may be used. It has the advantage of distracting the joint surfaces and allowing some restricted joint mobility. It has the disadvantage, however, of prolonged hospitalization and enforced supine positioning. The latter is a problem in the multiply injured or elderly patient. The primary use of traction is as a temporary splinting technique in the high energy fracture associated with severe soft tissue injury. When the soft tissues do not permit an early operative approach, it is difficult to keep the talus centred underneath the tibia in B3, C2 and C3 fractures. In these cases, a temporary calcaneal traction pin and elevation of the limb on a Bohler frame is indicated.

Rarely, primary or delayed primary arthrodesis may be indicated. Severe comminution, contaminated open wounds with soft tissue loss, and loss of cartilage on the bottom of the tibia or top of the talus may be indications for primary or delayed primary arthrodesis. Each case must be individualized based on the fracture, the condition of the soft tissues, other associated injuries, and goals and expectations of the patient. Although unreconstructable joint surfaces will inevitably lead to a poor radiographic result, if the distal tibia heals with good alignment, the subjective result can be better than the radiographic result and, therefore, in most cases it is better to defer arthrodesis. If necessary, late arthrodesis can be performed after the tissues have improved and some bone stock has been restored. When early arthrodesis is chosen, length is maintained with an external fixator and fusion supplemented by bone grafts. Sanders *et al.* (1989) have published a method of stabilization using an anterior reconstruction plate.

Internal fixation

Techniques of internal fixation have advanced considerably since the original publications in the 1970s, but the basic principle as outlined by Rüedi and Allgöwer still apply. Their step-by-step approach to tibial plafond fractures was:

1 Secure length and overall alignment by open reduction and internal fixation of the fibula.
2 Through an anteromedial approach, reduce and provisionally fix the articular fragments of the tibia.
3 Obtain rigid fixation with an anterior or medial buttress plate.
4 Bone graft the metaphyseal defect.
5 Begin early motion/long-term non-weight bearing.

If internal fixation is chosen, great attention must be given to soft tissue technique. Implants should not be placed under the tenuous subcutaneous anteromedial surface of the tibia. In addition, small implants should be used. Multiple screws with or without small buttress plates, sometimes supported by external splinting, are capable of doing the job that was once felt to require the larger implants.

Indirect reduction techniques should be utilized. This includes extensive preoperative planning, distractors to aid in reduction by ligamentotaxis, fluoroscopically assisted reductions, and various reduction forceps and aids. These techniques assist the surgeon in obtaining reduction without stripping the major fragments. The soft tissues become an aid to anatomical reduction rather than a barrier. In fractures with metaphyseal comminution, the reconstructed articular surface can be bridged to the diaphysis with a plate. This limits stripping and speeds healing in the metaphyseal area. If these techniques are adhered to, and the amount of soft tissue damage from the injury is not excessive, the complications of open reduction and internal fixation can be minimized (Figure 13.2).

Internal fixation techniques are indicated for B1 fractures. These are low energy rotational injuries usually associated with a fibular fracture and the tibial plafond component is fixed with one or two 3.5 or 4.0 screws. B2 and C1 fractures are also generally amenable to internal fixation with or without buttress plating with small plates and with or without bone grafting. B3, C2 and C3 fractures without excessive soft tissue injury may be successfully internally fixed in expert hands, but it is these fractures for which the complications are excessively high (see Complications). Careful consideration must be given before attempting wide open reduction and rigid internal fixation in these fractures. Fractures with significant articular com-

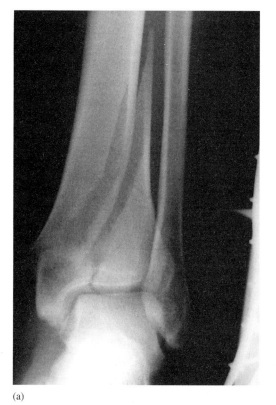

(a)

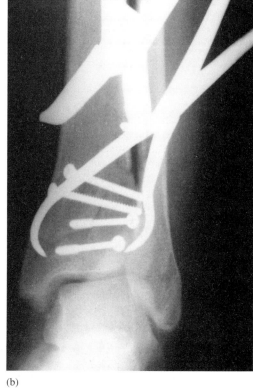

(b)

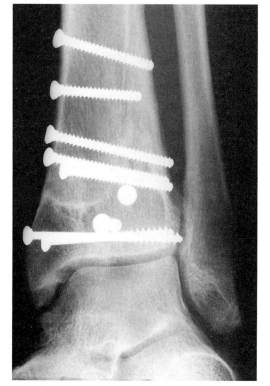

(c)

Figure 13.2 (a) An AP radiograph of a type C1 fracture; (b) indirect reduction techniques to aid reduction while minimizing soft tissue stripping; (c) 2-year follow-up after internal fixation with large screws only

minution and soft tissue injury are not amenable to ORIF under any circumstances. A very aggressive approach is to perform a primary free flap to avoid wound breakdown (Wiss, personal communication).

External fixation

External fixation has become popular for severe tibial plafond fractures, as a method to decrease the complication rate when compared with internal fixation techniques for similar fractures.

Ring fixators can obtain and maintain reduction on the same side of the joint, which permits early ankle movement. In this technique, an open reduction is performed to fix the articular surface with small screws, reconstructing the epiphyseal end of the bottom of the tibia. Cross-ankle distraction with a femoral distractor may aid this reduction. K-wires are then inserted into the distal fragment and tensioned on to a ring. These wires are small enough to obtain fixation around the screws even

in small distal articular sections. After tensioning, the wires provide distal fixation. This segment is then reduced to the tibia and fixed with further rings and tensioned wires or half pins. Ankle motion is possible beneath the reconstructed articular surface (Figure 13.3*a,b*).

This technique has the advantage that it allows joint mobility, and does not introduce any fixating components into the uninjured hindfoot. The disadvantages are that it is technically demanding, requires facility with ring fixator components, and still requires an open reduction of the articular surface. For the latter reason, this technique is probably best suited to A1, A2, A3, C1 and C2 fractures. Severe comminution of the articular surface in a B3 or C3 fracture with proximal displacement of the talus is still amenable to a ring fixator if a fixation segment is built distally to support the talus, but this eliminates the possibility for early motion.

A second external fixation strategy is to cross the joint with a distracting fixator as the first step in the

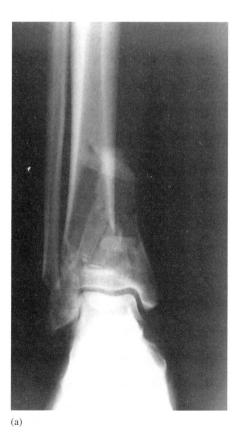
(a)

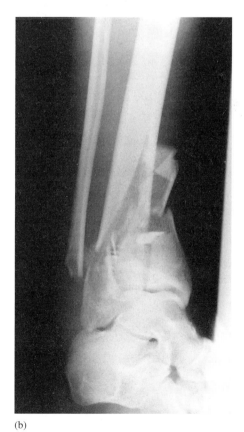
(b)

Figure 13.3   (a,b) AP and lateral radiographs of a C2 fracture; (c,d) mortise and lateral radiograph after reduction using a ring fixator; (e,f) AP and lateral radiographs at healing. (Case submitted by D. Covall, MD, Boston City Hospital)

Figure 13.3   *cont.*

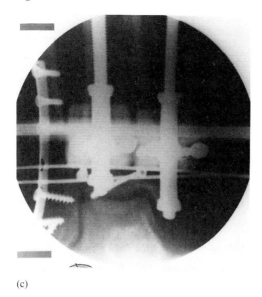

(c)

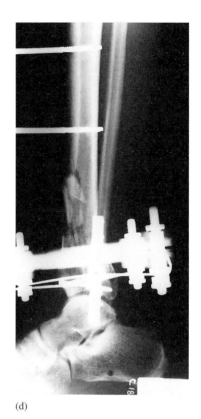

(d)

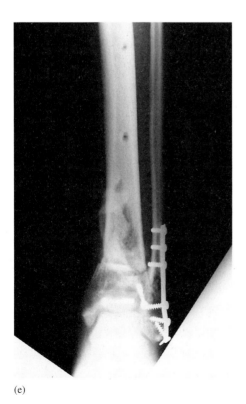

(e)

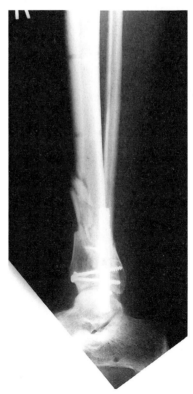

(f)

procedure. Distal screws may be fixed into the medial or lateral side of the talus or calcaneus, or both. Intraoperative distraction permits provisional reduction of articular fragments. If necessary, further joint realignment and/or bone grafting if necessary can then be accomplished by fluoroscopically assisted, minimally invasive or percutaneous techniques utilizing reduction forceps and cannulated screws. The advantages of this technique are ease of application, controlled intraoperative distraction and less invasive approaches to the distal tibia. The disadvantages include fixator screws into the hindfoot and ankle joint immobility.

An alternative technique involves the use of a hinged articulated external fixator for the ankle (Orthofix, SRL Verona, Italy) which potentially combines the advantages of ease of application, cross-ankle intra-operative distraction, and early postoperative motion (Ralston *et al.*, 1990). This is the authors' preferred method for the treatment of severe tibial plafond fractures. The fixator is applied to two screws distally, one in the calcaneus and one in the talus, and two screws proximally in the tibia. The hinge axis approximates the centre of rotation of the ankle joint.

The fixator is applied under fluoroscopic control. One screw is applied to the neck of the talus and one to the posterior angle of the os calcis straddling the neurovascular bundle and the subtalar joint. The talar screw is placed first. The screw is placed through the neck of the talus parallel to the dome. Depth of insertion must be checked on an AP fluoroscopic view of the foot to ensure bicortical purchase of the talus. A template is then applied to the talar screw, and all other screw insertion is done through the template. The calcaneal screw should be applied high in the posterior angle of the os calcis to allow ample room for postoperative dorsiflexion. Bicortical purchase of the calcaneal screw must also be obtained and is assured by visualizing an axial fluoroscopic view of the hindfoot. The proximal two tibial screws are similarly placed through the fixator template.

After screw placement the template is removed, the fixator is applied and the proximal ball joint is locked. The ankle is then distracted by applying a compression distraction apparatus to the fixator body, and the reduction is evaluated fluoroscopically. In some cases the reduction may be adequate at this stage. If so, the procedure is concluded without violating the soft tissue envelop around the fracture. This typically occurs in A2, C1 and C2 fractures.

In B2, B3 and C3 fractures further reduction of the articular surface is often needed. Based on pre-operative planning and intraoperative appearance after distraction, limited incisions are used to aid in reduction of the articular surface. These incisions should be located over a major fracture line so that the articular surface can be visualized through a 'fracture window'. This minimizes stripping of the articular fragments. Manipulation of large articular fragments percutaneously is aided by large tenaculum reduction forceps. Fixation of reduced fragments is obtained with 3.5 or 4.0 mm cannulated screws. Intraoperative distraction aids in visualization of the articular surface, and fracture lines. At the completion of the procedure, the distraction is decreased until the ankle takes on a normal symmetrical appearance on fluoroscopic images. The fixator then neutralizes the fracture (Figure 13.4).

In cases with a fibula fracture, the length and alignment of the fibula can often be controlled by the fixator, and internal fixation of the fibula is not necessary. However, in other cases, exact restoration of the fibula may assist in reduction of an anterolateral fragment of the tibial plafond or the distal fibula may become trapped posteriorly, and open reduction is necessary to restore its position. A lateral approach is made to the fibula, and it is plated with a one-third tubular plate.

At the completion of the procedure, the articulated hinge is locked with the ankle in a neutral position. When soft tissue swelling permits, patients are mobilized non-weight bearing and the articulated hinge is released to allow gentle active assisted ROM exercises. In these cases, a removable Orthoplast splint is fashioned to maintain the ankle in a neutral position while not doing ROM. Weight bearing is begun when early metaphyseal healing is likely, most commonly at 4–6 weeks or longer if there is a large metaphyseal defect. The fixator is removed when the fracture is radiographically and clinically healed. This occurred at an average of 13 weeks in our series. Healing times for these fractures tend to be quicker than with open reduction and internal fixation since the soft tissue envelope is kept largely intact.

Bone grafting is necessary when there is a significant metaphyseal defect. This can be accomplished through an incision used for limited open reduction or through a separate small incision. Bone grafting has been necessary in approximately 50% of our cases. The incidence of bone grafting is less with this technique because soft tissues are left intact on metaphyseal fragments and large

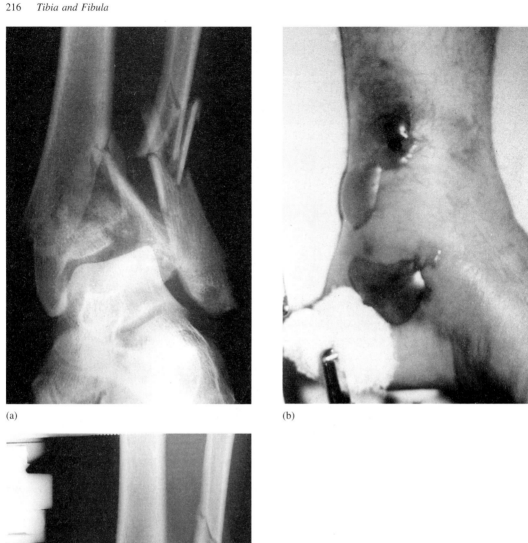

(a)

(b)

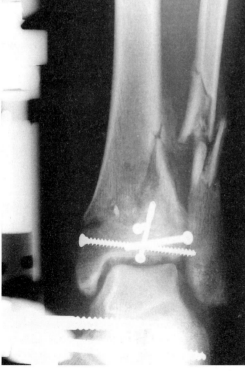

(c)

Figure 13.4   (a) AP radiograph of a type C3 fracture and (b) clinical photograph of the associated soft tissue injury and fracture blisters; (c) mortise radiograph after external fixation with limited internal fixation; (d,e) mortise and lateral radiographs at 8-month follow-up demonstrating solid healing with maintained position

Figure 13.4 *contd*

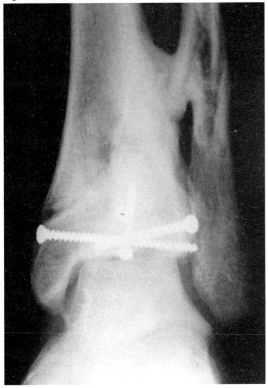

(d)

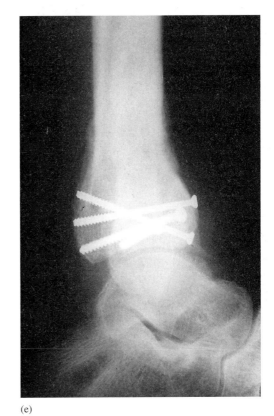

(e)

cavities are less frequently created than in wide open approaches.

Complications and treatment

Wound complications/infection

The majority of infections and wound breakdowns have occurred in closed fractures that underwent open reduction and internal fixation (Kellam and Waddell, 1979; Teeny *et al.*, 1990; Bonar *et al.*, 1992; McFerran *et al.*, 1992). This occurred most frequently in the high energy vertical compressive injuries. However, McFerran *et al.* found that 50% of their major complications occurred in the less severe Rüedi and Allgöwer type I and II fractures. This indicates that the soft tissue injury can be more severe than the fracture classification implies, and may lead to an underestimation of the risk of this complication.

The consequences of this complication can be devastating (Figure 13.5). Many series, including our own, include amputation as an eventual outcome. Even if the limb is salvaged, many addi-

tional procedures and prolonged courses of antibiotics are required. In McFerran's series, 21 patients required 77 additional operative procedures (McFerran *et al.*, 1992).

The best treatment of wound complications is to avoid them. Wound complications can be minimized by avoiding staples, keeping skin incisions more than 12 cm apart, and avoiding operation during the time of maximal wound ischaemia between 3–6 days (Trumble *et al.*, 1992). In addition, indirect reductions, avoiding the anteromedial surface of the tibia and not utilizing large plates, are important.

The treatment of wound complications/ osteomyelitis must be individualized and starts with recognizing a wound at risk. An early, aggressive approach to wound dehiscence, prior to infection setting in, is advisable. It is not wise to watch a superficial infection expectantly. While waiting and watching, the infection spreads and becomes harder to eradicate.

Significant areas of wound compromise with impending skin slough require appropriate debridement and soft tissue transfers. Stable internal fixation devices may be left in place. Local rotational

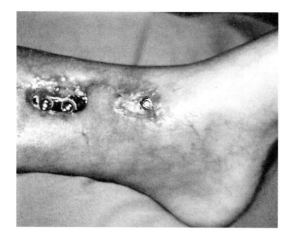

Figure 13.5   An example of wound breakdown over an anteromedial plate

flaps are not effective in the distal third of the tibia due to the low perfusion of the flap, which requires a large length to width ratio of 1:1 for flap viability (Trumble *et al.*, 1992). Free tissue transfer is therefore required. The possibilities include gracillis, latissimus, lateral thigh and radial forearm flaps. The defect is often small on the anterior tibia and larger flaps (latissimus and lateral thigh) may be too large to inset and may make shoe wear difficult. In addition, a long vascular pedicle is usually needed to span the zone of damaged tissue. Trumble *et al.* found that radial forearm fasciocutaneous flaps were highly suitable for the size and location of distal tibial soft tissue defects. However, there is some evidence that healing is better when bone is covered by muscle rather than fascia (Richards and Schemitsch, 1989).

Management is different once deep infection has become established. The involved soft tissue and bone must be extensively debrided and any involved hardware removed. Organism-specific antibiotics are begun and the fracture is usually stabilized with an external fixator. Once the bed is clean, soft tissue coverage is then obtained by free tissue transfer. Bone grafting is done to obtain union at 4–8 weeks after soft tissue coverage.

Green and Roesler (1987) called attention to the frequency of unsuspected chronic ankle joint infection causing persistent infection. The infection tracks down through fracture lines to the ankle joint and may be suspected by noting rapid narrowing on X-rays. The infection is not cleared until the ankle joint is debrided and fused.

A few authors have reported on ankle arthrodesis in the presence of ongoing infection and have attained high fusion rates (Green and Roesler, 1987; Cierny *et al.*, 1989; Sanders *et al.*, 1989), but all have emphasized the high cost in terms of time, money and emotional tolls on the patients. Most patients changed or lost their jobs and had significant stress on their personal relationships. The authors concluded that amputation should possibly have been encouraged early.

Non-union and delayed union

Non-union and delayed union and their treatment have been variably reported in the literature. The higher the energy of the fracture and the greater the soft tissue injury, the greater the incidence of delayed/non-union. The incidence appears to be about 5% regardless of treatment method, however Teeny *et al.* (1990) (8/60) and McFerran *et al.* (1992) (6/46) reported higher incidence in their series of patients treated by open reduction and internal fixation. Despite the fact that these fractures involve cancellous bone, the devascularization that occurs from the injury to the soft tissues can still lead to difficulties with healing. This problem is compounded when the soft tissues are further injured through an aggressive operative approach. For this reason, most advocates of internal fixation recommend routine bone grafting.

The treatment of a supramalleolar non-union secondary to an old tibial plafond fracture can be very challenging. If the condition of the soft tissues is good, there is no infection and there is no significant ankle joint arthrosis, a number of techniques may be successful. These techniques include grafting, internal fixation and external fixation.

If a supramalleolar non-union is well aligned an on-lay bone graft may obtain union. If this is done from a posterolateral approach, there is ample room to lay a graft on to the back of the tibia, and between the tibia and the fibula. This also avoids the anterior soft tissues which may have been previously injured or scarred from the original fracture or old surgical interventions.

In non-infected cases internal fixation techniques with plates and screws appear to be much safer than in acute plafond fractures. Hypertrophic non-unions will often heal with plate stabilization and compression alone without bone grafting (Wiss *et al.*, 1992).

External fixation techniques have particular utility in infected cases or when realignment is required. To obtain the stability necessary to heal a non-union, fixation should be into the distal tibial fragment rather than spanning the ankle joint.

This can be accomplished with monolateral fixators, but if the distal fragment is small, tension wire ring fixation is preferable. In infected non-unions, excision of the entire distal tibial segment, tibiotalar arthrodesis and then bifocal treatment to regain length through a proximal corticotomy may be the only salvage other than amputation.

When supramalleolar non-union is combined with ankle arthrosis, this becomes a difficult two-level reconstructive problem. Extensive stabilization and bone grafting are required to secure union and ankle arthrodesis at the same time. We have treated 8 cases with this combined problem with a variety of internal and external fixation techniques. Only 5 have healed without requiring additional surgery. Patients should be counselled about the difficulty of management. When accompanied with infection, unless the patient is willing to undergo resection and bone transport, amputation should be considered.

Arthrosis

The incidence of arthrosis has not been reported in many series and the criteria for diagnosis varied widely or were not specified. Up to 50% arthrosis rates have been reported. Two points have been emphasized. First, significant arthrosis, if it was going to develop, typically did so within the first 1–2 years (Rüedi, 1973; Rüedi and Allgöwer, 1979). Secondly, the presence or degree of arthro-sis radiographically did not correlate well with subjective clinical results, but did correlate with objective results of joint range of motion. The incidence of arthrosis requiring surgical management many years after injury was low (Rüedi, 1973; Rüedi and Allgöwer, 1979; Ovadia and Beals, 1986; Etter and Garz, 1991).

The origin of the arthrosis is debated and probably relates to several factors. The quality of reduction is thought to affect the development of arthrosis. In addition, articular cartilage damage at the time of injury contributes to the development of arthrosis irrespective of the quality of articular reduction. To this point, Etter and Ganz (1991) noted that 4 of 24 patients with anatomical reduction developed severe arthrosis. It has been our impression that arthrosis correlates more with the type of injury than the quality of reduction (Figure 13.6). Other contributing factors include, avascular necrosis of subchondral bone fragments and infection which can lead to rapid severe arthrosis. When rapid loss of articular cartilage occurs in the first 6 months after injury, infection should be considered.

The conservative treatment of post-traumatic ankle arthritis includes custom-moulded ankle–foot orthoses with rocker bottom soles and occasionally anterior clam shells or leather ankle lacers for further support. The surgical treatment of severe post-traumatic arthritis of the ankle is arthrodesis. Many techniques are available.

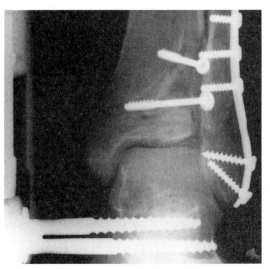

(a)

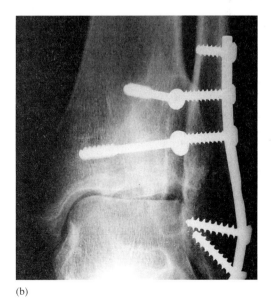

(b)

Figure 13.6 (a) Postoperative AP radiograph of a type C3 fracture after external fixation, combined with limited internal fixation showing a good reduction with associated anterolateral comminution. A 2-year follow-up radiograph (b) shows post-traumatic arthrosis, despite the good reduction

Damaged soft tissues and previous incisions must be taken into account in planning the surgery. The presence of old hardware may vary the approach. Bone grafting is necessary if there is extensive loss of distal tibial bone stock. Combined arthrosis of the subtalar and midfoot joints may be treated with extensive fusion, but this must be looked at as a salvage procedure. Papa and Myerson *et al.* (1992) have described extended fusion of the ankle and hindfoot in 5 old plafond fractures utilizing an extended posterior approach. They point out that exact positioning of the foot is critical to minimize gait disturbance and callus formation.

Conclusion

Tibial plafond fractures remain one of the most challenging injuries facing the traumatologist. Detailed classifications to substratify fractures are now available. The appreciation of the soft tissue injury in this tenuous location of the distal tibia has become paramount. The incidence of complications has been exceedingly high leading to an evolution of management. Extensive exposure and retraction of soft tissues needs to be avoided during treatment. The use of large anteromedial buttress plates has been increasingly condemned. Newer methods of treatment emphasize some form of external fixation with limited fixation for reducing the articular surface in treating the more severe injuries. In less severe fractures without significant soft tissue damage it may be that limited internal vs. external fixation may work equally well.

The treatment of complications of tibial plafond fractures is challenging and best handled by avoidance in the first place. A wound at risk for breakdown should be recognized early and treated aggressively with soft tissue transfer prior to deep infection setting in. After osteomyelitis has developed, the treatment options are limited and costly in terms of time, money and emotion. Experts in this area have advocated consideration for early amputation. In addition, a certain number of patients will go on to develop post-traumatic arthrosis and it is not yet known whether any of the different treatment methods will affect the incidence of this outcome.

References

Ayeni, J.P. (1988) Pilon fractures of the tibia: a study based on 19 cases. *Injury*, **19**, 109–114

Bonar, S.B. and Marsh J.L. (1993) Unilateral external fixation for severe pilon fractures. *Foot Ankle*, **14**,: 57–64

Bonar, S.B., Marsh, J.L. and Andre, M. (1992) Unilateral external fixation compared to open reduction and internal fixation for severe tibial plafond fractures. *Orthop. Trauma Assoc.*, October

Bone, L., Stegemann, P., McNamara, K. and Seibel, R. (1990) The use of external fixation in severe fractures about the ankle. *Orthop. Trans.*, **14**, 265

Bourne, R.B., Rorabec, C.H. and Macnab, J. (1983) Intra-articular fractures of the distal tibia: the pilon fracture. *J. Trauma*, **23**, 591–5

Chau, A.F. and Catagni, M.C. (1992) Pilon fractures: treatment by the Ilizarov method. *Am. Assoc. Orthop. Surg.* p. 66

Cierny, G., Cook, W.G. and Mader, J.T. (1989) Ankle arthrodesis in the presence of ongoing sepsis. *Orthop. Clin North Am.*, **20**, 709–21

Destot, E. (1911) *Traumatismes du pied et ryon x malleoles, astralage, calcaneus, avant-pied.* Masson, Paris

Dillin, L. and Slabaugh, P. (1986) Delayed wound healing, infection and non-union following open reduction and internal fixation of tibial plafond fractures. *J. Trauma*, **26**, 1116–19

Etter, C. and Ganz, R. (1991) Long-term results of tibial plafond fractures treated with open reduction and internal fixation. *Arch. Orthop. Trauma Surg.*, **210**, 277–83

Friel, J.P. (1974) *Dorland's Illustrated Medical Dictionary*, 25th edn, W.B. Saunders, Philadelphia

Giachino, A.A. and Hammond, D.I. (1987) The relationship between oblique fractures of the medial malleolus and concomitant fractures of the anterolateral aspect of the tibial plafond. *J. Bone Joint Surg.*, **69A**, 381–4

Green, S.A. and Roesler, S. (1987) Salvage of the infected pilon fracture. *Techniques Orthop.*, **2**, 37–41

Gustilo, R.B. and Anderson, J.T. (1976) Prevention of infection in the treatment of one-thousand and twenty-five open fractures of long bones. Retrospective and prospective analyses. *J. Bone Joint Surg.*, **58A**, 453–8

Kellam, J.F. and Waddell, J.P. (1979) Fractures of the distal tibial metaphysis with intra-articular extension-the distal tibia explosion fracture. *J. Trauma*, **19**, 593–601

Lauge-Hansen, N. (1948) Fractures of the ankle. *Arch. Surg.*, **56**, 259–317

Maale, G. and Seligson, D. (1980) Fractures through the distal weight-bearing surface of the tibia. *Orthopaedics*, **3**, 517–21

Marsh, J.L., Bonar, S., Nepola, J. *et al.* (1991) Fractures of the tibial plafond – treatment with articulated external fixation. Orthopaedic Trauma Association, Seattle, Washington, 1 November 1991

Mast, J.W., Spiegel, P.G. and Pappas, J.N. (1988) Fractures of the tibial pilon. *Clin. Orthop.*, **230**, 68–82

McFerran, M.A., Smith, S.W., Boulas, H.J. and Schwartz, H.S. (1992) Complications encountered in the treatment of pilon fractures. *J. Orthop. Trauma*, **6**, 195–200

Murphy, C.P., D'Ambrosia R. and Dabezies E.J. (1992) The small pin circular fixator for distal tibial pilon fractures with soft tissue compromise. *Orthopaedics*, **14**, 283–90

Ovadia, D.N. and Beals, R.K. (1986) Fractures of the tibial plafond. *J. Bone Joint Surg.*, **68A**, 543–51

Papa, J.A. and Myerson, M.S. (1992) Pantalar and tibiotalocalcaneal arthrodesis for post-traumatic osteoarthrosis of the ankle and hindfoot. *J. Bone Joint Surg.*, **74A**, 1042–9

Pierce, F.O. Jr and Heinrich, J.H. (1979) Comminuted intra-articular fractures of the distal tibia. *J. Trauma*, **19**, 828–32

Ralston, J.L., Brown, T.D., Nepola, J.V., Williams, D.R. and Marsh, J.L. (1990) Mechanical analysis of the factors affecting dynamization of the orthofix dynamic axial fixator. *J. Trauma*, **4**, 449–57

Richards, R.R. and Schemitsch, E.H. (1989) Effect of muscle flap coverage on bone blood flow following devascularization of a segment of tibia; an experimental investigation in the dog. *J. Orthop. Res.*, **7**(4), 550–8

Rüedi, T. (1973) Fractures of the lower end of the tibia into the ankle joint: results 9 years after open reduction and internal fixation. *Injury*, **5** 130–4

Rüedi, T.P. and Allgöwer, M. (1969) Fractures of the lower end of the tibia into the ankle joint. *Injury*, **1**, 92–9

Rüedi, T.P. and Allgöwer, M. (1979) The operative treatment of intra-articular fractures of the lower end of the tibia. *Clin. Orthop.*, **138**, 105–10

Ruoff, A.D. and Snider, R.K. (1971) Explosion fractures of the distal tibia with major articular involvement. *J. Trauma*, **11**, 866–73

Saleh, M., Shanahan, M.D.G. and Fern, E.D. (1993) Intra-articular fractures of the distal tibia: surgical management by limited internal fixation and articulated distraction. *Injury*, **24**, 37–40

Sanders, R., Pappas, J., Mast, J. and Helfet, D. (1992) The salvage of open grade IIIB ankle and talus fractures. *J. Orthop. Trauma*, **6**, 201–8

Scheck, M. (1965) Treatment of comminuted distal tibia fractures by combined dual-pin fixation and limited open reduction. *J. Bone Joint Surg.*, **47A**, 1537–53

Teeny, S., Wiss, D.A., Hathaway, R. and Sarmiento, A. (1990) Tibial plafond fractures: errors, complication and pitfalls in operative treatment. *Orthop. Trans.*, **14**, 265

Tornetta, P. III, Weiner, L., Bergman, M. *et al.* (1993) Pilon fractures: treatment with combined internal and external fixation. *J. Orthop. Trauma*, **7**, 489–96

Trumble, T.E., Benirschke, S.K. and Vedder, N.B. (1992) Use of radial forearm flaps to treat complications of closed pilon fractures. *J. Orthop. Trauma*, **6**, 358–65

Tscherne, H. and Goetzen, L. (ed.) (1984) *Fractures with Soft Tissue Injuries*, Springer-Verlag, Berlin

Tscherne, H. and Schatzker, J.: (1992) *Major Fractures of the Pilon, Talus, and Calcaneus*, Springer-Verlag, Berlin

Webster's Ninth New Collegiate Dictionary (1980) G. and C. Merrian Co.

Williams, C.W., Langston, J. and Sanders, A. (1967) Comminuted fractures of the distal tibia into the ankle joint. Proceedings of the Western Orthopaedic Association. *J. Bone Joint Surg.*, **49A**, 192

Wiss, A., Johnson, D. and Miao, M. (1992) Compression plating for nonunion after failed external fixation of open tibial fractures. *J. Bone Joint Surg.*, **74A**, 1279–1285

14

Ankle fractures

C. Court-Brown

Ankle fractures have been extensively studied over the years. They are the commonest intra-articular fracture that orthopaedic surgeons regularly operate on and they comprise about 60% of all fractures of the tibia and fibula. Surprisingly, there is greater uniformity of opinion as regards their management than is encountered with fractures of the tibial diaphysis. This is probably because of two main reasons. First, it has become accepted that intra-articular fractures should be treated by accurate fragment reduction and rigid fixation, and as virtually all ankle fractures are intra-articular, the teachings of the AO group (Müller *et al.*, 1991) and others have been adopted by most surgeons. In addition, it is impossible to fix ankle fractures adequately except by internal fixation techniques, and although intramedullary nailing techniques, usually in the form of Rush pins (see Figure 14.15), can be used, most ankle fractures will be fixed using AO techniques (Müller *et al.*, 1991) or occasionally by the use of Kirschner wires, bone staples or cerclage wiring. Thus most surgeons have adopted conventional AO techniques to treat ankle fractures and therefore practise rigid fixation, this being frequently associated with early joint mobilization.

Despite this apparent uniformity of view, there are a number of arguments regarding the management of ankle fractures, and this chapter will concentrate on these current controversies rather than repeat the excellent descriptions of ankle surgery that are contained in other texts (Müller *et al.*, 1991; Browner *et al.*, 1992).

The role of classification systems in ankle fractures

The relative frequency with which surgeons encounter ankle fractures has meant that the classification systems are probably better understood and applied than classifications dealing with other tibial fractures. As detailed in Chapter 1, there are two principal classifications of ankle fractures in current use. The Lauge-Hansen (1948–54) classification is an aetiological classification based on the position of the foot at the time of injury and the direction of the deforming force. The AO classification (Müller *et al.*, 1990) is a morphological classification based on the radiological features of the different fracture types. The division of ankle fractures into three types based on the position of the fracture in relation to the syndesmosis is easy to understand but there is debate about the prognostic significance of the AO classification (Broos and Bisschop, 1991).

At first sight it would appear that the two classifications are compatible and that they have merely used different methods of arriving at the same end-product. However, there are a number of differences. There is general agreement that most ankle fractures follow supination–eversion injuries (Lindsjö, 1981). Lauge-Hansen believed that the first stage of a supination–eversion injury was tearing of the anterior tibiofibular ligament. The equivalent AO B1.1 fracture apparently has an intact ligament, although it is torn in the B1.2 and B1.3 fractures. The A1.1, A1.2 and A1.3 fractures all correspond well to variations of the supination–abduction type I fracture and the A2.2 fracture is a type II supination–abduction fracture. The AO B2.1 isolated malleolar fracture is associated with a rupture of the fibular collateral ligament. Isolated medial malleolar fractures in the Lauge-Hansen classification are seen with pronation–eversion type I injuries or pronation–abduction type I injuries. In both cases the fibular collateral ligament is intact.

It is difficult to be certain about the AO classification of a number of fractures where there is said to be ligamentous disruption in association with an obvious fracture. For example, the distinction between the B1.1 and B1.2 fractures or the presence of a lateral ligamentous rupture associated with an A2.1 medial malleolar fracture can only be based on accurate clinical examination or MRI scanning. The latter is rarely performed in simple ankle fractures and the former is often unobtainable in the acute situation. Thus it is not always possible to classify fractures with complete accuracy. The same criticism may be levelled at the Lauge-Hansen classification where, for example, it may be difficult to diagnose a supination–eversion type III fracture with rupture of the posterior syndesmosis. The Lauge-Hansen classification is probably most useful if one is considering non-operative fracture management but despite its aetiological advantages it is probably now been superseded by the surgically orientated AO classification. However, there will be reference to both classifications in this chapter.

Incidence and epidemiology

Bengner *et al.* (1986) studied two 3-year periods in 1950–52 and 1980–2 comparing the incidence of a number of different fractures in Malmo, Sweden. They examined the comparative incidence of ankle fractures in these two periods, showing that there were 383 fractures between 1950 and 1952 compared with 739 in the 1980–2 period. The age-specific incidence of certain fractures had changed in the 30-year intervening period. In the isolated lateral malleolar fracture, which consisted of AO type B lateral malleolar fractures, there was an increase in men up to 45 years of age and in women over 75 years of age. For bimalleolar and trimalleolar fractures, there was no increase in men but there was an increase in women over the age of 45, this being more pronounced over 65 years of age. The authors also showed an increase in the proportion of ankle fractures associated with severe injuries and with sports injuries.

There are very few studies of the epidemiology of ankle fractures from one centre dealing with all different types of pathology. The epidemiological characteristics of ankle fractures in the Edinburgh population were presented in Chapter 2. A similar study was undertaken in the Mayo Clinic, USA (Daly *et al.*, 1987). They also examined the different types of ankle fractures seen over a 3-year period. In their study 15% of the ankle fractures followed road traffic accidents or falls from a height compared with 16% in Edinburgh. In contrast, they found that 33% of their fractures occurred in sports injuries and 40% occurred after relatively minor injuries such as twists or falls. These figures differ from the Edinburgh series, where the comparative figures are 15.6% and 63.6%. The cause of these differences is not known. The Mayo group considered fractures that did not involve the lateral malleolus to be unclassifiable according to the Weber (AO) system, but if the 77% of the fractures that they considered classifiable by the AO system is extrapolated, then they found that 53.2% of their fractures were type B, 35.1% were type A and 11.7% were type C. These figures correspond almost exactly with the Edinburgh figures in Chapter 2 and are very similar to those of Lindsjö (1985), who analysed 611 ankle fractures, stating that 56% were type B, 25% were type A and 13% were type C. In the Mayo series 69% of ankle fractures were unimalleolar, 19% were bimalleolar and 12% were trimalleolar. Again this showed surprising similarity to the Edinburgh figures, which show 69.8% unimalleolar fractures, 20.5% bimalleolar and 9.7% trimalleolar fractures. These epidemiological figures demonstrate the clinical and economic importance of isolated malleolar fractures and for this reason it is important that orthopaedic surgeons appreciate how to deal with these injuries.

Treatment of infra- and trans-syndesmotic fractures

Unimalleolar fractures

The commonest ankle fractures dealt with by orthopaedic surgeons are those involving the medial or lateral malleoli. Table 2.24 shows that the A2.1 medial malleolus fracture (Figure 14.1) has different epidemiological characteristics when compared with lateral malleolar fractures, these being the A1.2 (Figure 14.2), A1.3 (Figure 14.3) and B1.1 (Figure 14.4) fractures. Fractures of the

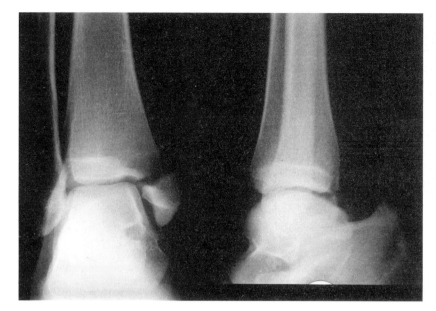

Figure 14.1
The anteroposterior and lateral X-rays of an A2.1 medial malleolar fracture. This radiological appearance is produced in the Lauge-Hansen PEI or PAI fractures. Isolated medial malleolar fractures carry a worse prognosis than isolated lateral malleolar fractures. Their epidemiological characteristics also differ (Table 2.23)

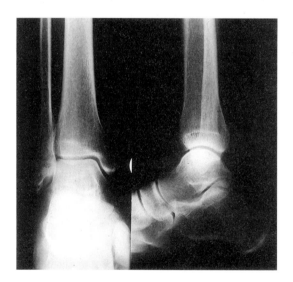

Figure 14.2   The A1.2 fracture. This is an avulsion fracture and is equivalent to the Lauge-Hansen SAI injury. The fractures is rarely displaced and rarely requires operative treatment

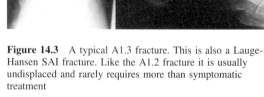

Figure 14.3   A typical A1.3 fracture. This is also a Lauge-Hansen SAI fracture. Like the A1.2 fracture it is usually undisplaced and rarely requires more than symptomatic treatment

medial malleolus occur in younger patients and are associated with higher velocity injuries than lateral malleolar fractures. Chapter 2 shows a high proportion of road traffic accidents, falls from a height and sporting injuries in medial malleolar fractures and a lower incidence of twisting injuries and simple falls.

In recent years, little has been written about the treatment of isolated fractures of the medial malleolus. Most authors have concentrated on fractures of the lateral malleolus and fractures which involve more than one malleolus when discussing the relative merits of operative and non-operative management. The general view of clinicians is that accurate repositioning of the medial malleolus is essential and that all displaced medial malleolar fractures should be reduced and internally fixed. The question of what constitutes an undisplaced

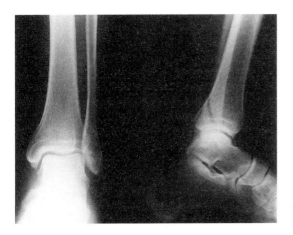

Figure 14.4 A typical B1.1 fracture. This corresponds to the Lauge-Hansen SEII fracture. The management of this fracture is discussed in the text, but it is crucial to distinguish it from the B2.1 or Lauge-Hansen SEIV fracture which is inherently unstable. (see Figure 14.7)

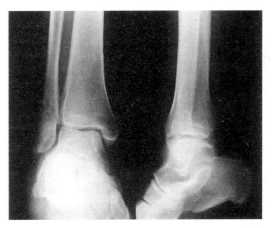

Figure 14.5 A B1.3 lateral malleolar fracture. The distinction from the B1.1 fracture lies in the degree of comminution at the fracture site. The treatment is, however, the same as for a B1.1 fracture although significant comminution might be associated with shortening or external rotation

fracture is often difficult to answer (Joy *et al.*, 1974). Pettrone *et al.* (1983) used a gap of 1 mm on the anteroposterior X-ray when considering medial malleolar displacement. There is little to prove or disprove this figure, but surgeons should be aware that fractures which are apparently undisplaced on one X-ray view may show greater displacement on another view. Great care must be taken in assessing medial malleolar displacement, and if there is doubt about displacement it is better to operate. Minor fractures of the tip of the medial malleolus should be considered as equivalent to deltoid ligament strains or ruptures and need not be reattached.

Lateral malleolar fractures

There has been considerable interest in the management of isolated fractures of the lateral malleolus in recent years, probably because there is now mounting evidence that non-operative management of the AO B1.1 (Lauge-Hansen SEII) fracture gives results that are at least equivalent to operative management. The B1.1 fracture (Figure 14.4) constitutes almost 20% of all the ankle fractures seen by orthopaedic surgeons (see Table 2.23). These fractures are caused by an external rotation force acting on the supinated foot and are usually displaced at the time of presentation. In addition to rotational displacement there may also be comminution, as in the AO B1.3 fracture (Figure 14.5) and a degree of shortening. Obviously rotation and shortening leads to articular incongruity and many

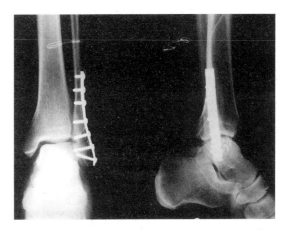

Figure 14.6 Anteroposterior and lateral postoperative X-rays of an internally fixed B1.1 fracture. The use of a curved lateral AO plate is demonstrated. Alternative techniques are to use multiple lag screws for a long spiral fracture or an anti-glide plate

surgeons believe that such incongruity should be treated by open reduction and rigid internal fixation (Figure 14.6). Again there is difficulty in defining displacement, with Pettrone *et al.* (1983) accepting up to 2 mm displacement on the anteroposterior or lateral X-rays.

Other surgeons take the view that if osteoarthritis and ligamentous insufficiency were common sequelae of the AO group B1 fractures, then large numbers of patients would be complaining of these sequelae, and this does not appear to be the case.

Kristensen and Hansen (1985) and Bauer *et al.* (1985) both carried out retrospective long-term studies to investigate the prognosis of these fractures. Kristensen and Hansen (1985) followed up 94 non-operatively managed patients, 16–25 years after their fracture. The primary displacement of these fractures was poor in 89 cases according to Cedell's (1967) radiological criteria, but despite this, 73 patients were symptom-free and the remaining 16 had negligible symptomatology. No patient showed a reduced capacity for unprotected work or exercise and no patient showed radiological signs of osteoarthritis.

Bauer *et al.* (1985) also carried out a retrospective study examining 143 patients at an average of 29 years after fracture. They included AO type A, B and C fractures, although they studied 49 patients with Lauge-Hansen SEII fractures. They only found one patient with this fracture who had developed osteoarthritis and noted that primary displacement of up to 3 mm was compatible with treatment success. Their conclusions were that AO group B1 fractures did not require operative fixation. Attention has been drawn to the fact that these observations were made on patients less than 50 years of age (Cedell, 1985), but there is no evidence that older patients are subjected to a greater number of complications. A recent study by Michelson *et al.* (1992) pointed out the difficulty in accurately measuring radiographs and therefore the problems that arise when trying to assess fibular shortening, rotation and displacement. They examined 26 ankle fractures, of which 21 were supination–eversion injuries. They found that despite the fact that every patient had an apparent external rotation deformity of the lateral malleolus on plain X-ray, CT evaluation rarely demonstrated external rotation of the distal fibula with respect to the talus or the distal tibia. These results support the findings of Bauer *et al.* (1985) and Kristensen and Hansen (1985), and suggest that Lauge-Hansen SEII or AO group B1 fractures do not usually require operative treatment. Occasionally the surgeon will encounter significant displacement of the lateral malleolar fracture and surgery will then be required.

The role of non-operative management in the treatment of AO group B fractures has been expanded by a number of surgeons to the extent that very little treatment is actually given to these injuries. Zeegers *et al.* (1989) examined the use of a supportive sports shoe in 23 patients with Lauge-Hansen SEII injuries in which displacement was said to be less than 2 mm. Initially a supportive

bandage was applied for one week following which the supportive sports shoe was worn for a further 5 weeks. Their results were good and they concluded that this type of treatment was successful and in particular diminished the time off work.

Ryd and Bengtsson (1992) extended this type of treatment philosophy treating SEII fractures with up to 2 mm of displacement in an elastic bandage and advocating immediate weight bearing. In 49 patients only 4 had minor symptoms and patients were back at normal activities in 4 months, this being somewhat less than the equivalent time following surgery.

There seems little doubt that SEII fractures can be treated non-operatively. The amount of displacement, shortening or rotation that is acceptable has not been accurately defined, but it would appear from the long-term studies of Bauer *et al.* (1985) and Kristensen and Hansen (1985) that the amount of displacement commonly encountered makes little difference to the prognosis. Fractures associated with gross displacement should be internally fixed.

The alternative lateral malleolar fractures are the AO A1.2 (Figure 14.2) and A1.3 (Figure 14.3) configurations, these being variants of the Lauge-Hansen supination–adduction type I injury. They are avulsion fractures and rarely displace significantly. Little has been written about the management of these injuries, as in general the prognosis is good and 4–6 weeks in a below-knee walking cast or supportive strapping is all that is required.

One of the problems in treating the common B1.1 fracture is that the deltoid ligament may be ruptured. This converts the fracture into an AO B2.1 or Lauge-Hansen SEIV fracture. Occasionally there may be fibular comminution, making the fracture a B2.3 in the AO classification (Figure 14.7). The B2.1 or B2.3 fractures, unlike the B1.1 fracture, are unstable. The patient usually presents with lateral talar shift and an increased gap between the medial wall of the talus and the medial malleolus on X-ray. This may be difficult to detect and the surgeon should look carefully to see if the joint space is wider medially than superiorly. If there is any doubt as to the presence of a B2.1 or B2.3 fracture, an examination under anaesthesia should be performed.

The problem of talar shift was highlighted by Ramsey and Hamilton (1976). They showed that a 1 mm lateral displacement of the talus was associated with a mean decrease in contact area of 42%. Increasing displacements were associated with a greater decrease in contact area, although the

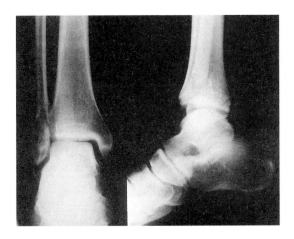

Figure 14.7   A B2.3 or Lauge-Hansen SEIV fracture. The comminuted nature of the fibula seen particularly on the lateral view makes this a B2.3 fracture in the AO classification. Lateral talar shift is noted and this must be reduced accurately if a good result is to be obtained. This was the most common fracture configuration seen in the Edinburgh series of open ankle fractures

incremental rise lessens after 1 mm of shift. Their results clearly point to the importance of accurate repositioning of the talus in the ankle mortice, showing that even minor discrepancies will considerably alter the loading across the ankle joint.

Pettrone *et al.* (1983) confirmed the importance of accurate reduction of the ankle joint in these injuries, showing statistically better results after internal fixation of SEIV injuries compared with

non-operative management. Similar findings were also shown by Yed and Kristensen (1980). It is recommended that the B2.1 and B2.3 fracture should be treated by accurate fibular reduction and rigid internal fixation using AO techniques. The question always arises as to the importance of suturing the deltoid ligaments. There is no clinical evidence that this is necessary (De Souza *et al.*, 1985) but an X-ray should be taken after fibular plating to check on the reduction of the ankle joint. If the medial side remains open, the deltoid ligament should be removed from the joint and sutured. This is, however, rare.

Bimalleolar fractures

These fractures are classified in the AO, A2, A3 and B2 groups, the B2.2 fracture representing the commonest bimalleolar fracture (Figure 14.8). This fracture represents a variant of the Lauge-Hansen SEIV fracture and is merely a variant of the B2.1 fracture previously discussed. These fractures are unstable and difficult to treat non-operatively. There may be considerable displacement of the ankle joint on initial presentation and skin ischaemia may be a problem. An initial closed reduction to relieve pressure on the skin should be performed unless immediate surgery is undertaken (Watson and Hollingdale, 1992). Few surgeons use closed reduction and the application of a cast for definitive management and internal fixation is indicated for these fractures unless the medical condition of the patient precludes surgery.

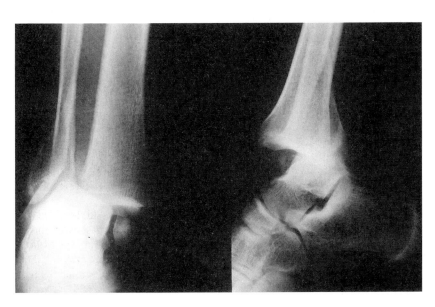

Figure 14.8   A B2.2 fracture. The spiral nature of the fibular fracture and the transverse medial malleolar fracture show that this is a Lauge-Hansen SEIV fracture. The ankle is dislocated and this represents a classic example of the low Dupuytren's fracture

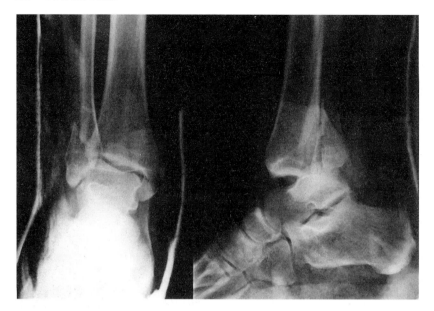

Figure 14.9 (a) A B3.3 trimalleolar fracture. Again this is a variant of the SEIV where, instead of a rupture of the posterior tibiofibular ligament, there has been an avulsion fracture from the posterior malleolus. The avulsed posterior malleolar fragment corresponds to about 25% of the distal articular surface

The argument about the method of fixation of bimalleolar fractures centres around whether the lateral malleolus should be internally fixed as well as the medial malleolus. Ashurst and Bromer (1922) advocated reduction of the medial malleolus. They and many other surgeons believed that the lateral malleolar fragment could be subsequently treated by plaster immobilization. However, Yablon *et al.* (1977) suggested that this method of management was associated with a significant degree of osteoarthritis. They demonstrated that mere fixation of the medial malleolus did not correct talar rotation and they strongly advocated accurate reduction and internal fixation of both medial and lateral malleoli regarding the lateral malleolus as the key to the anatomical reduction of displaced bimalleolar fractures. This view is now widely held. Pettrone *et al.* (1983) showed statistically significantly improved results following internal fixation of both malleoli when compared with fixation of only the medial malleolus. Limbird and Aaron (1987) dealt with the problem of bimalleolar fractures associated with significant fibular comminution. They pointed out the inherent instability of this fracture and the advantages of open reduction and internal fixation associated with bone grafting of the fibular defect.

Trimalleolar fractures

Trimalleolar fractures are represented in the AO classification by the B3.2 and the B3.3 fractures.

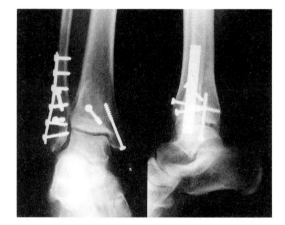

Figure 14.9 (b) The fracture has been reduced and fixed using conventional AO technique and has healed well. Lag screws were used prior to the application of a fibular plate and one screw was used to secure the medial malleolus and the posterior malleolus, this screw being inserted from the anterior aspect

The B3.3 fracture is almost as common as the B2.2 bimalleolar fracture (Table 2.21). The B3.3 trimalleolar fracture (Figure 14.9) is a variant of the Lauge-Hansen SEIV fracture, where the posterior malleolus is avulsed during the third stage. The posterior malleolar fragment can vary in size from a small peripheral rim fracture to a fracture fragment that may involve more than half of the articular surface.

The treatment of the trimalleolar fracture is essentially the same as the bimalleolar fracture. The controversy concerns the need for operative fixation of the posterior malleolus. The classical teaching is that posterior malleolar fragments that involve less than 25% of the articular surface do not require reduction and fixation (Miller, 1974; De Souza *et al.*, 1985). This view has been supported by Harper and Hardin (1988), who carried out a retrospective review of 38 patients in whom there was a posterior malleolar fragment involving more than 25% of the joint surface. They included external rotation and abduction injuries and compared operative treatment of the posterior malleolus with non-operative treatment. They emphasized the importance of accurate lateral malleolar reduction but felt that fixation of the posterior malleolus was unnecessary. They showed that the incidence of anatomical reduction in both groups was similar and this is an important point. Accurate reduction of large posterior malleolar fragments is surprisingly difficult and involves considerable soft tissue dissection. It is not unusual to see residual articular deformity after fixation.

Jaskulka *et al.* (1989) examined the size of the posterior malleolar fragment and the usefulness of surgery. They looked at all posterior malleolar fractures, including rim fractures, and showed that even small rim fractures were associated with an increased incidence of osteoarthritis and they concluded that some of the problems of the management of posterior malleolar fractures were related to articular damage and could not be treated. They also showed that the results associated with fractures of less than 5% of the articular surface were similar to the results seen with larger fracture fragments. However, they did conclude that at least in the case of larger fragments, operative treatment affected the prognosis. They felt that anatomical reduction led to a decrease in the incidence of osteoarthritis, although they did not feel able to detail a particular size of fracture fragment that required operative fixation. On balance, it does seem reasonable to fix posterior malleoli fractures if a good reduction cannot be achieved by closed means (Figure 14.9), but care must be taken to ensure that an accurate reduction of the posterior malleolus is achieved.

Treatment of supra-syndesmotic fractures

Supra-syndesmotic ankle fractures are classified in the AO classification as type C fractures. In the Lauge-Hansen classification they can occur following an external rotational force on a pronated foot, the PEIII fracture (Figure 14.10), or with a pronation–abduction fracture, the PAIII fracture (Figure 14.11). It is important to distinguish between supra-syndesmotic fibular fractures caused by external rotation and those which are

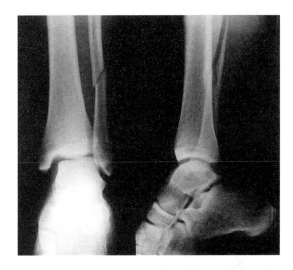

Figure 14.10 A C1.1 fracture with spiral supra-syndesmotic fibular fracture and an obvious disruption of the deltoid ligament. This fracture corresponds to a Lauge-Hansen PEIII fracture. As with the B2.1 fracture, it is important adequately to reduce the talus

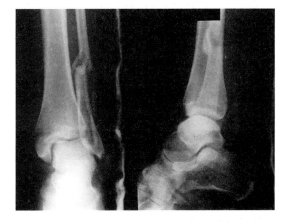

Figure 14.11 A C2.2 fracture. The comminution and transverse nature of the fibular fracture demonstrated that this is a Lauge-Hansen PAIII fracture.

caused by an abduction injury. In abduction injuries the anterior and posterior components of the syndesmosis and the interosseous membrane up to the level of the fibular fracture will be disrupted. In the external rotation supra-syndesmotic fracture the posterior syndesmosis acts as the fulcrum of rotation and under these circumstances the damage to the posterior syndesmosis and the interosseous membrane may be very much less, making the PEIII fracture more stable than the PAIII fracture.

In the AO classification there is a separate group (C3) for Maissoneuve fractures. These are, however, produced by the same forces as the supra-syndesmotic fractures associated with lower fibular fractures. Their importance lies in the fact that the presence of a high fibular fracture is often either missed or misinterpreted (Figure 14.12). If such a fracture is seen, the surgeon must always carefully examine the ankle clinically and radiologically to make sure that an ankle fracture or ligamentous disruption is not missed.

Pankovich (1978) has suggested that supra-syndesmotic fractures may occur in supination–eversion injuries although Lauge-Hansen (1948–54) did not mention the possibility. Pankovich suggests that rupture of the interosseous membrane and a supra-syndesmotic fibular fracture follow rupture of the anterior tibiofibular ligament and it is possible for a type C fracture combination to occur in the presence of an intact deltoid ligament. This conclusion is not supported by either of the AO or Lauge-Hansen classifications, which suggest that there must be a rupture of the deltoid ligament or a medial malleolar fracture to allow for a supra-syndesmotic fibular fracture. However, there seems little doubt that the association of a spiral supra-syndesmotic fibular fracture without a deltoid rupture does exist (Figure 14.13), although it is probably uncommon, the classical PAIII and PEIII injuries being seen more frequently. Table 2.21 shows that the C1.1 and C1.2 fractures occur with approximately equal frequency, with the C2.2 and C2.3 fractures being the only other type C fracture, occurring with a frequency of at least 1%.

Supra-syndesmotic fractures of the proximal fibula are rare, accounting for only 0.9% of the Edinburgh series. These were discussed by

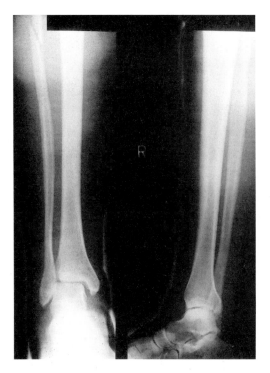

Figure 14.12 A C3.3 ankle fracture with a high fibular fracture, rupture of the deltoid ligament and a posterior malleolar fragment. This is a variant of the Maissoneuve fracture

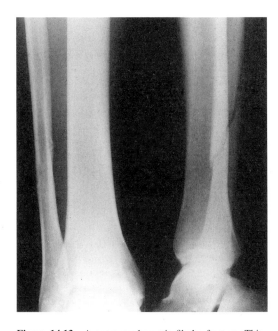

Figure 14.13 A supra-syndesmotic fibular fracture. This was caused by rotational force on the fixed ankle. On clinical examination there was no evidence of discomfort on the medial side of the joint, suggesting that the deltoid ligament was intact, and there was no evidence of ankle instability on fluoroscopy, showing that the posterior syndesmosis and the interosseous membrane were intact

Pankovich (1976). Again, he believed that these fractures were caused by supination–eversion injuries and he stressed that it was possible to have the equivalent injury without an ankle fracture. The AO classification also allows for this by suggesting that there may be a proximal tibiofibular dislocation rather than a proximal fibular fracture.

There is agreement that it is important to understand and diagnose the mechanisms of supra-syndesmotic ankle fractures. Failure to recognize the presence of an inferior tibiofibular diastasis and associated intraosseous membrane rupture may lead to inadequate treatment of an unstable fracture with consequent instability, pain and osteoarthritic change.

The variant described by Pankovich (1978), with an intact deltoid ligament, is stable and providing there is no significant fibular disruption it can be treated non-operatively by the application of a below-knee cast. Other supra-syndesmotic fractures should be recognized as potentially unstable and the surgeon should be aware of the importance of accurate reduction and internal fixation. Pronation–abduction injuries (see Figure 14.11) will always disrupt the entire inferior tibiofibular syndesmosis, which must then be reduced and held by a syndesmosis screw. If the supra-syndesmotic fibular fracture is relatively low, a syndesmosis screw may not be required. Boden *et al.* (1989) showed that if the fibular fracture was between 3 cm and 4.5 cm proximal to the ankle and was rigidly plated, then the residual intact interosseous membrane in combination with the rigid plate would permit sufficient stability to manage without a syndesmosis screw. If a screw is to be placed across a syndesmosis it can either be placed through one of the screw holes in the plate or separately. The presence of a high fibular fracture and a complete disruption leaves the surgeon with the choice of reducing and plating the fibular fracture or inserting a diastasis screw or both. The key problem is the diastasis and therefore it is logical to treat the high supra-syndesmotic fracture with a diastasis screw and only plate the fracture if it is significantly displaced. If a syndesmosis screw is inserted in the presence of a displaced high fibular fracture the fibula will be fixed in a malreduced position. If there is doubt, it is wise to plate the fibular fracture and then insert a diastasis screw.

Supination–external rotation injuries appear to be somewhat different. It is likely that the posterior syndesmosis acts as a fulcrum around which rotation takes place and the interosseous membrane and posterior syndesmosis may well be considerably less damaged than they would be in the presence of an abduction injury. It is therefore suggested that the surgeon performs an examination under anaesthesia, including stress views, to investigate the integrity of the syndesmosis. If there is a low supra-syndesmotic fibular fracture, direct palpation of the intraosseous membrane and syndesmosis can be undertaken. If the posterior fibres of the syndesmosis are found to be intact, a diastasis screw is not required. In all cases the medial malleolus fracture, if present, should be accurately reduced and rigidly fixed.

Syndesmosis fixation

The objective behind inserting a syndesmosis screw is to restore as well as possible the relationship between the fibula and the tibia. There is a tendency to overclose the syndesmosis and this must be avoided. Olerud (1985) demonstrated that dorsiflexion was lost in proportion to the degree of plantarflexion that existed when the syndesmosis was fixed. For this reason it seems sensible to fix the syndesmosis with the foot in dorsiflexion.

There is debate about the number and the technique of insertion of the screws used to fix the syndesmosis. One or two screws can be used and the screws may penetrate all four cortices of the fibula and tibia or may only penetrate the lateral tibial cortex. It is likely that these debates are somewhat academic and that in the clinical situation it seems that there is no real advantage in any particular technique. One screw placed in all four cortices such that the correct relationship of the fibula and tibia is maintained is sufficient. A fully threaded screw is preferred as this avoids the possibility of over-tightening but it does require accurate reduction of the syndesmosis prior to screw insertion.

Most surgeons believe that the syndesmosis screw should be removed after 6 or 8 weeks to allow for correct motion between the distal fibula and tibia. This can usually be done under local anaesthetic. If it is not done, the screw frequently loosens or breaks and there seems to be remarkably little morbidity from leaving the syndesmosis screw in position.

Postoperative management

The treatment of ankle fractures managed non-operatively is straightforward. The cast, brace or splint is usually kept in position for about 6 weeks and then a course of rehabilitation exercises instituted. Where the fracture is operatively managed, there is debate about the usefulness of early joint mobilization and weight bearing.

If AO techniques are used to treat the ankle fracture and all components of the fracture are fixed, then early mobilization of the ankle and subtalar joints can be instituted. A number of different treatment regimes have been suggested. Burwell and Charnley (1965) advocated postoperative joint mobility exercises in bed until motion was restored followed by full weight bearing in a cast. Lund-Kristensen *et al.* (1982) either used no cast or applied one for a few days postoperatively and then allowed full joint mobilization out of the cast. They advocated the use of crutches to maintain a non-weight bearing status. Meyer and Kumler (1980) used a postoperative cast but only for an average of 3.8 weeks followed by non-weight bearing mobilization until fracture union.

In a busy unit with patients who sometimes do not cooperate with complicated postoperative regimes, it can be an advantage to apply a cast postoperatively and maintain it for the treatment period, but this philosophy should be balanced against any morbidity inherent in the use of a cast. Søndenaa *et al.* (1986) randomized internally fixed ankle fractures into a group treated in a cast for 6 weeks and a second group who had a cast for 3 days followed by a joint mobilization regime. They found a significant reduction of dorsiflexion, plantar flexion and inversion at 6 weeks in the cast-managed group but no difference from 12 weeks onwards. At neither postoperative period did they see differences in muscle strength, osteoporosis or ankle joint cartilage height. However, they did find the early mobilization group to have less pain up to 18 weeks after fracture, although the results between these two groups were similar at one year.

Cimino *et al.* (1991) compared the use of an ankle foot orthosis (AFO) and a cast following operative management of ankle fractures. They showed that the AFO group contained a greater number of patients who had ankle dorsiflexion that exceeded 15°. They also demonstrated no loss of reduction with early mobilization in the AFO group or from early weight bearing in either group. They suggested that the tendency that some surgeons showed to promote non-weight bearing following ankle fixation was incorrect, and this view is confirmed by the work of Ahl *et al.* (1986, 1987). They used stereophotogammatry to analyse fracture movement in isolated lateral malleolar fractures (1986) and bimalleolar and trimalleolar fractures (1987). They used less rigid fixation in the form of pins, staples and cerclage wire and despite this showed no loss of fracture position.

Overall, it is probably advantageous to allow early ankle and subtalar movement after surgery, although the benefits seem to be relatively little. Cast management carries little morbidity and can be used without significant loss of movement. Early weight bearing should be encouraged and non-weight bearing should never be substituted for poor surgical technique.

Open ankle fractures

Open fractures of the ankle are relatively rare, accounting for only 1% of the series detailed in Chapter 2. The distribution of AO types is similar for both closed and open ankle fractures, the only difference being that where the B2.1 fracture accounts for 6.7% of the overall series, 30.8% of the open fracture group showed a B2.1 configuration. Only 23.8% of the open fractures were Gustilo type III in severity (Figure 14.14). The epidemiology of open ankle fractures differs in other series. The Edinburgh figures are from a unit taking all types of pathology from the community. More specialized centres orientated towards the management of severe trauma may show a different spectrum of open fractures. Franklin *et al.* (1984) analysed their experience of the management of open ankle fractures in Seattle, USA, in a level 1 trauma centre. They had a 42.1% incidence of Gustilo type III open fractures in a group of patients where road traffic accidents accounted for 60% of the cases.

The management of open fractures has changed over the past 10–15 years, with improved fixation and plastic surgery techniques. There has also been an increased awareness of the importance of an early radical debridement, and in general the result of the management of open fractures in all areas of the body has improved in recent years. Chapman and Mahoney (1979) reported no infections in grade I open ankle fractures, with 11.1% infection in grade II fractures and 100% infection in 3 grade III fractures.

By way of contrast, Franklin *et al.* (1984), in a review of 38 open ankle fractures treated by aggressive early debridement, early rigid internal fixation and appropriate soft tissue management, reported only one possible infection, although there were no sequelae from osteomyelitis in this case. They had no non-unions and reported excellent functional results in 74.3% of the patients.

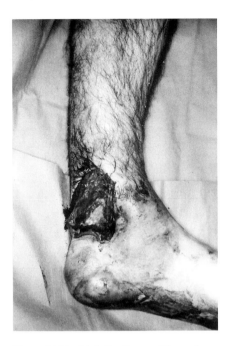

Figure 14.14 (a) A Gustilo type III open fracture-dislocation of the ankle with considerable bony contamination and soft tissue damage

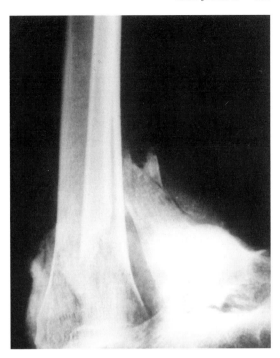

Figure 14.14 (b) Showing that this is a C2.2 or Lauge-Hansen PAIII fracture. Reduction was difficult and fixation was undertaken medially and laterally. Postoperatively a distally based fasciocutaneous flap was required to close the skin defect

Bray *et al.* (1989) compared immediate internal fixation versus closed immobilization and delayed fixation in a retrospective study of 31 open ankle fractures. They showed significantly better dorsiflexion and inversion of the primarily fixed fractures as well as significantly decreased hospitalization time, although the pain and function scores were similar between the two groups.

The management of open ankle fractures should follow the same guidelines suggested for the management of open tibial diaphyseal fractures. The key to success in the management of any open fracture is the adequacy of the initial debridement and the later handling of the soft tissues, including the speed and adequacy of flap cover if this is required. Debridement should remove all dead and devitalized tissue as well as all vestiges of contamination. It is suggested that saline lavage is used during the debridement. Rigid internal fixation should be undertaken using AO techniques and the primary skin wound should never be closed, although the skin extensions can be closed if this can be done without any tension.

It is recommended that all open ankle fractures are re-examined 36–48 hours after the initial surgery and that flap cover, if required, should be carried out at this time. The overall principles are well summarized by Franklin *et al.* (1984).

Prognosis

There are a number of evaluation systems to allow assessment of the success of the treatment of ankle fractures (Mazur *et al.*, 1979; Lindsjo, 1981; Olerud and Molander, 1986; Baird and Jackson, 1987). Table 14.1 shows the system produced by Baird and Jackson, with that of Olerud and Molander shown in Table 14.2. Baird and Jackson's evaluation criteria are self-contained with reference to pain, stability, function, ankle motion and radiological changes. Olerud and Molander include references to pain, stiffness, swelling and function but do not refer to radiological changes. The authors use the Cedell (1967) classification of radiological displacement.

Lindjso (1981) analysed 310 ankle fractures and showed statistically better results in men than

Table 14.1   The ankle scoring system of Baird and Jackson (1987)

	Points
Pain	
A No pain	15
B Mild pain with strenuous activity	12
C Mild pain with activities of daily living	8
D Pain with weight bearing	4
E Pain at rest	0
Stability of ankle	
A No clinical instability	15
B Instability with sports activities	5
C Instability with activities of daily living	0
Ability to walk	
A Able to walk desired distances without limp or pain	15
B Able to walk desired distances with mild limp or pain	12
C Moderately restricted in ability to walk	8
D Able to walk short distances only	4
E Unable to walk	0
Ability to run	
A Able to run desired distances without pain	10
B Able to run desired distances with slight pain	8
C Moderate restriction in ability to run, with mild pain	6
D Able to run short distances only	3
E Unable to run	0
Ability to work	
A Able to perform usual occupation	10
B Able to perform usual occupation with restrictions in some strenuous activities	8
C Able to perform usual occupation with substantial restrictions	6
D Partially disabled; selected jobs only	3
E Unable to work	0
Motion of the ankle	
A Within 10° of uninjured ankle	10
B Within 15° of uninjured ankle	7
C Within 20° of uninjured ankle	4
D < 50% of uninjured ankle, or dorsiflexion < 5°	0
Radiographic result	
A Anatomic with intact mortise (normal medical clear space, normal superior joint space, no talar tilt)	25
B Same as A with mild reactive changes at the joint margins	15
C Measurable narrowing of superior joint space, with superior joint space > 2 mm, or talar tilt 2 mm	10
D Moderate narrowing of the superior joint space, with superior joint space between 2 and 1 mm	5
E Severe narrowing of the superior joint space, with superior joint space < 1 mm, widening of the medial clear space, severe reactive changes (sclerotic subchondral bone and osteophyte formation)	0
Maximum possible score	100

Excellent = 96–100 points, good = 91–95 points, fair = 81–90 points, poor = 0–80 points

women except for women aged between 65 and 74 years, where the results were similar. He noted that the poorest results were in women of ages 45–64 years. Interestingly, he found that better clinical results were obtained with AO type B and C fractures than with type A fractures. He did not find that suture of the deltoid or anterior tibiofibular ligaments influenced the results, but he did stress the importance of accurate reduction in obtaining good clinical results. In terms of function, he showed that 90% of the patients returned to the same occupation and 82% returned to their previous sports and other physical activities. Overall, 89% were able to walk normally and 85% managed

Table 14.2 **The ankle score of Olerud and Molander (1986)**

			Points
I	Pain (25 points)	None	25
		While walking on uneven surfaces	20
		While walking on even surface outdoors	10
		While walking indoors	5
		Constant and severe	0
II	Stiffness (10 points)	None	10
		Stiffness	0
III	Swelling (10 points)	None	10
		Only evenings	5
		Constant	0
IV	Stair climbing (10 points)	No problems	10
		Impaired	5
		Unable	0
V	Running (5 points)	Possible	5
		Impossible	0
VI	Jumping (5 points)	Possible	5
		Impossible	0
VII	Squatting (5 points)	No problems	5
		Unable	0
VIII	Supports (10 points)	No support	10
		Taping, wrapping	5
		Stick or crutch	0
IX	Work, activities of daily life (20 points)	Same as before injury	20
		Loss of tempo	15
		Change to a simpler job/half-time	10
		Disabled, strongly impaired work capacity	0

stairs easily. Seventy-eight per cent of patients were completely pain-free. Olerud and Molander (1986) examined the outcome of bimalleolar and trimalleolar ankle fractures. Their average ankle score (see Table 14.2) was 80.2 ± 20.6 (range 10–100). The score varied directly with the degree of fracture displacement measured on the post-operative X-rays, with significantly better results being obtained in perfectly reduced fractures. With reference to joint movement they showed a restriction of less than 5° of dorsiflexion in 34% of the patients, 6–10° in 27% of the patients, 11–15° in 24% of the patients and more than 15° restriction of dorsiflexion in 16% of their fracture population. Radiological evaluation showed osteoarthritic change in 32% of the ankles. Again the degree of osteoarthritis varied directly with the adequacy of fracture reduction.

Broos and Bisschop (1991) analysed 612 surgically treated ankle fractures. They concluded that isolated malleolar fractures have a better prognosis than trimalleolar fractures. They also showed that an isolated medial malleolar fracture has a worse prognosis than an isolated lateral malleolar fracture and multi-malleolar fractures, including the medial malleolus, have a worse prognosis than if the medial malleolus is not involved. Further,

they observed larger fixed posterior malleolar fragments resulted in a worse prognosis than small unfixed fragments.

The conclusions to be gained from the literature are that ankle fractures are similar to other intra-articular fractures. The prognosis depends on the degree of bone, cartilage and in particular soft tissue damage. The adequacy of reduction is vital and high energy injuries result in a worse prognosis than low energy injuries. This accounts for the prognostic difference between medial and lateral malleolar fractures.

Ankle fractures in the elderly

As with other fractures, the incidence of fracture of the ankle in the elderly is increasing. Not only are the numbers of fractures secondary to osteoporosis increasing in the population but the elderly are physically fitter and demand a higher standard of treatment than might have been expected in the past. In the Edinburgh series 41.5% of the ankle fractures occurred in patients of 50 years or older, with 27.7% occurring in patients at least 60 years. Obviously in the elderly population the requirement for surgical management may be dictated by

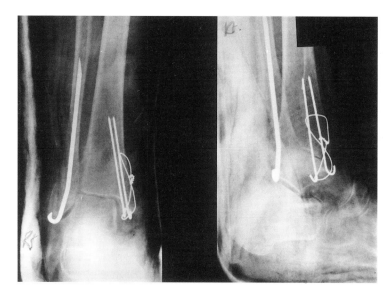

Figure 14.15 Examples of a B2.2 fracture in an elderly woman with osteoporotic bone. A Rush pin has been used to stabilize the lateral fracture and Kirschner wires with cerclage wires have been employed on the medial side. Postoperative casting is essential and a good result was obtained

the physical state of the patient, but it is strongly recommended that unless there are strong reasons to the contrary, ankle fractures in the elderly should be treated according to the same criteria applied to younger patients.

Beauchamp *et al.* (1983) examined 126 patients over 50 years of age, comparing operative fixation with non-operative management. They showed that operative management results in a significantly better reduction than non-operative management but at final follow-up the incidence of pain, swelling, weakness, instability and patient satisfaction was similar between the two groups. In addition they pointed out the increased complication rate associated with ankle fracture fixation in this elderly group.

Anand and Klenerman (1993) retrospectively reviewed a series of 80 patients over the age of 60 years treated by either non-operative or operative management. They showed quite clearly that only the undisplaced fractures did well with non-operative management. In their displaced fracture group 96.4% of the patients were either symptomatic or dissatisfied at final follow-up. In the operative group 88.5% of the patients were satisfied with their treatment. They did find soft bone in 54.2% of the patients that were operated on and although they used AO techniques they felt that a number of 'innovative adaptations' needed to be used to achieve stability in some patients. They emphasized that rigid internal fixation was not their aim and they used a below-knee plaster to protect the fixation in all cases. Their conclusions were

that age should not dictate the treatment of ankle fractures in the elderly and that the maintenance of anatomical congruity is as important in the elderly as in the young.

One of the problems about using screws and plates in osteoporotic bone is that they tend to pull out. To avoid this, meticulous adherence to surgical technique is important but occasionally the bone will be so porotic that other techniques must be used and indeed the 'innovative adaptations' of Anand and Klenerman (1993) may well be necessary. As long as the surgeon realizes that rigid internal fixation is not being achieved, the use of intramedullary devices such as the Rush pin to stabilize the fibula and Kirschner wires with or without tension banding supplemented by a postoperative cast can achieve excellent results (Figure 14.15).

Biodegradable fracture fixation

The use of metallic implants for internal fixation of ankle fractures has been successful but their use frequently means that a second operation is required to remove the implant. This has led to the investigation of biodegradable implants made of polyglycolide or polylactide. Initially good results were reported with the use of biodegradable implants in the management of simple displaced unimalleolar and bimalleolar fractures (Rokkanen *et al.*, 1985) and the technique has been extended to investigate the use of these implants in more severe ankle fractures. Hirvensalo (1989) used polyglycolide rods to stabilize Lauge-Hansen III and IV, PAIII and PEIII and IV fractures. He used polyglycolide rods to fix the fibula and medial fractures as well as using rods to stabilize the syndesmosis. He found good results but reported 6 cases of accumulation of a polyglycolide mass behind the scar. In one case this was associated with a sinus.

Recently more doubt has been cast on the use of biodegradable implants. Frøkjaer and Møller (1992) reported sinus formation, osteolysis, pseudoarthrosis and secondary fracture displacement. They suggested that polyglycolide fixation be abandoned. Böstman *et al.* (1992) also recorded transient local non-bacterial inflammatory reactions in 11.1% of patients treated with polyglycolide screws. They did not detect any deleterious effects from the implant, but stressed that the long-term consequences were not known.

References

Ahl, T., Dalen, N., Holmberg, S. and Selvik, G. (1986) Early weight bearing of malleolar fractures. *Acta Orthop. Scand.*, **57**, 526–9

Ahl, T., Dalen, N., Holmberg, S. and Selvik, G. (1987) Early weight bearing of displaced ankle fractures. *Acta Orthop. Scand.*, **58**, 535–8

Anand, N. and Klenerman, L. (1993) Ankle fractures in the elderly: NVA versus ORIF. *Injury*, **24**, 116–20

Ashurst, A.P.C. and Bromer, R.S. (1992) Classification and mechanism of fractures of the leg bones involving the ankle. *Arch. Surg.*, **4**, 51–129

Baird, R.A. and Jackson, S.T. (1987) Fractures of the distal part of the fibula with associated disruption of the deltoid ligament. *J. Bone Joint Surg.*, **69A**, 1346–52

Bauer, M., Bergstrom, B., Hemborg, A. and Sandegard, J. (1985) Malleolar fractures: nonoperative versus operative treatment: a controlled study. *Clin. Orthop.*, **199**, 17–27

Bauer, M., Johnsson, K. and Nilsson B. (1985) Thirty year follow up of ankle fractures. *Acta Orthop. Scand.*, **56**, 103–6

Beauchamp, C.G., Clay, N.R. and Thexton, P.W. (1983) Displaced ankle fractures in patients over 50 years of age. *J. Bone Joint Surg.*, **65B**, 329–32

Bengner, U., Johnell, O. and Redlund-Johnell, I. (1986) Epidemiology of ankle fracture 1950 and 1980. *Acta Orthop. Scand.*, **57**, 35–7

Boden, S.D., Labropoulos, P.A., McCowin, P. *et al.* (1989) Mechanical consideration for the syndesmosis screw. *J. Bone Joint Surg.*, **71A**, 1548–55

Böstman, O., Partio, E., Hirvinsac, E. and Rokkanen, P. (1992) Foreign body reactions to polyglycolide screws. Observations in 24/216 malleolar fracture cases. *Acta Orthop. Scand.*, **63**, 173–6

Bray, T.J., Endicott, M. and Capra, S.E. (1989) Treatment of open ankle fractures: immediate internal fixation versus closed immobilization and delayed fixation. *Clin. Orthop.*, **240**, 47–52

Broos, P.L.O. and Bisschop, A.P.G. (1991) Operative treatment of ankle fractures in adults: correlation between types of fracture and final results. *Injury*, **22**, 403–6

Browner, B.D., Jupiter, J.B., Levine, A.M. and Trafton, P.C. (1992) *Skeletal Trauma*, Saunders, Philadelphia

Burwell, H.N. and Charnley, A.D. (1965) The treatment of displaced fractures at the ankle by rigid fixation and early joint movement. *J. Bone Joint Surg.*, **47B**, 634–60

Cedell, C.A. (1967) Supination outward rotation injuries of the ankle. A clinical and roetgenological study with special reference to the operative treatment. *Acta Orthop. Scand.*, Suppl. 110

Cedell, C.A. (1985) Is closed treatment of ankle fractures advisable? *Acta Orthop. Scand.*, **56**, 101–2

Chapman, M.W. and Mahoney, M. (1979) The role of early internal fixation in the management of open fractures. *Clin. Orthop.*, **138**, 120–31

Cimino, W., Ichtertz, D. and Slabaugh, P. (1991) Early mobilisation of ankle fractures after open reduction and internal fixation. *Clin. Orthop.*, **267**, 152–6

Daly, P.J., Fitzgerald, R.H., Melton, L.J. and Ilstrup, D.M. (1987) Epidemiology of ankle fractures in Rochester, Minnesota. *Acta Orthop. Scand*, **58**, 539–44

De Souza, L.J., Gustilo, R.B. and Meyer, T.J. (1985) Displaced external rotation–abduction fractures of the ankle. *J. Bone Joint Surg.*, **67A**, 1066–74

Franklin, J.L., Johnson, K.D. and Hansen, S.T. (1984) Immediate fixation of open ankle fractures. *J. Bone Joint Surg.*, **66A**, 1349–56

Frøkjaer, J. and Møller, B.N. (1992) Biodegradable fixation of ankle fractures. *Acta Orthop. Scand.*, **63**, 434–6

Harper, M.C. and Hardin, (1988) Posterior malleolar fractures of the ankle associated with external rotation-abduction injuries. *J. Bone Joint Surg.*, **70A**, 1348–56

Hirvensalo, E. (1989) Fracture fixation with biodegradable rods. *Acta Orthop. Scand.*, **60**, 601–6

Jaskulke, R.A., Ittner, G. and Schedl, R. (1989) Fractures of the posterior tibial margin: their role in the prognosis of malleolar fractures. *J. Trauma*, **29**, 1565–70

Joy, G., Patzakis, N.J. and Harvey, P.J. (1974) Precise evaluation of the reduction of severe ankle fractures. *J. Bone Joint Surg.*, **56A**, 979–93

Kristensen, K.D. and Hansen, T. (1985) Closed treatment of ankle fractures. Stage II supination–eversion fractures followed for 20 years. *Acta Orthop. Scand.*, **56**, 107–9

Lauge-Hansen, N. (1950) Fractures of the ankle: II. Combined experimental-surgical and experimental-roentgenologic investigations. *Arch. Surg.*, **60**, 957–85

Limbird, R.S. and Aaron, R.K. (1987) Laterally comminuted fracture-dislocation of the ankle. *J. Bone Joint Surg.*, **69A**, 881–5

Lindsjö, U. (1981) Operative treatment of ankle fractures. *Acta Orthop. Scand.*, **52**, Suppl. 189

Lund-Kristensen, J., Grieff, J. and Riegels-Nielson, P. (1982) Malleolar fractures treated with rigid internal fixation and immediate mobilization. *Injury*, **13**, 191–5

Mazur, J.M., Schwartz, E. and Simon, S.R. (1979) Ankle arthrodesis. Long-term follow-up with gait analysis. *J. Bone Joint Surg.*, **61A**, 964–75

Meyer, T.L. and Kumler, K.W. (1980) ASIF technique and ankle fractures. *Clin. Orthop.*, **150**, 211–6

Michelson, J., Magid, D., Ney, D.R. and Fishman, E. (1992) Examination of the pathologic anatomy of ankle fractures. *J. Trauma*, **32**, 65–70

Miller, A.J. (1974) Posterior malleolar fractures. *J. Bone Joint Surg.*, **56B**, 508–12

Müller, M.E., Allgöwer, M., Schneider, R. and Willenegger, H. (1991) *Manual of Internal Fixation*, 3rd edn, Springer-Verlag, Berlin

Muller, M.E., Nazarian, S., Koch, P. and Schatzker J. (1990) *The Comprehensive Classification of Fractures of Long Bones*, Springer-Verlag, Berlin

Olerud, C. (1984) The effect of the syndesmotic screw on the extension capacity of the ankle joint. *Arch. Orthop. Trauma Surg.*, **102**, 201–2

Olerud, C. and Molander, H. (1986) Bi- and trimalleolar ankle fractures operated with non-rigid internal fixation. *Clin. Orthop.*, **206**, 253–60

Pankovich, A.M. (1976) Maisonneuve fracture of the fibula. *J. Bone Joint Surg.*, **58A**, 337–42

Pankovich, A.M. (1978) Fractures of the fibula proximal to the distal tibio-fibular syndesmosis. *J. Bone Joint Surg.*, **60A**, 221–9

Pettrone, F.A., Mitchell, G., Pee, D. *et al.* (1983) Quantitative criteria for prediction of the results after displaced fracture of the ankle. *J. Bone Joint Surg.*, **65A**, 667–77

Ramsey, P.L. and Hamilton, W. (1976) Changes in the tibio-talar area of contact caused by lateral talar shift. *J. Bone Joint Surg.*, **58A**, 356–7

Rokkanen, P., Bostman, O., Vainionpaa, S. *et al.* (1985) Biodegradable implants in fracture fixation: early results of treatment of fractures of the ankle. *Lancet*, **1**, 1422–4

Ryd, U. and Bengtsson, S. (1992) Isolated fracture of the lateral malleolus requires no treatment. *Acta Orthop. Scand.*, **63**, 443–6

Søndenaa, K., Høigaard, V., Smith, D. and Alho, A. (1986) Immobilisation of operated ankle fractures. *Acta Orthop. Scand.*, **57**, 59–61

Watson, J.A.S. and Hollingdale, J.P. (1992) Early management of undisplaced ankle fractures. *Injury*, **23**, 87–8

Yablon, I.G., Heller, F.G. and Shouse, L. (1977) The key role of the lateral malleolus in displaced fractures of the ankle. *J. Bone Joint Surg.*, **59A**, 169–73

Yde, J. and Kristensen, K.D. (1980) Ankle fractures: supination–eversion fractures of stage IV. *Acta Orthop. Scand.*, **51**, 981–90

Zeegers, A.V.C.M., Van Raay, J.J.A.M. and Vander Werken, C. (1989) Ankle fractures treated with a stabilising shoe. *Acta Orthop. Scand.*, **60**, 597–9

15

Isolated fractures of the tibia and fibula

C. Court-Brown and S. Sjolin

Isolated fractures of the tibia have provoked a surprising amount of controversy amongst orthopaedic surgeons. Even the most basic aspect of these fractures provokes disagreement. There was considerable dispute until recently as to whether the presence of an intact fibula improved or worsened the prognosis of the tibial fracture in terms of time to union and the incidence of malunion. Jackson and Macnab (1959) analysed 45 isolated tibial fractures and noted that while the transverse tibial fractures maintained alignment this was not the case with oblique fractures. They stated that lateral angulation in an oblique isolated tibial fractures caused fracture site distraction and they suggested that internal fixation should be employed using an intrafragmentary screw for this type of isolated fracture. Charnley (1961) took the same view about oblique isolated tibial fractures. He also noted a tendency of the tibial fragments to 'float' so that they separated in the lateral direction. He pointed out the high incidence of varus deformity and felt that the apparent simplicity of the fracture masked considerable soft tissue disruption with separation of the bone fragments from the interosseous membrane and disruption of the normal pathway for callus formation.

Teitz *et al.* (1980) also felt that the isolated tibial fracture was associated with significant problems. They divided their patient population according to age and noted a much higher complication rate in patients of at least 20 years of age. In this group they documented a 26.0% incidence of non-union or delayed union as well as a 26% incidence of varus malunion. They also found that 8.6% of the group had pain or X-ray changes in the ipsilateral ankle. In the patients who were aged less than 20 years, they noted the same incidence of varus malunion, but only 2.2% showed delayed or non-union and 4.4% had ankle problems. They undertook some biomechanical studies which pointed to the presence of a tibiofibular length discrepancy and altered strain patterns in the tibia and fibula. They attributed the improved results in the younger group to the greater compliance of the fibula and soft tissues.

In contrast to the somewhat pessimistic views expressed by these authors, other surgeons have suggested that the isolated tibial fracture is a benign variant of the group of fractures affecting the tibia and fibula. Nicoll (1964) reported an incidence of delayed union of 9% in isolated tibial fractures compared with 29% when the fibula was fractured. Hoagland and States (1967) noted that the median cast time for the treatment of isolated tibial fractures was 4 months compared with 5.5 months when both bones were fractured. Hooper *et al.* (1980) only had a 2% incidence of non-union with non-operative management of isolated tibial fractures, but as with Teitz *et al.* (1980), they noted a 25% incidence of varus malunion which they attributed to dorsiflexion of the ankle. They suggested that as the foot is dorsiflexed the ankle mortise widens, causing a varus tilt at the fracture. They found wedging of the plaster to be unsatisfactory and suggested applying the cast with the foot in equinus. Recently there has been almost uniform agreement that isolated tibial fractures carry a better prognosis than those of the tibia and fibula. Allum and Mowbray (1980) examined the cumulative percentage curves for fracture healing and showed that not only was union faster with an intact fibula, but the non-union rate was less.

Epidemiology

The data presented in Chapter 2 show that 22.4% of tibial fractures seen in the Edinburgh Orthopaedic Trauma Unit are associated with an intact fibula. This figure probably represents an accurate overall picture of the incidence of the isolated tibial fracture as the unit takes all the pathology in its area. Similar figures were seen by Teitz *et al.* (1980) and Sarmiento *et al.* (1989), with 20% and 24% respectively. Other authors have documented lower figures, between 10.7% (Hoagland and States, 1967) and 17% (O'Dwyer *et al.*, 1992). This figure is obviously influenced by the type of trauma admitted to the hospital, and in a busy German trauma unit admitting a high proportion of younger patients following severe trauma only 12% of tibial fractures were associated with an intact fibula (Pennig, Unpublished data, 1994). In children isolated tibial fractures are extremely common, with Briggs *et al.* (1992) reporting an incidence as high as 38%.

It is possible that many of the different opinions and results about isolated fractures in the literature relate to the fact that no series of these fractures has been adequately classified. O'Dwyer *et al.* (1992) separated their fractures into low and high velocity injuries as well as open and closed fractures, and in a later series (O'Dwyer *et al.*, 1993) they also referred to the orientation of the fracture and the degree of comminution as well as the degree of displacement. However, there has as yet been no breakdown of the isolated tibial fracture according to the AO classification.

Table 15.1 shows the breakdown of the isolated tibial fractures in the series detailed in Chapter 2 using the AO classification. Isolated tibial fractures fill six separate subgroups in the A and B groups in the AO classification, although the status of the fibula does not enter into the criteria used for inclu-

sion of fractures into the C groupings. Despite this, there were 4 (3.4%) type C tibial fractures associated with an intact fibula (Figure 15.1). It is obvious from Table 15.1 that the commonest configuration is the A3.1 fracture (Figure 15.2), with about half of the series showing a transverse tibial fracture. Table 2.6 indicates that the A3.1 fracture and A3.3 fractures are in fact the most common subgroups of tibial fractures seen by surgeons. The spiral A1.1 fracture (Figure 15.3) and the oblique A2.1 fracture (Figure 15.4) are the only other fractures occurring with an incidence of greater than 10%. The B2.1 intact bending wedge fracture is the commonest type B, with the B1.1 spiral wedge and the B3.1 fragmented bending wedge (Figure 15.5) fractures occurring with equal frequency. All of the type C isolated fractures, except one, were C1.1 complex spiral fractures (Figure 15.1).

Table 15.1 The relative incidence of the different types of isolated tibial fractures with relation to each other and the whole tibial fracture group

AO subgroup	No.	% of isolated tibial fractures	% of all tibial fractures
A1.1	19	16.3	3.7
A2.1	15	12.8	2.9
A3.1	57	48.7	11.0
B1.1	6	5.1	1.2
B2.1	10	8.5	1.9
B3.1	6	5.1	1.2
C1.1	3	2.6	1.9
C2.2	1	0.8	4.8

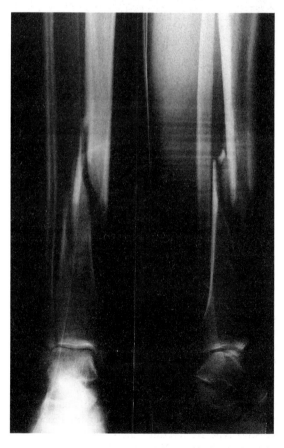

Figure 15.1 A C1.1 fracture of the tibia associated with an intact fibula. This illustrates that complex tibial fractures can occur in the presence of an intact fibula

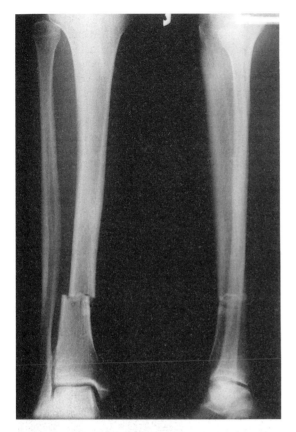

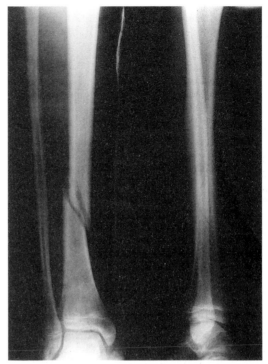

Figure 15.3   An A1.1 fracture. This is an unstable configuration which shows a tendency to varus malalignment, as seen in this X-ray

Figure 15.2   An A3.1 fracture. This is by far the commonest fracture configuration of isolated tibial fractures

The causes of isolated tibial fractures are listed in Table 2.14. This indicates that these tend to be low velocity fractures and this view is confirmed by examining the comparative descriptors of isolated tibial fractures and fractures of both bones (Table 15.2). This table indicates that there are obvious differences between isolated tibial fractures and fractures of both the tibia and fibula, with a different spectrum of AO fracture types, percentage of open fractures, percentage of severe closed fractures and incidence of severe comminution. In addition, there was a much lower incidence of road traffic accidents and a higher incidence of soccer injuries in the isolated group. Interestingly, despite the significantly lower incidence of open fractures in the isolated fracture group, there was a very similar incidence of Gustilo type III fractures amongst the open fractures in each group. However, there were no grade IIIb fractures in the isolated tibial group, and indeed this is not surprising given the severity of these injuries. None of the AO type C isolated fractures was open. The data in Table 15.2 regarding isolated fractures differ a little from other series.

Hoagland and States (1967) noted that 61% of their isolated fractures followed high energy trauma, and O'Dwyer *et al.* (1992) found that

Table 15.2   Comparative analysis of characteristics of isolated tibial fractures and fractures of both the tibia and fibula

	Isolated tibia fractures	*Tibia and fibula fractures*
Incidence (%)	22.4	77.6
Average age (yr)	30.4	39.2
AO type A	77.8	47.6
AO type B	18.8	29.1
AO type C	3.4	23.3
Open fractures (%)	7.7	28.1
Gustilo type III (%)	66.6	59.6
Tscherne type C2 and C3	12.8	45.2
Winquist–Hansen type 3 and 4 (%)	6.0	29.9
Road traffic accidents (%)	21.4	42.0
Soccer (%)	46.1	18.5

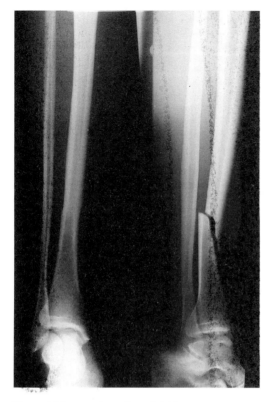

Figure 15.4   An A2.1 oblique tibial fracture

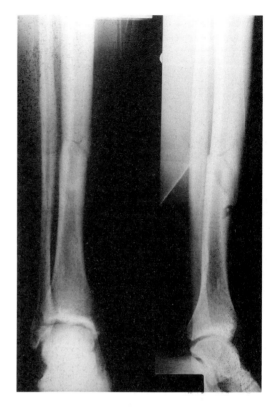

Figure 15.5   A B3.1 fragmented wedge fracture

49.5% of their series were associated with high energy injury. In the Edinburgh series, 26.6% of the injuries followed road traffic accidents, falls from a height, or a direct blow to the leg. Hoagland and States (1967) and O'Dwyer *et al.,* (1992) also reported a higher incidence of open fractures, with 39% and 17% respectively. These differences presumably reflect different patient populations.

Treatment

Until recently the management of most tibial fractures and virtually all low velocity tibial fractures was non-operative. In recent years, however, there has been increased interest in the use of plates, intramedullary nails and external fixation in the management of all types of tibial fractures. With isolated tibial fractures the main reason for surgery was to avoid non-union and significant varus deformity (Jackson and Macnab, 1959; Charnley, 1961; Burwell, 1971) and there have been very few references to limb or patient function after isolated tibial fractures. Recently Van der Werken *et al.*

(1993) reported good functional results after external fixation of isolated tibial fractures.

As previously stated, both Jackson and Macnab (1959) and Charnley (1961) agreed that the oblique isolated tibial fracture had a poor prognosis. This has recently been confirmed by Den Outer *et al.* (1990), who reported that 58% of oblique isolated tibial fractures healed with significant malalignment. Jackson and Macnab (1959) suggested the use of intrafragmentary screw fixation with a supplementary cast, but Charnley (1961) did not support this idea. It is of interest that Charnley felt that the A1.1 spiral fracture did not displace and had a good prognosis. Unfortunately, as Figure 15.3 indicates, this is not always the case. Burwell (1971) thought that the isolated tibial fracture was an indication for plating, and more recently Court-Brown *et al.* (1990) suggested that locked intramedullary nailing was indicated for all displaced tibial fractures, including those associated with an intact fibula. Van der Werken *et al.* (1993) have documented the advantages of a simple unilateral external fixator.

Of the 117 patients with isolated tibial fractures detailed in the Edinburgh study, 77 were followed up on a retrospective basis. Most of the remaining patients followed were resident in other parts of the country with a few having inadequate documentation. Angulation and fracture displacement was assessed on the initial X-rays. The method of management was decided by the attending surgeon. Fifty-one of the fractures were treated non-operatively, 20 were treated by Gross–Kempf intramedullary nailing, and the remaining 6 were treated with an external fixation device. Of the 51 fractures treated non-operatively, 18 showed initial displacement and 33 were undisplaced. Twenty-one of the undisplaced fractures healed in their original position. Of these, 18 were A3.1 fractures and none was a type B or C fracture. Of the remaining 12, 5 were internally fixed secondarily because of varus or recurvatum deformities. The remaining 7 fractures all healed in 5° of varus. Five of the conservatively managed undisplaced fractures refractured between 7 and 12 months after the initial injury.

Only 3 of the 18 non-operatively managed displaced fractures healed in acceptable alignment. Eleven of the remaining 15 fractures healed with between 5 and 15° of varus and the remaining 4 were internally fixed secondarily because of varus malalignment. The mean time to union was 11 weeks for the initially undisplaced group and 14 weeks for the group that presented initially with displaced fractures. Two of the non-operatively managed displaced fractures refractured between 4 and 6 months after the initial injury. Thus 13.7% of the fractures that were primarily managed non-operatively refractured.

Twenty-six fractures were treated operatively. Twenty were treated by Gross–Kempf intramedullary nailing and 6 with external fixation. There were a number of complications seen with the intramedullary nailing series. Two patients had compartment syndrome. Both were picked up using compartment pressure monitoring and after fasciotomy there were no long-term sequelae. One patient had a septic arthritis of the knee, this being the only such case in over 600 tibial nailings in the Edinburgh unit. The mean time to union for this group was 16 weeks. There were no refractures. In the externally fixed group, 3 eventually healed in varus malalignment and 2 of the externally fixed group had tibial refractures after 8 and 19 months.

The conclusions to be drawn from the Edinburgh series are that the mean time to union for these fractures is less than the mean time to union for fractures of both the tibia and fibula. The non-operatively managed undisplaced fractures healed in less than 12 weeks and in young people such fractures can usually be treated non-operatively with every chance of preserving excellent joint function (Court-Brown, 1993). The undisplaced AO type A fractures tend to remain undisplaced, although care must be taken to monitor the fracture position for the first few weeks after the initial injury. The AO type 3.1 fracture (Figure 15.2) carries the best prognosis as regards maintenance of position.

The prognosis for the displaced type A fracture is worse. Most of these fractures will remain displaced and it is preferable to treat these fractures operatively. All type B and C fractures should be fixed as otherwise a varus malunion can be expected. The principle complication of non-operative management was refracture and the high non-union rates noted by Teitz *et al.* (1980) were not seen. These conclusions agree with those of O'Dwyer *et al.* (1993), who state that isolated tibial shaft fractures are relatively 'benign' injuries and that the majority will heal satisfactorily in plaster. They state that the features that should suggest poor prognosis to the surgeon are open injuries, oblique or comminuted fractures, high velocity injuries and angulation or displacement. They also believe that any fracture that requires manipulation should probably be fixed internally. The optimal method of fracture fixation will depend on the experience of the surgeon, but it is suggested that either intramedullary nailing (Court-Brown *et al.*, 1990) or external fixation with a simple unilateral external fixator be used. Van der Werken *et al.* (1993) maintained an external fixator for an average of 6 weeks, following which they used a functional brace for an average of four more weeks. All of their fractures healed in alignment and they reported excellent limb and patient function. Failure to treat isolated tibial fractures adequately primarily often leaves the surgeon with a difficult secondary operation. At first sight it would appear straightforward to reduce and fix a varus non-union of the tibia. However, a partial fibulectomy has to be performed and it may be surprisingly difficult to mobilize all the soft tissues adequately to permit proper reduction of the tibial fracture. This is particularly true of spiral fractures, but regardless of the type of tibial fracture, an open reduction will almost certainly be required.

Isolated fractures of the fibula

The surgeon will encounter isolated fractures of the fibula under three circumstances. Two of these are best described as 'apparent' isolated fractures, these being the avulsion fracture of the proximal fibula associated with ligamentous disruption of the knee (AO 41 A1.1, Chapter 1) and the high supra-syndesmotic fibular fracture associated with AO type C ankle fractures (see Figure 14.12).

The presence of an avulsion fracture of the head of the fibula suggests an association with severe ligamentous disruption of the knee. This usually involves the collateral ligaments but there may also be cruciate damage. Usually the bone fragments are comparatively small and no specific treatment beyond the repair of the appropriate ligaments is required. Occasionally, however, the avulsed fragment is large enough so that internal fixation will aid knee stability and under these circumstances intrafragmentary screw fixation or a figure-of-eight wire repair can be undertaken.

Apparently isolated fractures of the fibula are most commonly seen in association with ankle fractures. These fractures are not uncommon (Chapter 14) and should never be confused with true isolated fibula fractures. Examination of the ankle will show associated fractures or ligamentous injuries. The surgeon should be aware of the fracture described by Pankovich (1978), where the supra-syndesmotic fibula fracture is associated with an intact deltoid ligament. There will, however, be discomfort over the anterior syndesmosis secondary to rupture of the anterior tibiofibular ligament and this clinical sign will prevent confusion with a true isolated fibular fracture. The management of supra-syndesmotic fibula fractures is detailed in Chapter 14.

True isolated fibular fractures (Figure 15.6) that have no other bony or ligamentous components are surprisingly rare, comprising only 0.5% of the overall tibia and fibula fracture group detailed in Chapter 2. Of the 11 fractures, 5 occurred in the proximal third, 5 in the middle third and only one in the distal third of the diaphysis. They are low velocity injuries and analysis of the cause of these fractures shows a very wide spectrum. Two occurred after a simple fall, one as a result of a fall downstairs and 2 as a result of a direct blow to the lateral aspect of the lower leg. Three occurred as a result of sporting injuries, 2 from soccer and one from rugby football. The remaining 2 fractures occurred in elderly pedestrians (68 and 71 years) involved in road traffic accidents.

Treatment of true isolated fibula fractures is symptomatic. Usually supportive strapping or an elastic bandage is all that is required, but a below-knee walking cast, functional brace or air cast can

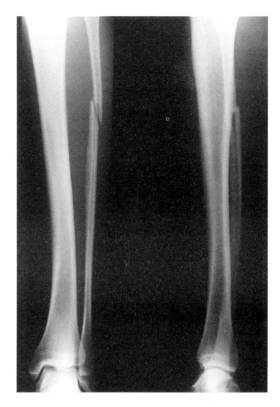

Figure 15.6   A true isolated fracture of the fibula. This occurred following a sporting injury

be used for pain control and to facilitate mobilization. The fracture usually unites in 6–8 weeks and complications are few. Should non-union occur it is suggested this be treated by conventional means using an AO plate supplemented by bone grafting for atrophic non-union.

Few complications of true fibula fractures are reported. Fractures around the neck of the fibula may cause damage to the superficial peroneal nerve and late entrapment of this nerve by callus has been reported (Mino and Hughes, 1984).

References

Allum, R.L. and Mowbray, M.A.S. (1980) A retrospective review of the healing of fractures of the shaft of the tibia with special reference to the mechanism of injury. *Injury*, **11**, 304–8

Briggs, T.W.R., Orr, M.M. and Lightowler, C.D.R. (1992) Isolated tibial fractures in the shoulder. *Injury*, **23**, 308–10

Burwell, H.N. (1971) Plate fixation of tibial shaft fractures. *J. Bone Joint Surg.*, **53B**, 258–71

Charnley, J. (1964) *The Closed Treatment of Common Fractures*, Churchill Livingstone, Edinburgh

Court-Brown, C.M., Christie, J. and McQueen, M.M. (1990) Closed intramedullary tibial nailing: its use in closed and type I open fractures. *J. Bone Joint Surg.*, **72B**, 605–11

Court-Brown, C.M. (1993) Fractures of the tibial diaphysis. *Int. J. Orthop. Trauma*, **3**, 40–6

Den Outer, A.J., Meeuwis, J.D., Herman, J. and Zwaveling, A. (1990) Conservative versus orthopaedic treatment of displaced non-comminuted tibial shaft fractures. *Clin. Orthop.*, **252**, 231–6

Hoagland, F.T. and States, J.D. (1967) The factors influencing the rate of healing of tibial shaft fractures. *Surg. Gynecol. Obstet.*, **124**, 71–6

Hooper, G., Buckstone, R.A. and Gillespie, W.J. (1980) Isolated fractures of the shaft of the tibia. *Injury*, **12**, 283–7

Jackson, R.W. and Macnab, I. (1959) Fractures of the shaft of the tibia. A clinical and experimental study. *Ann. J. Surg.*, **97**, 543–7

Mino, D.E. and Hughes, E.C. (1984) Bony entrapment of the superficial peroneal nerve. *Clin. Orthop.*, **184**, 203–6

Nicoll, E.A. (1964) Fractures of the tibial shaft. A survey of 705 cases. *J. Bone Joint Surg.*, **46B**, 373–87

O'Dwyer, K.J., Devriese, L., Feys, H., Ver Creysse, L. and Jameson-Evens, D.C. (1992) The intact fibula. *Injury*, **23**, 314–16

O'Dwyer, K.J., Devriese, L., Feys, H. and Ver Creysse, L. (1993) Tibial shaft fractures of the intact fibula. *Injury*, **24**, 591–4

Pankovich, A.M. (1978) Fractures of the fibula proximal to the distal tibiofibular syndesmosis. *J. Bone Joint Surg.*, **60A**, 221–9

Teitz, C.C., Carter, D.R. and Frankel, V.H. (1980) Problems associated with tibial fractures and intact fibulae. *J. Bone Joint Surg.*, **62A**, 770–6

Van der Werken, C., Meeuwis, J.D. and Oostvogel, H.J.M. (1993) The simple fix: external fixation of displaced isolated tibial fractures. *Injury*, **24**, 46–8

16

Tibial fractures in children

D. Pennig

Introduction

Fractures of the tibia in children and adolescents do occur but are rare (Van Laer, 1986). Birth fractures have not been reported. In an analysis of 8682 children's fractures collected in Sweden fractures of the tibial diaphysis accounted for only 5% of the group and were the sixth most common fracture (Landin, 1983). The age distribution tended to be uneven with peaks around 7 years, 10 years and 15 years in boys and 7 years and 14 years in girls. The fractures were usually either related to activities within the home or sports activities including bicycle riding (Henderson et al., 1992). In Landin's statistics the overall refracture rate was 0.5% with the tibial refracture rate being 0.4%, this being somewhat less than the average. An analysis of Landin's data over 30 years suggests that there appears to be a gradual increase in the incidence of tibial fractures (Landin, 1983).

Classification

Injuries of the epiphysis and the metaphysis are classified according to Salter Harris (1963) and Aitken (1965). The relationship between the two classification systems is explained in Chapter 1 and the Salter Harris classification system is illustrated in Figure 1.10.

Proximal tibial fractures

Proximal tibial fractures in childhood are rare. Whereas epiphysiolysis in the distal femur is relatively common the equivalent injury in the proximal tibia is unusual. The explanation for this can be seen in the morphology of the proximal tibial physis which is a biplanar structure. A complete epiphysiolysis (Salter Harris type I) (Figure 16.1) requires forceful hyper-extension or flexion. Aitken type I, II and III fractures are exceedingly rare.

Treatment

Salter Harris type II/Aitken type I injuries (Figure 16.2a) are usually seen just prior to growth arrest, and if they are displaced open reduction with internal fixation is advisable (Harris et al., 1983). The choice of implants lies between screws and wires. Postoperative long-leg cast immobilization for 4–6 weeks is recommended. Salter Harris type III/Aitken type II (Figure 16.2c) as well as Salter Harris type IV/Aitken type III (Figure 16.2e) injuries with displacement are almost always indications for operative treatment (Burkhardt and Peterson, 1979; Canale and Shelton, 1979; Ehrlich and Strain, 1979; Hansen, 1990). Anatomical reduction is of paramount importance and screw fixation with screws placed parallel to the growth plate is advisable (Skak et al., 1987). Again immobilization with a long-leg cast for 4–6 weeks is necessary.

Avulsion of the inter-condylar eminence

Lesions of the cruciate ligaments in childhood are uncommon (Hyndman and Brown, 1979) and are usually associated with an avulsion fracture of inter-condylar eminence (Lee, 1937; Meyers and McKeeves, 1970). Treatment depends on the degree

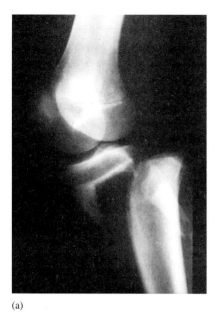

(a)

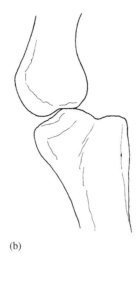

(b)

Figure 16.1 (a) Radiograph of a 15-year-old boy showing epiphysiolysis. A popliteal artery lesion was present

Figure 16.1 (b,c) With anterior displacement of the epiphysis a popliteal artery injury may occur

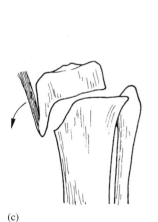

(c)

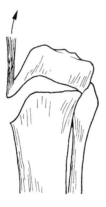

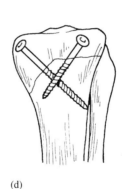

(d)

Figure 16.1 (d) Treatment by open reduction and internal fixation with two or three 4.5 mm lag screws

of displacement of the fragments. Technically a complete avulsion of the inter-condylar eminence is a Salter Harris type III/Aitken type II fracture and is associated with an equivalent prognosis (Figure 16.3). Arthroscopic examination may be performed (Eilert, 1976; Morrissy *et al.*, 1982; Eiskjar and Larsen, 1987) to document accurately the extent of the fracture displacement, the soft tissue injury, and consequently the mobility of the fragment, as well as the size of the fragment (Kennedy, 1979). If the fragment is undisplaced conservative treatment with long-leg cast immobilization for 6 weeks is sufficient. Should the intercondylar eminence be displaced arthroscopically assisted reduction screw fixation or cerclage wiring through a parapatella incision is recommended.

Again immobilization in a long-leg cast for 6 weeks is recommended.

Avulsion of a tibial tuberosity

This injury (Hand *et al.*, 1971; Christie and Dvonch, 1981; Ogden, 1982; Wiss *et al.*, 1991) is caused by the pull of the quadriceps on the flexed knee during sport (Figure 16.4). It is a Salter Harris type III/Aitken type II fracture. The treatment should be operative since a malunion may cause a partial epiphysiodesis and a secondary genu recurvatum (Pennig *et al.*, 1990). Open reduction and cerclage wiring or tension band fixation is performed. Long leg cast immobilization for 6 weeks is recommended. In metaphyseal fractures (Figure

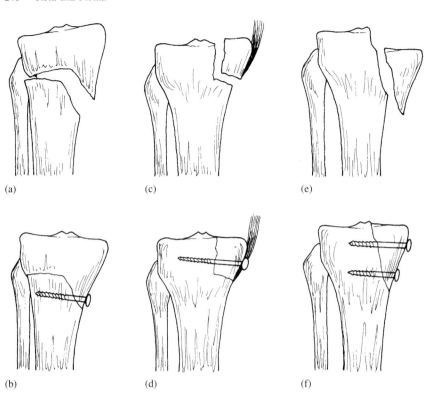

(a)   (c)   (e)

(b)   (d)   (f)

Figure 16.2 Proximal tibial fractures. (a) Salter–Harris type II/Aitken type I injury; (b) anatomical reduction is followed by open or percutaneous insertion of a 4.0 or 4.5 mm lag screw; (c) Salter–Harris type III/Aitken type II injury; (d) anatomical reduction is followed by lag screw fixation (4.0/4.5 mm); (e) Salter–Harris type IV/Aitken type III injury; (f) anatomical reduction is followed by lag screw fixation in the epiphysis and metaphysis

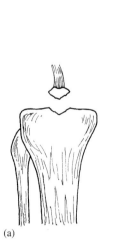
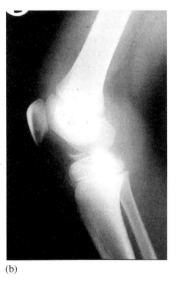
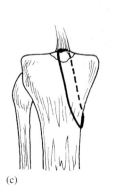

(a)   (b)   (c)

Figure 16.3 (a) Avulsion of the intercondylar eminence. (b) Radiograph of an 11-year-old boy showing an avulsion of the intercondylar eminence. (c) Arthroscopically assisted reduction is followed by insertion of a cerclage wire or, in larger fragments, of a short screw not crossing the growth plate

16.5) the vertical part of the growth plate may be damaged. If the growth plate is not affected a reduction under general anaesthetic should be performed and conservative treatment instigated using a long-leg cast which should be kept in position for 6 weeks. If however the growth plate is affected (Figure 16.5a) and displaced, open reduction and internal fixation with crossed Kirschner wires is recommended. Again long-leg cast immobilization for 6 weeks is required.

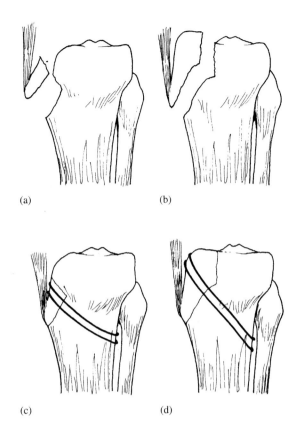

(a)　　　　　　　　(b)

(c)　　　　　　　　(d)

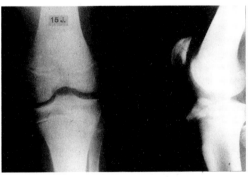

(e)

Figure 16.4 (a) Avulsion of a smaller fragment of the tibial tuberosity; (b) open reduction is followed by K-wire fixation supplemented with a figure-of-eight tension bend;
(c) avulsion of a larger size fragment of the tibial tuberosity;
(d) open reduction is followed by stabilization with the same technique; (e) radiograph of a 15-year-old boy showing an avulsion of a larger size fragment of the tibial tuberosity

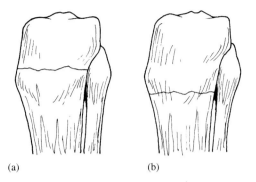

(a)　　　　　　　　(b)

Figure 16.5 Proximal tibial fracture: (a) the vertical portion of the proximal tibial growth plate is crossed by the fracture line which may lead to premature fusion; (b) fracture line is not crossed in the growth plate with good prognosis

Proximal metaphyseal fractures

A metaphyseal fracture of the tibia (Figure 16.6) whether or not it is associated with a fracture of the fibula, may lead to a progressive valgus deformity (Coates, 1977; Bahnson and Lovell, 1980; Weber *et al.*, 1980). A number of explanations have been suggested, none of which seem fully to explain the different aspects of the valgus deformity. In operatively treated fractures of the tibial metaphysis interposition of the periosteum or the pes anserinus in the fracture may be found (Weber *et al.*, 1980) (Figure 16.7*a*). Only after the interposed soft tissues are removed from the fracture can an anatomical reduction be achieved (Figure 16.7*b*). The periosteum and pes anserinus are sutured (Figure 16.7*c*) and cast immobilization for 6 weeks is advisable. Since direct primary treatment is more successful and straightforward than the correction of a late valgus deformity it is important that the surgeon understands the problems associated with this injury and is prepared to undertake operative management.

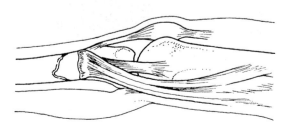

Figure 16.6 Proximal metaphyseal fracture of the tibia with valgus deformity

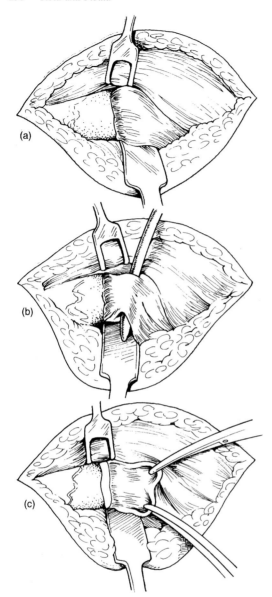

Figure 16.7 (a) Operative finding in a proximal metaphyseal tibial fracture with the periosteum and the pes anserinus interposed. (b) The interposed soft tissue is elevated. (c) Suturing of the soft tissues as the final step in the operation

Tibial shaft fractures

Fractures of the tibial diaphysis in children mainly occur during sporting activities (Blount, 1955; Pollen, 1973; Morrissy *et al.*, 1982). The fracture pattern tends to vary with the age of the child (Van Laer, 1986).

Subperiosteal and greenstick fractures

These fractures are mainly seen in children up to the age of 6 years (Weber *et al.*, 1980). Subperiosteal fractures may occur following a torsional movement which fractures the cortex but leaves the periosteal sleeve intact (Figure 16.8). These are stable fractures and are not associated with a significant risk of late deformity.

Greenstick fractures are caused by a bending force which causes a rupture of the periosteum on the tension side (Figure 16.9) (Briggs *et al.*, 1992).

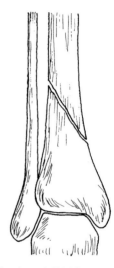

Figure 16.8 Subperiosteal tibial fracture with periosteal sleeve intact

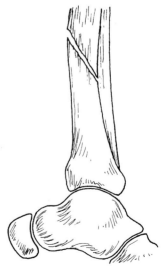

Figure 16.9 Greenstick fracture of the tibia with dorsal periosteum ruptured

Again this is a stable fracture and displacement is virtually unknown. These fractures most commonly occur in the distal metaphysis. They should be treated by immobilization in a long-leg cast for 2 weeks followed by the use of a Sarmiento type of cast brace for a further 4 weeks. Greenstick fractures may require reduction to correct the angle of deformity (Briggs *et al.*, 1992). The surgeon may have to fracture the intact cortex during manipulation to allow for correct positioning of the fragments (Weber *et al.*, 1980).

Displaced diaphyseal fractures

These fractures occur more commonly in older children. They can be stable or unstable and the injuries to the soft tissues may be as severe as those observed in adults (Ogden, 1992). Stable fractures (Figures 16.10, 16.11) are reduced and a long-leg cast is applied. Unstable fractures often benefit from an initial period of traction using about 10% of the body weight. The traction should be maintained for a week and subsequently a long-leg cast can be applied. It is important to assess whether there is rotational deformity of the tibia (Figure 16.12) as spontaneous correction of a rotational deformity is limited in the tibia (Weber *et al.*, 1980; Van Laer, 1986). The surgeon should compare the injured side to the uninjured side to assess the degree of rotational deformity.

In children older than 12 years treatment in a Sarmiento-type functional brace can be employed after about 2 weeks in a long-leg cast. In unstable fractures there is always a risk of shortening and to prevent this Russell traction can be used making use of an os calcis Kirschner wire or Steinmann pin (Figure 16.13). One to 3 kg of traction is usually sufficient unless the child is very obese (Weber *et al.*, 1980). The minimum time for traction is 7 days and it should not exceed 2 weeks (Weber *et al.*, 1980). A long-leg cast can then be applied for a further 2–3 weeks and a walking cast for 3–4 weeks after that. Shortening of up to 1 cm is acceptable (Van Laer, 1986).

In tibial diaphyseal fractures it is important to realize that the radiological callus response is less pronounced than in adults. Clinical assessment of fracture stability is as important as radiological

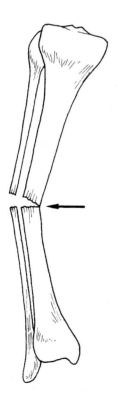

Figure 16.10 Greenstick fracture of the tibia with lateral periosteum ruptured

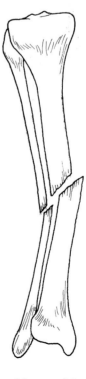

Figure 16.11 Displaced fracture of the tibia with circumferential disruption of the periosteum

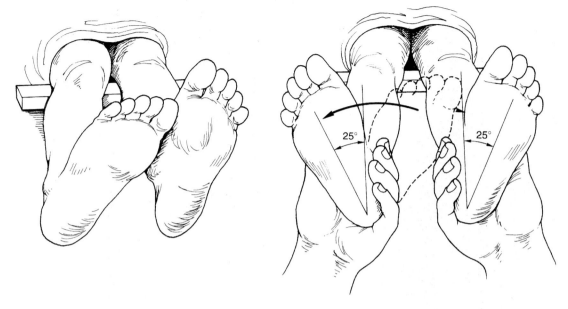

Figure 16.12   Clinical correction of a torsional deformity in the tibia. The foot position on the uninjured side is used as an indicator of the correct position of the injured side

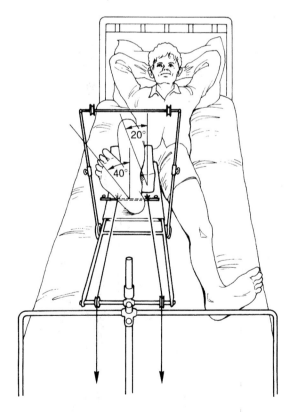

Figure 16.13   Russell-type extension with correct positioning of the tibial axis. The opposite side is used as a reference

assessment. Because of the difficulty in assessing callus it is important that, where possible, X-rays should be performed without a cast.

Open fractures

Open tibial diaphyseal fractures are usually unstable and should be treated in a similar manner to open fractures in adults (Cramer *et al.*, 1992). Thorough soft tissue debridement is important in the management of these injuries and stabilization is best performed with an external fixator on the anteromedial side (Weber *et al.*, 1980) (Figure 16.14). Compartment syndromes occur in children and can develop more quickly than in adults (Weber *et al.*, 1980). It is important to monitor adequately the development of the compartment syndrome and to undertake early fasciotomy to avoid late sequelae.

The soft tissue defect that exists after debridement is usually treated with a split-skin graft or a mesh graft. Healing of the soft tissues in children is good because of their excellent vascularity and free flaps will rarely be required. Late correction with soft tissue expansion techniques can be used instead of free flaps in children.

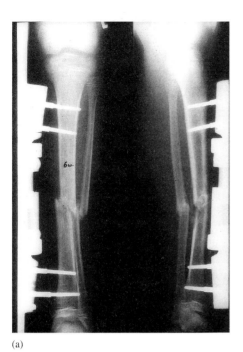

(a)

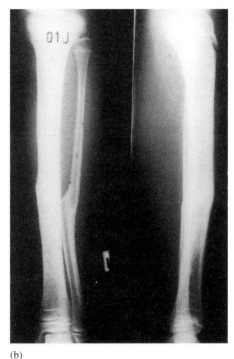

(b)

Figure 16.14   Second-degree compound tibial fracture in a multiply injured 9-year-old child. (a) Stabilization with the unilateral external fixator showing early callus formation 6 weeks after the injury; (b) complete bone remodelling one year after the fracture

Distal metaphyseal fractures

This fracture used to be relatively common in skiing because of the position of the boot top. With modern equipment however a fracture of the tibial diaphysis is now more frequent (Weber *et al.*, 1980). Displaced distal metaphyseal fractures (Figure 16.15) should be reduced so that anatomical alignment is achieved. There may be a recurvatum or antecurvatum deformity and the surgeon may find that it is necessary to place the foot in an equinus position for a short period to facilitate reduction. This can be maintained for about 3 weeks. Subsequently a weight bearing cast can be applied for a further 3 weeks with the foot in the neutral position.

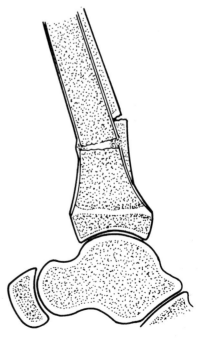

Figure 16.15   (a) Distal tibial fracture. The anterior periosteum is ruptured, there is minor posterior comminution

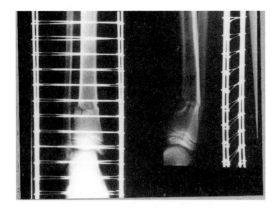

Figure 16.15   (b) Radiograph of an 8-year-old girl with a distal tibial fracture showing comminution of the anterior cortex and an angulation of 15%

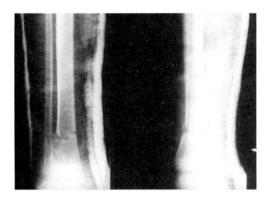

Figure 16.15   (c) Reduction and cast fixation in a temporary equinus position

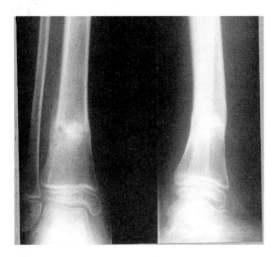

Figure 16.15   (d) Radiograph 9 weeks after the injury with a minor recurvation which can be expected to correct spontaneously

Malleolar fractures

Injuries to the tibio-talar joint always affect the growth plate. The injury is usually indirect and forceful external rotation in abduction with pronation of the foot can cause an epiphysiolysis (Salter Harris type I) or a fracture with a metaphyseal fragment (Salter Harris type II/Aitken type I). With internal rotation, adduction and supination more severe injuries may result. In children younger than 8 years of age injuries to the tibio-talar joint are rare. Ligamentous injuries without associated bony avulsions are also unusual (Crenshaw, 1965; Izant *et al.*, 1969; Cooperman *et al.*, 1978; Dias and Tachdjian, 1978; Kärrholm *et al.* 1981; Dias and Giegerich, 1983; Grace, 1983; Kling *et al.*, 1984).

Epiphysiolysis and fractures with a metaphyseal fragment

These are the most common injuries to the tibio-talar joint and are usually benign. The growth plate itself is not injured and the articular surface remains intact. However the periosteum may be interposed between the bone ends and consequently closed reduction may be impossible (Figure 16.16). This may also occur in fractures that present with a metaphyseal fragment (Salter Harris type II/Aitken type I) (Figure 16.17). Growth disturbance is very unusual in these injuries.

Management of Salter Harris type I and type II injuries is conservative but it is important to secure anatomical alignment. In adolescents however the

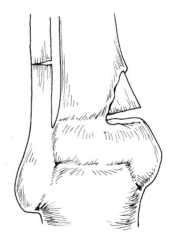

Figure 16.16   Epiphysiolysis in the distal tibia (Salter–Harris type I). Interposition of the periosteum

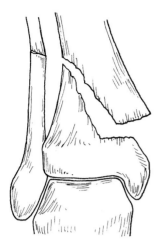

Figure 16.17 Epiphysiolysis in the distial tibia with a metaphyseal fragment (Salter–Harris type II/Aitken type I)

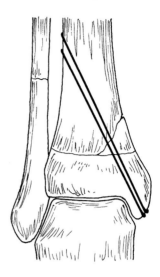

Figure 16.19 With small metaphyseal fragments K-wire fixation is advisable. Note the K-wires crossing the growth plate

potential for the growth plate to compensate for any minor residual malalignment is almost exhausted and anatomical reduction is mandatory. If the surgeon cannot reduce the displacement the interposed periosteum has to be removed from the growth plate and fracture reduction thereby achieved. If the metaphyseal fragment is large (more than 50% of the cross sectional area of the distal tibia) open reduction is required. The fragment may be fixed using either a lag screw or Kirschner wires (Figures 16.18, 16.19).

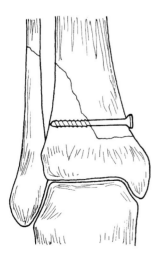

Figure 16.18 Anatomical reduction is followed by lag screw fixation with a 4 or 4.5 mm implant

Initially a back slab is applied but after the swelling has reduced a complete non-weight bearing cast can be applied. Within 2–3 weeks a walking cast can be used, this remaining in place for between 4 and 6 weeks depending on the age of the patient. It is important to remember that repetitive attempts at reduction may cause more injury to the growth plate than a small incision and open reduction. If after reduction the fracture is stable and redisplacement is considered unlikely fixation is unnecessary. Otherwise Kirschner wire fixation is recommended to achieve stability.

Fractures with epiphyseal fragments or epimetaphyseal fragments

Fractures with epiphyseal fragments (Salter Harris type III/Aitken type II fractures) and fractures with epimetaphyseal fragments (Salter Harris type IV/Aitken type III fractures) are more difficult to treat as they are intra-articular fractures and the growth plate is more commonly injured. Not only do these fractures traverse both the growth plate and the articular surface of the tibia but the surgeon should be aware of the possibility of a compression injury of the growth plate as well. It is also possible that the epiphyseal vascular supply may have been damaged causing local ischaemia. Both displaced epiphyseal (Figure 16.20) as well as epimetaphyseal (Figure 16.21) fractures require open reduction and internal fixation. The implants

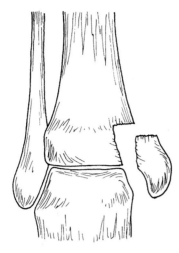

Figure 16.20   Salter–Harris type III/Aitken type II fracture of the medial malleolus. Both the articular surface and the growth plate are crossed

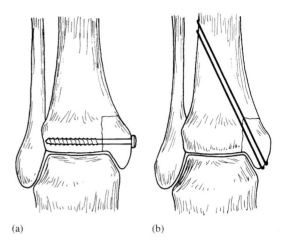

(a)   (b)

Figure 16.22   (a) Open reduction and internal fixation of the fracture shown in Figure 16.21 with a 4 or 4.5 mm lag screw. (b) In smaller children with bony dimensions unsuitable for screw fixation K-wires may be used after anatomical reduction. Note the K-wires crossing the growth plate

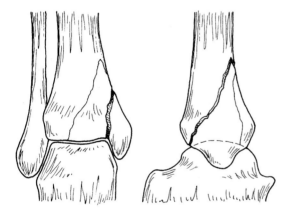

Figure 16.21   Salter–Harris type IV/Aitken type III epimetaphyseal fracture in the distal tibia

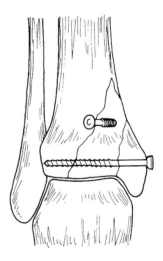

Figure 16.23   Stabilization of the epimetaphyseal fracture shown in Figure 16.22. Two lag screws are used for the epiphyseal and the metaphyseal fracture line: 4 or 4.5 mm implants are used

of choice are Kirschner wires and lag screws. In smaller children a 4 mm lag screw may be used with a 4.5 mm malleolar screw in larger children. Adequate exposure of the fracture fragments and the anatomical reduction is essential. After reduction temporary K-wire fixation can be used and anteroposterior and lateral intraoperative X-rays should be taken to check the fracture position. The K-wires are subsequently replaced by one or two screws lying parallel to the joint line (Figure 16.22*a*). If the medial malleolus has to be reattached to the metaphysis parallel Kirschner wires crossing the growth plate are employed (Figure 16.22*b*). Figure 16.23 shows the fixation for an

epimetaphyseal injury. Postoperatively a back slab is applied for one week. After the swelling has reduced a below knee cast is applied but weight bearing should not be allowed for about 3 weeks. The total immobilization time lasts for 4–6 weeks and the implants are removed after 6–8 weeks.

Physiological growth arrest of the physis starts in its centre followed by the medial part with the lateral part of the physis remaining open longest.

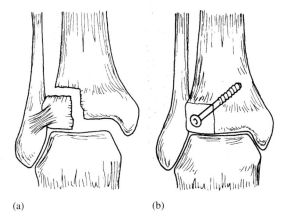

(a)   (b)

Figure 16.24 (a) Transition fracture of the lateral epiphysis in the distal tibia. The fracture line crosses both the articular surface and the growth plate. (b) Lag screw stabilization after anatomical reduction with a 4 or 4.5 mm screw

During this phase an avulsion of the lateral epiphyseal area with the attached syndesmotic ligaments may occur (Figure 16.24) (Kleiger and Mankin, 1964). Surgery is indicated as there is intra-articular malalignment. Open reduction and internal fixation with a screw should be performed. Postoperative immobilization is similar to the protocol suggested for other distal epiphyseal fractures.

Weber *et al.* (1980) analysed 53 fractures of the malleoli treating 12 non-operatively and the other 41 by open reduction. In the more benign Salter Harris type I and II fractures non-operative treatment was usually employed. Complications included overgrowth, valgus malposition, loss of motion and pain. In the more demanding Salter

Harris type III and IV fractures there were a number of unsatisfactory results. Amongst the complications were varus deformity and post-traumatic osteoarthritis. Surprisingly the Salter Harris type IV fractures had a better outcome than the Salter Harris type III fractures.

Shortening in tibial fractures

Shortening is frequently associated with non-operative treatment of tibial fractures. In children up to 5 years of age 10–15 mm of shortening is acceptable. In children from 5 to 10 years of age 5–10 mm of shortening can be accepted and in children from 10 to 15 years of age only 5 mm of shortening is permissible.

Bone overgrowth is another possible result of tibial fracture. This appears to be less frequent and less significant than in the femur but the surgeon should be aware of it and maintain careful supervision (Figure 16.25).

Axial malalignment should be corrected if at all possible. The surgeon should remember that a valgus deformity is less of a problem for the ankle joint. Recurvatum and antecurvatum should be avoided as they are not corrected and rotational deformity must be corrected at all costs since spontaneous correction of such deformity is very limited if it occurs at all.

Conclusions

Injuries to the proximal and distal growth plates of the tibia require careful attention and the surgeon

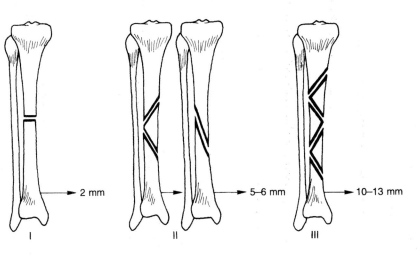

2 mm   5–6 mm   10–13 mm

I   II   III

Figure 16.25 Overgrowth depending on the fracture type. With a transverse fracture the resultant overgrowth is about 2 mm, with oblique and third fragment fractures 5–6 mm, whereas in comminuted fractures it is 10–15 mm

should be familiar with the potential outcome of these fractures and their complications. Benign injuries must be distinguished from potentially difficult fractures. When the articular surface is involved anatomical reduction is required to avoid later problems such as post-traumatic osteoarthritis. Multiple attempts at closed reduction may be harmful to the growth plate and should not be undertaken. Treatment of these injuries requires considerable experience.

Whenever open reduction and internal fixation is performed careful attention must be paid to the surgical technique. Implants must be selected according to the patient's age and the dimensions of the skeleton.

In tibial shaft fractures varus deformities up to 15° can be accepted in a child of less than 6 years. These may be expected to correct spontaneously whereas valgus deformities as well as antecurvatum and recurvatum are incompletely corrected. Rotational deformities usually persist. Overgrowth after tibial diaphyseal fractures which are treated non-operatively is unusual. Operative stabilization should be limited to specific indications such as the multiply injured or a combination of ipsilateral tibial and femoral fractures. In these conditions as well as in open fractures external fixation is a useful treatment method (Klein *et al.*, 1989).

Tibial non-union is unusual. Marti did not encounter any non-unions in 638 fractures (Weber *et al.*, 1980). However in a similar period a number of non-unions were encountered after failed attempts at internal fixation of the tibial diaphysis. Internal fixation was generally inappropriate and non-union was the consequence. Thus open reduction and internal fixation cannot be recommended. If stabilization of diaphyseal fractures is necessary external fixation is the appropriate choice.

References

Aitken, A.P. (1965) Fractures of the proximal tibial epiphyseal cartilage. *Clin. Orthop.*, **41**, 92

Bahnson, D.N. and Lovell, W.W. (1980) Genu valgum following fractures of the proximal tibial metaphysis in children. *Orthop. Trans.*, **4**, 306

Blount, W.P. (1955) *Fractures in Children*, Williams & Wilkins, Baltimore

Briggs, T.W., Orr, M.M. and Lightowler, C.D. (1992) Isolated tibial fractures in children. *Injury*, **23**, 308

Burkhardt, S.S. and Peterson, H.A. (1979) Fractures of the proximal tibial epiphysis. *J. Bone Joint Surg.*, **61A**, 996

Canale, S.T. and Shelton, W.R. (1979) Fractures of the tibia through the proximal tibial epiphyseal cartilage. *J. Bone Joint Surg.*, **61A**, 167

Christie, M.J. and Dvonch, V.M. (1981) Tibial tuberosity avulsion fracture in adolescents. *J. Pediatr. Orthop.*, **1**, 391

Coates, R. (1977) Knock-knee deformity following upper tibial 'greenstick' fractures. *J. Bone Joint Surg.*, **59B**, 516

Cooperman, D.R., Spiegel, P.G. and Laros, G.S. (1978) Tibial fractures involving the ankle in children: the so-called triplane epiphyseal fracture. *J. Bone Joint Surg.*, **60A**, 1040

Cramer, K.E., Limbird, T.J. and Green, N.E. (1992) Open fractures of the diaphysis of the lower extremity in children. *J. Bone Joint Surg.*, **74A**, 218

Crenshaw, A.H. (1965) Injuries of the distal tibial epiphysis. *Clin. Orthop.*, **41**, 98

Dias, L.S. and Giegerich, C.R. (1983) Fractures of the distal tibial epiphysis in adolescence. *J. Bone Joint Surg.*, **65A**, 438

Dias, L.S. and Tachdjian, M.O. (1978) Physeal injuries of the ankle in children. *Clin. Orthop.*, **136**, 230

Ehrlich, M.G. and Strain, R.E. Jr (1979) Epiphyseal injuries about the knee. *Orthop. Clin. North Am.*, **10**, 91

Eilert, R. (1976) Arthroscopy of the knee joint in children. *Orthop. Rev.*, **5**, 61

Eiskjar, S. and Larsen, S.T. (1987) Arthroscopy of the knee in children. *Acta Orthop. Scand.*, **58**, 273

Grace, D.L. (1983) Irreducible fracture separations of the distal tibial epiphysis. *J. Bone Joint Surg.*, **65B**, 160

Hand, W.L., Hand, C.R. and Dunn, A.W. (1971) Avulsion fractures of the tibial tubercle. *J. Bone Joint Surg.*, **53A**, 1579

Hansen, S.T. (1990) Internal fixation of children's fractures of the lower extremity. *Orthop. Clin. North Am.*, **21**, 353

Harries, T.J., Lichtman, D.M. and Lonon, W.D. (1983) Irreducible Salter–Harris II fracture of the proximal tibia. *J. Pediatr. Orthop.*, **3**, 92

Henderson, R.C., Kemp, G.J. and Campion, E.R. (1992) Residual bone-mineral density and muscle strength after fractures of the tibia and femur in children. *J. Bone Joint Surg.*, **74A**, 211

Hyndman, J.C. and Brown, D.C. (1979) Major ligamentous injuries of the knee in children. *J. Bone Joint Surg.*, **61B**, 245

Izant, R.J., Rothman, B.F. and Frankel, V. (1969) Bicycle spoke injuries of the foot and ankle in children: an underestimated 'minor' injury. *J. Pediatr. Surg.*, **4**, 654

Kärrholm, J., Hansson, L.I. and Laurin, S. (1981) Computed tomography of intraarticular supination-eversion fractures of the ankle in adolescents. *J. Pediatr.*, **1**, 181

Kennedy, J.R. (1979) *The Injured Adolescent Knee*, Williams & Wilkins, Baltimore

Kleiger, B. and Mankin, H.J. (1964) Fracture of the lateral portion of the distal tibial epiphysis. *J. Bone Joint Surg.*, **46A**, 25

Klein, W., Pennig, D. and Brug, E. (1989) Die Anwendung eines unilateralen Fixateur externe bei der kindlichen Femurschaftfraktur im Rahmnen des Polytraumes. *Unfallchirurg*, **92**, 283

Kling, T.F., Bright, R.W. and Hensinger, R.M. (1984) Distal tibial physeal fractures in children that may require open reduction. *J. Bone Joint Surg.*, **66A**, 647

Landin, L.A. (1983) Fracture patterns in children. *Acta Orthop. Scand.*, Suppl. 202, vol. 54

Lee, H.G. (1937) Avulsion fracture of the tibial attachments of the crucial ligaments: treatment by operative reduction. *J. Bone Joint Surg*, **19**, 460

Meyers, M.H. and McKeever, F.M. (1970) Follow-up notes: fracture of the intercondylar eminence of the tibia. *J. Bone Joint Surg.*, **52A**, 167

Morrissy, R.E., Eubanks, R.G., Park, J.P. *et al.* (1982) Arthroscopy of the knee in children. *Clin. Orthop.*, **162**, 103

Odgen, J.A. (1982) *Skeletal Injury in the Child*, Lea & Febiger, Philadelphia

Pennig, D., Klein, W. and Baranowski, D. (1990) Die Anwendung der Kallusmodulation zur Korrektur des posttraumatischen Genu recurvatum. In *Verletzungen der unteren Extremität bei Kindern und Jugendlichen* (eds Rahman and Breyer) Springer-Verlag, Berlin, p. 220

Pollen, A.G. (1973) *Fractures and Dislocations in Children*, Williams & Wilkins, Baltimore

Reynolds, D.A. (1981) Growth changes in fractures of the long bones. *J. Bone Joint Surg.*, **63B**, 83

Salter, R.B. and Harris, W.R. (1963) Injuries involving the epiphyseal plate. *J. Bone Joint Surg.*, **45A**, 587

Skak, S.V., Jensen, T.T. and Poulsen, T.D. (1987) Fracture of the proximal metaphysis of the tibia in children. *Injury*, **18**, 149

Spiegel, P.G., Cooperman, D.R. and Laros, G.S. (1978) Epiphyseal fractures of the distal ends of the tibia and fibula: a retrospective study of 237 cases in children. *J. Bone Joint Surg.*, **60A**, 1046

Van Laer, L. (1986) Frakturen und Luxationen im Wachstumsalter, Thieme-Verlag, Stuttgart

Von Vinz, H. (1972) Operative Behandlung von Knochenbrüchen bei Kindern. *Zentralbl. Chir.*, **97**, 1377

Weber, B.G., Brunner, Ch. and Freuler, R. (eds) (1980) *Treatment of Fractures in Children and Adolescents*, Springer-Verlag, Berlin

Weinberg, A.M., Reilmann, H., Lampert, C. *et al.* (1994) Erfahrungen mit dem Fixateur externe bei der Behandlung von Schaftfrakturen im Kindesalter. *Unfallchirurg.*, **97**, 107

Wiss, D.A., Schilz, J.L. and Zionts, L. (1991) Type III fractures of the tibial tubercle in adolescents. *J. Orthop. Trauma*, **5**, 475

Index